THE BRAIN SUPREMACY

The Brain Supremacy

Notes from the frontiers of neuroscience

KATHLEEN TAYLOR

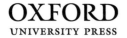

OXFORD

UNIVERSITY PRESS

OXFORD
UNIVERSITY PRESS

Great Clarendon Street, Oxford, OX2 6DP,
United Kingdom

Oxford University Press is a department of the University of Oxford.
It furthers the University's objective of excellence in research, scholarship,
and education by publishing worldwide. Oxford is a registered trade mark of
Oxford University Press in the UK and in certain other countries

First Edition published in 2012

Impression: 1

British Library Cataloguing in Publication Data
Data available

Library of Congress Cataloging in Publication Data
Data available

ISBN 978-0-19-960337-4

Printed in Great Britain by
Clays Ltd, St Ives plc

This book is dedicated,
with thanks for all her help,
to Gillian

Table of Contents

List of Figures

List of Tables

Acknowledgments

Among the many who have assisted me, I would first like to thank the anonymous readers, together with the Delegates of Oxford University Press, who approved the book for publication. They were most helpful with suggestions, and my ideas are much clearer in consequence. John Stein (University of Oxford) and Peter Hansen (University of Birmingham) were also helpful and instructive, and I am grateful to the University of Oxford's Department of Physiology, Anatomy and Genetics for granting me the status of research visitor.

My thanks to the Alzheimer's Disease Education and Referral Center (a service of the National Institute of Aging), the Bodleian Library, Piers Cornelissen (University of York), Benjamin Crowell (Fullerton College), Mark Dow (University of Oregon), Peter Hansen, Bob Jacobs (Colorado College), Alyse Jacobson (of the Society for Neuroscience, SfN), Malcolm Kendall (University of Birmingham), the National Institute of Mental Health, Robert Sekuler (Brandeis University), the Science Photo Library, Laszlo Seress (University of Pécs), John Stein, and Joanne Wyles (University of Birmingham) for their generosity, advice, and help with images, whether or not the images made it into the final version. I would also like to thank Michelle Roberts and Karen Pine of the BBC, for permission to reproduce the segment discussed in Chapter 14; Jackie Perry of SfN, for permission to reproduce excerpts from the *Journal of Neuroscience*; Audrey Springer and Diane Sullenberger, for permission to reproduce excerpts from PNAS; and Michael Diamond (Wayne State University), for answering my query about a conference presentation.

I am especially grateful to René Hen (Columbia University) for reading and commenting on a large section of Chapter 12.

My parents, as ever, offered vital moral support, as did my friend, patient critic, and extensive proofreader Gillian Wright. My thanks to all three for their thoughtful comments on the text.

Last, though definitely not least, I owe a great deal to the University of Oxford, and to the excellent team at Oxford University Press (Emma Marchant, Phil Henderson, Fiona Vlemmiks, Jenny Lunsford, and others), and especially to *The Brain Supremacy*'s editor, Latha Menon.

1

Introducing the Brain Supremacy

Neuroscience is coming of age

(The Royal Society)

Welcome to the future. This is a book about the way we live now, and the way we'll live soon. As the twenty-first century gathers pace, science and technology are changing the world ever faster. From quantum mechanics to electronics, from materials science to robotics, the physical sciences have allowed us to reshape the planet, manipulate electrons, build micromachines and create today's information society. My niece and nephew are growing up in a very different environment from my own childhood, extraordinarily different from my parents' youth, and quite alien to the world my grandmother grew up in a century ago.

Science and technology are also changing their nature—and ours. Since their beginnings they have been dominated by our increasing control of matter and energy, but now, for the first time, our control of the physical world will extend to precise and systematic control of some particularly special bundles of matter: us. Science is already approaching the era of what I call the brain supremacy: a change in its power dynamics as currently dominant sciences like physics are joined and then surpassed by neuroscience. The brain supremacy will offer human beings—some human beings—the power to manipulate human nature mechanically and directly, by changing the brain.

Depending on whether or not you think that scientists are a) heroes of the modern age who will solve all our problems, b) dangerous monomaniacs, on no account to be trusted with anything really important, or c) somewhere in between, you will find the possibilities suggested by current brain research either a) a fuss about nothing, b) indescribably alarming, or c) completely confusing. Respondents in all three categories, however, are liable to agree that whatever the truth behind the neurohype, that truth is important. Brains matter. They matter because they're so central to the meaningful, virtual, abstract and experiential aspects of our existence—the ones we value most.

Brain research is already changing our sense of what being human involves, rejecting the age-old idea of a spiritual essence in favour of an organic approach. This is what the feared materialism of modern science tells us. Brains are the pieces of meat which give us our selves, allowing you and me to exist as the people we are. Without them there would be no music, beauty, poetry, or science. There would be no vicious murder or despairing suicide either; but also no joy of sex, no delight in nature, no pleasure in getting lost in a really good book. Everything meaningful in your life and mine needs a cranial pudding to express itself, and each of those puddings is unique, irreplaceable and still mysterious. Brains are astonishing, beautiful, intricate, delicate marvels. Like human lives, they are good things in and of themselves.

If you were ill, and needed a heart transplant to save your life, would you accept one? Most people would; they feel that having a different heart wouldn't disrupt their sense of personal identity. How about a brain transplant? If your brain were removed and put into storage to make room for a new, younger cerebrum, would you be in the body or in the storage? What if all your former synaptic settings were copied across to the new brain? Or if only part of it—the cortex—were transplanted? These thought-experiments and others suggest that we identify ourselves with our brains in a way we don't with other parts of our bodies. Practical experiments, ethical and otherwise, suggest that we are right to do so. We can swap hearts, lose a kidney, cope without hands or eyes, and still be human, but remove the brain and what's left is a kind of desecration: man made meat.

The power of self-fashioning

As well as shaking up our ideas of what we are, the brain supremacy promises unparalleled techniques for changing brains directly: not with language or images or drugs, or new gadgets to play with, but by altering the behaviour of neurons and the function of their genes. Of course, brain manipulation isn't novel; we do it indirectly all the time and we always have. The social power which bends others to your will is so greatly valued that pursuing it is one of humanity's great occupations.[1] With tongues and guns, ideals and incentives, persuasion and pressure and sheer propaganda, human beings have had a lot of practice in treating others, *pace* the strictures of Immanuel Kant, instrumentally: as means to an end, objects to be utilized and adjusted, rather than individuals who are ends in themselves. And the methods we use affect our brains and bodies. Drugs change your genes. So do stressful events, meals eaten, conversations.

Yet we often fail to achieve the changes we want. To date, attempts to control other human beings have faced a mighty obstacle: the bony castle of the skull. That barrier has never been invincible—bullets or an axe will penetrate it—but it has kept out many less violent and crude attacks. Barred from the inner sanctuary of the brain, we were left with the evolved skills of social interaction and the knowledge built upon them: psychology, anthropology, history, literature. That, plus rare neurological patients, years of detailed observation of human behaviour, and what we had learned from studying the brains and behaviours of other species. The idea of an equivalent capacity to that of, say, modern chemistry applied to the management of other human beings is therefore a tremendously attractive prospect, particularly for those people and institutions tasked with managing or predicting human behaviour.

The level of control which will be made possible by the brain supremacy is the stuff of science fiction dreams, or nightmares. With advances in reproductive technology, we can already adjust a person's genes before he or she is even born, but only in the crudest of ways. In the future, we may be able to change more subtle features of thought, mood, belief and personality, tweaking brains gene by gene and protein by protein, at any stage in life, and possibly without the person realizing. We have barely begun to grasp the implications of the powers we are about to gain. Yet we are already living in the shadow of the brain supremacy. The study of human brains has undergone colossal growth in recent years, and it's time to think hard about the brave new world that researchers are starting to map out—a world in which neuroscience can change not only the technologies we use to live, but the beliefs and desires of the people who use them. *The Brain Supremacy* offers a guide to that world: a questioning look at the issues raised by our growing understanding of ourselves.

The change is well under way. Today it seems that everywhere you look there are debates about neuroscience's impact on society. Neuroscience and the law; what brain research tells us about child development; how brain-based technologies will transform entertainment and communications; and much else neurofuturist besides. Brain research apparently shows how addicts' or criminals' (or fat people's or anorexics') brains, or even the brains of left- and right-wing voters, are different from medium-weight, unaddicted, law-abiding, politically indecisive types.[2] Brain research, it seems, explains—or will soon explain—everything from love of music to love of money, from spirituality to bullying, from artistic genius to alcoholism.

A recent headline from the *Daily Telegraph* claims that a 'Telepathic computer can read your mind'.[3] The BBC, describing the new field of neuromarketing ('sell-to-cell'?), asks, 'Can brain scans help companies sell more?'[4] These media stories are fuelled by science journals and press releases. They encourage a feeling that brain research is rapidly advancing—or encroaching—on core aspects of human nature.

Are you, for instance, religious? The eminent journal *Neuron* features a paper called 'The spiritual brain'; and *Trends in Cognitive Sciences* one on 'The origins of religion'.[5] Perhaps you're concerned about crime, justice and moral responsibility? The new field of neurolaw addresses those issues.[6] Do you have a phobia? Relax: a recent piece from *Nature* is titled 'Editing out fear', while the *Daily Telegraph* quotes a researcher as claiming that an 'Injection could cure phobias', implying that it's only a matter of time before we leave such dysfunctions behind.[7] Do you think of consciousness or intelligence as central to what makes us human? Brain scientists are tackling both topics: *Science* reports on how researchers can distinguish conscious from non-conscious brain activity, while *Nature Reviews Neuroscience* recently summarized 'The neuroscience of human intelligence differences'.[8] As for the softer sides of human nature—empathy, cooperation, love and so on—social neuroscience has had them in its sights for quite some time.[9]

Already, terms such as 'neuromarketing' and the prospects of drugs to improve concentration, memory and exam performance are raising hackles. Those hackles are likely to go on rising, because these days neuroscience is reaching far beyond the cure of disease, towards understanding and even, perhaps, improving healthy brains. The message behind the excitable headlines is that our skulls are becoming metaphorically see-through, our actions ever more predictable, our brain activity ever more interpretable, and our thoughts and feelings there for the taking by anyone with a clever enough machine.

Figure 1a gives a visual impression of the brain supremacy's development so far, showing how often the term 'neuroscience' was used in books in English published in the years 1900–2008 (and digitized by the US corporation Google). The upward trend begins in the mid-1970s, climbs steadily through the 1980s and accelerates thereafter. (For comparison, Figures 1b and 1c show equivalent plots for another science, biochemistry, and for the term 'science'.) Figure 1d reflects the extent to which neuroscience has penetrated popular media in the last two decades, showing the number of mentions of the word 'neuroscience' in newspaper headlines for the years 1991–2010.[10] Clearly, in so

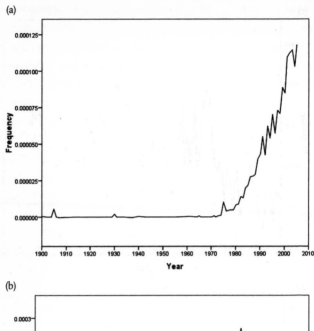

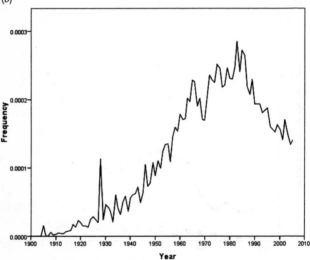

FIGURE 1: The brain supremacy illustrated.

Figure 1a shows the frequency of the term 'neuroscience', over the years 1900–2008. Figures 1b (lower image) and 1c (next page) show frequencies for the terms 'biochemistry' and 'science', respectively. Figure 1a illustrates the upward trend in the use of 'neuroscience' in published books, which begins in the mid-1970s, rises steeply in the following decades, and is still ongoing. Figures 1b and 1c show that this is not a general cultural trend for all sciences, or for science in general. (For more details see the Appendix.)

(c)

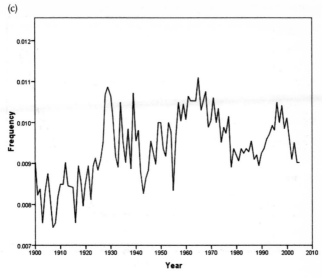

(d)

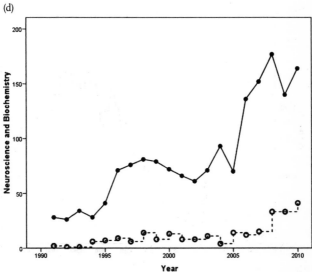

Figure 1d uses a different measure of the extent to which awareness of neuroscience and biochemistry has percolated into popular culture: US newspaper headlines for the years 1991–2010 (there are after all many science books published which very few people read, compared with those who read newspapers). The US was selected because of its position as world leader in neuroscience. Once again, the trend for 'neuroscience' (solid line, closed circles) is rising, suggesting that mainstream media awareness of brain research increased sharply in the mid-1990s and again in the mid-2000s. The graph for 'biochemistry' (dashed line, open circles) is flatter.

far as the headlines reflect the stories, neuroscience has become increasingly talked-about, especially within the last five years. The years 1990–1999 were declared by US President George H.W. Bush to be the 'Decade of the Brain'; but it is since that decade that the brain supremacy has really begun to take shape. Over the last five years for which data are available (2004–8), the number of neuroscience articles published has grown by 18%. The figures for related research fields are even higher: clinical neurology 23%, psychiatry 25%, psychology 39% and behavioural sciences 48%.[11] Brain research is a growth industry.

Your opinion counts

As citizens whose taxes fund much of this research, we stand on the brink of a future in which the human race could change itself for the better, or make our collective situation very much worse. The coming changes will be relevant to all of us, just as the development of the Internet has altered our lives. The choices we make now will affect what we do with the gifts, the superpowers, which the brain supremacy will give us. Those choices have implications for our children and grandchildren, since the brain supremacy will be established by the time they grow up.

The speed of scientific advance, however, is accelerating so fast that today's adults will also be affected. Like it or not, governments, companies and military organizations in the West, and no doubt elsewhere, look set to acquire sophisticated new methods of changing other people's thinking, feelings and even existence. This will happen subtly at first, as adverts become more effective and governments smarter at persuading us to do what they prefer. Later, medicine may offer treatments, far more effective than current psychotherapies, for those of us plagued by negative thoughts or traumatic memories.[12] Doctors may be able to ease an abused child's suffering, or help a war victim escape her memories of seeing her family killed. Later still, we may be able to change our own memories, record our own dreams and read people's thoughts. Companies may be able to boost our desire for

8

products by stimulating our brains directly. In war, soldiers may take a pill to help them do their brutal work more effectively, while their weapons induce overwhelming fear or sickness in their enemies, or control them remotely, or burn out their brains from a distance. The prospects for future terrorism are also horrifying. Some developments we may not know about at all, unless some courageous war correspondent breaks the news of their use against our enemies.

We need to be careful when it comes to developing technologies which can slip through the skull to directly manipulate the brain. They cannot be morally neutral, these world-shaping tools; when the aspect of the world in question is a human being, morality inevitably rears its hydra heads. Technologies which profoundly change our relationship with the world around us cannot simply be tools, to be used for good or evil, if they alter our basic perception of what good and evil are.

They already have. An example is the development of fighter bombers, which has allowed the destruction by fire of innocent civilians to feel less like mass murder and more like a high-adrenaline game. Intellectually, a pilot knows those explosions, far below, are annihilating other human beings. Distance and technology, however, prevent this truth from being felt as well as known, so that the deaths seem less like real events with human consequences. This makes killing much easier for the killers, psychologically as well as physically.

Tools have always been able to change the minds which wield them. What the brain supremacy offers is the power to change those human minds directly and systematically. Neuroscience and psychology, more than ever before, can offer profound manipulations of human nature. To date, our methods of controlling people have lagged far behind our ability to world-shape (i.e. to change our surroundings to conform to someone's idea of how they should be).[13] That gap is now closing. We need to stop and think about what's coming, and in which directions we want—and don't want—developments to go.

What we can be sure of is that governments around the world, and especially their military institutions, are extremely interested in certain current neuroscientific research. Work on the pharmacology of extreme stress, which has obvious relevance to soldiers' performance, is one example among many.[14] The growing power of neuroscience to manipulate human brains directly offers capacities beyond the dreams of the most totalitarian government. Your skull is not the fortress it once was.

So far we have developed many ways to kill as well as achieving some success in healing. The brain supremacy could expand our ability to help other people, but it also offers seductive new ways to make use of them. Which approaches we adopt, which technologies we reject, that's up to us. We are the citizens of the coming neuroworld, and ours are the brains that are likely to be changed.

In other words, this is not an optional discussion. The pace of scientific discovery is now so rapid that the kinds of choices outlined in *The Brain Supremacy* will be forced on us whether we like it or not. To ask in advance what kind of society we want gives us some control over our future. It also requires, however, that we change our own attitudes and behaviour voluntarily, before we are compelled to do so in the service of someone else's interests. We need to think about how best to make those changes.

Exploring the brain supremacy

This book offers snapshots of current brain research, revealing how it achieves its remarkable results and gains its remarkable power to improve human lives. Praise is not unadulterated, since one of my aims is to highlight some queries about where the science roller-coaster may be taking us, but I want to show you the beauty of brains and brain science. There is cause for concern, but also much to celebrate. Neuroscience is a discipline of great and growing power, and it offers much to delight and fascinate. Used wisely, it could help to solve our hardest problems: mental health and other brain disorders, violence, overconsumption, addiction and many more.

To make choices about how to shape the brain supremacy we need to know what's likely to be on the menu. That means exploring the realm of the brain. Many pioneers have preceded us, and the brain supremacy's impact on our culture has already made the language of neuroscience familiar to some extent. That impact has largely been via the media, and I will have more to say on the relationship between source and interpreter later.

Neuroscience itself has produced a vast amount of knowledge about our brains. It has unravelled the structure of synapses and traced the fibre tracts which bind brain regions together. It has deconstructed many of the receptor proteins by which neurons take information from their environs, and the neurotransmitter molecules that carry that information. It has seen how brain areas, and individual cells, communicate; how proteins twist to let neurons turn on a gene; and how ions flow to send electrical charges along a cell's axon, in order to activate a synapse.

Is this not evidence of a discipline settling into maturity, its core problems mostly dealt with, the rest to be mopped up in steady middle age? Anything but. One of the themes of this book is that the excitement of brain research is only just beginning. Neuroscience is passing out of its childhood, starting to reach for the power of adolescence, but it's got a long way to go before it settles into adulthood, and the next few decades will be transformative. As I hope you will see in later chapters, the amount we have learned is far outweighed by what we still don't know. Studying the brain has proved far more complicated than anyone expected, back in the days when computer scientists confidently talked of modelling its function on machines so feeble that today's low-end word-processing software would overwhelm them. We have better computers now, but we still can't simulate anything approaching the brain's capacities.

Science's revisionist tendencies also need to be taken into account. Much of the neuroscience I learned as an undergraduate has been proved wrong. No doubt some of what I read in the research literature in the year 2010, when most of this book was drafted, will also be found to be incorrect. What we have learned about brains has revealed immense new complications. We have many hypotheses to explain them, but we do not have the overarching simplifications of a mature theory. Not yet.

It is worth bearing in mind, incidentally, that to scientists a hypothesis is much more preliminary than a theory. Theories are well-established frameworks, built up over the course of many experiments: relativity, evolution and synaptic transmission are theories. Hypotheses are explanations which may have some support, but have not yet reached the level of acceptance of theories; a current example is the claim that the hormone oxytocin, acting in the brain, plays a role in social cognition. One of the commonest frictions between scientists and the media results from the journalistic habit of describing a floundering response to a curveball question—'Dr Taylor has written a book on cruelty. So, Dr Taylor, is the Internet making us cruel?'—as a theory. Desperate off-the-cuff fudging like Dr Taylor's answer shouldn't even be called a hypothesis.

What do we have after all those decades of work? Knotty problems still to solve. More types of brain cells, more chemicals by which they communicate, more varieties of responses to the hormones in our blood and the products of our guts, more intricate networks of genes and proteins in neurons, more factors affecting the synapses through which neurons send their signals.[15] Oh, and I haven't mentioned the additional dimensions of difficulty offered up by neurons' ability to synchronize and adapt their behaviour by adjusting their connections, therefore demanding we understand them through time as well as across the space of the brain's different regions.[16] Or the disconcerting recent developments which suggest that brains are closely bound to our immune systems, hormones and gut function—more closely than scientists, understandably impressed by the protective prowess of the blood–brain barrier, had hitherto assumed.[17] As research advances, complexities multiply.

One can't help thinking that if brain research ever chooses to acquire a motto it shouldn't go for triumphalism, gimmickry or smart-alec humour (temptations all scientists would do well to resist), but for a tone of mild apology: 'Actually, it's more complicated than that...'

Since I'll be needing to make this statement from time to time, I hereby abbreviate it to IMCOTT. In neuroscience, It's always More COmplicated Than That.[18] As the writer John Buchan opined, in another context, 'There is no simple key to complex things.'[19]

Yet not all is chaos. Neuroscience and psychology have had over a century to establish some basic principles of how brains and their concomitant minds operate. Science works by accretion (like oysters slowly building up pearls around a piece of grit) as well as by revolution (like hermit crabs changing shells). Though even basic principles can prove wrong, they're a lot more trustworthy than the cutting-edge research that makes the headlines. Like a coral reef, the well-established core may take your weight where the edges would crumble beneath you.

To be able to shape the path of the brain supremacy we do not need to be scientists. However, politicians, citizens and the media do need guidance on when, and how much, to trust the findings with which they are presented—often second-hand, since science journals are not exactly emblems of popular culture. Although neuroscience has proved a rich mine for the media, learning about it is not as simple as reading journalists' coverage of science. Many claims that appear in the science news are made for non-scientific reasons, and not all of them accurately reflect the research on which they are reporting.[20] To be able to assess speculation about mind-reading machines, for instance, we need to understand not only what the scientific studies tell us but how the researchers came to their conclusions, and this information is often not made available.

A couple of spare decades in which to learn neuroscience is unrealistic, unless you have no other plans for your retirement. There are, however, shortcuts. While working on my doctorate, I was asked to give two undergraduates eight tutorials on neurophysiology to prepare them for an exam. The catch was that they were supposed to have had eight tutorials already, but a system failure meant that we had to start from scratch. The undergraduates passed the exam—one with distinction—and they did it by focusing not on the facts of brain research but on its methods and principles. Once that framework was in place, they had no problem making sense of individual data and remembering the facts they needed for the exam.[21] In its emphasis on the methods of brain research, this book is designed to offer a similar framework, making sense of the science which will pave the way for the brain supremacy.

The keys to power

What we need, in short, is to venture into a relatively unexplored region of neuroscience: the fascinating territory of scientific methods. That term, 'fascinating', is used neither lightly nor ironically. Methods are science's great unspoken secret, its keys to power, far more than the findings splashed across the media. Findings are often revised and sometimes retracted; methods are refined. Learning about findings teaches us particular facts, which may later change. Learning about methods allows us to understand not only current but future brain research. (As in studying any language, vocabulary alone is not enough; you need grammar as well.) There are also relatively few kinds of methods, whereas the slew of data is already impossible for any one human to track.

How will the brain supremacy gain its formidable power to change our natures? What will let loose these visions of redesigning human-kind, bringing them from mere dreams to exciting—or alarming—possibilities? No single finding, eye-catching though it may be. What makes science so astoundingly capable is not what it knows, but how it knows it: the famous scientific method which tests ideas (hypotheses) against reality (data) using carefully designed experiments. Likewise, the key to the brain supremacy is in the methods researchers use to do their studies: the neurotech arsenal which drives its onward march. From histology to electrophysiology, from two-photon uncaging to optogenetics, it is the technology of brain research which underpins its astonishing promises.

There are so many steps between the brain itself and the resulting data that these techniques have a huge effect on how researchers see and understand their subject matter. Knowing more about the methods and interpretations which lie behind, say, a picture of the brain obtained with fMRI (functional magnetic resonance imaging) is therefore essential for assessing the claims which that picture helps to make, some of which are decidedly dubious.[22]

Of humans and their tools

Another advantage of understanding the methods is that it reminds us that no machine is actually miraculous, amazing though neurotech can seem. In fact, each technology is defined as much by what it can't do as what it can. Consider the much-quoted wisdom of the psychologist Abraham Maslow:

> I remember seeing an elaborate and complicated automatic washing machine for automobiles that did a beautiful job of washing them. But it could do only that, and everything else that got into its clutches was treated as if it were an automobile to be washed. I suppose it is tempting, if the only tool you have is a hammer, to treat everything as if it were a nail.[23]

Understanding how hammers work is a necessary prerequisite for understanding what they can and cannot do. Of course, their limitations may not matter for the task in hand; if all you want to do with your hammer is hit nails, you may not care that it's useless for painting walls. Early neuroimaging studies often seemed to embrace this approach, as if their authors were thinking (which they may well have been): 'We have this toy, it cost a bomb, we're damn well going to use it'.

If, however, you want to paint a wall, you need to think about what hammers can't do and what other tools you need. A facile truism, for a hammer, but worth noting for an fMRI or PET (positron emission tomography) scanner, because of the human tendency to treat any sufficiently complicated machine as if it were a minor deity. (If you have ever found yourself begging an uncooperative gadget to work you will know the syndrome.) It is easy, as research has shown, to be cajoled by those pretty pictures of brains into lending the results of imaging studies an authority and truth they may not deserve.[24] For examples of pretty pictures, see the colour plates.

We greatly discount the extent to which the machines we use to look at the brain determine what we see there. Of course, we know that opening a human skull would not reveal bright colours crawling like amoebae over the surface of the brain. But we may be tempted to think that if, say, certain parts of the brain 'light up' when people are lying, then we can use fMRI as a lie detector (of which more later). Part of that temptation results from not knowing what is actually going on when a brain is scanned. Understanding the technology, and the considerable amount of interpretation involved, may seem like a tough way of immunizing you against being misled, but as with vaccination the rewards are worth any minimal discomfort.

Neuroscience methods, the many and varied ways of seeing and manipulating the brain, have been honed to astonishing levels of precision. They are testaments to extraordinary skill and smart thinking, deserving of far more attention than they get. In chapters to come I will set out some of the most intriguing and important of the many developments in brain research. Intriguing, because they show the creative genius of scientific problem-solving. Important, in that without them modern neuroscience would not exist and the brain supremacy would never happen.

Yet it is happening, and debating its implications is too vital to be left to experts. Like my previous books *Brainwashing* and *Cruelty*, therefore, *The Brain Supremacy* is not written for specialists but for anyone interested in the topic.[25] My approach is to lay out what may soon be possible and then look at what neuroscience has already achieved and how it has achieved it. That means including a variety of subject matter, from neuroscience to chemistry, and physics to ethics. I have tried to keep language accessible and jargon minimal, so prior study of either neuroscience or psychology is not required—though readers familiar with protons, molecules and cells may be at an advantage.

One of the features of this book is its use of very recent scientific research. The major papers I discuss are from high-impact, peer-reviewed journals and were published in 2010. I will be describing their work, and the methods employed, in some depth, but don't be deterred. Brains are so much to do with us that their sciences are a treasure house of interest, and that is especially true of the neurotech which drives brain exploration. The deeper you go, the more fascinating things become. Neuroscience, despite the concerns I'll be confronting in these pages, is a subject worth exploring, admiring, even loving, as I hope you'll agree.

Chapters 2, 3 and 4 consider what future technologies may be possible. They also set out my main themes: the motives for research, its interdisciplinary nature, some of the problems which need to be resolved if the brain supremacy is to reveal its full potential, and the importance, for solving those problems, of understanding that science is at base about methods more than it is about data.

Since to understand brains it helps to know what they look like, Chapter 5 roams through some of the most memorable data and images produced in the endeavour to understand brain structure. One key approach was to adopt the science of anatomical dissection. This may sound even duller than methods, but the impression is misleading: to open up the skull is to delve into a realm of wonders. That enterprise, neuroanatomy, is one of the loveliest in neuroscience, full of beautiful names and spectacular images. It gave the modern discipline its vocabulary and grammar, the foundation of brain science ever since.

From grasping the brain's structure, the next step is to try to understand its function. To do this, scientists have developed ways of seeing living brains in action. Examples of neuroimaging and brain manipulation use their technologies to give us different understandings of what brains are and how they work. Each method has its pros and cons, and each its own implications for the brain supremacy. The elderly but still-informative technology of positron emission tomography (PET, Chapter 6) demonstrates one way of interfering with brains: by adding a molecular hijacker that subverts their natural biochemical mechanisms. Functional magnetic resonance imaging (fMRI) offers another, as we shall see in Chapter 7, adding not molecules but energies to the system under study to change its subatomic properties. A third approach aims for greater naturalism, simply observing the brain as it goes about its business; these are the electromagnetic recording technologies described in Chapters 8 and 9.

The lenses may look different, but the neurotechnologies described in Chapters 5 to 9 are all ways of seeing the brain.[26] Observation and description, however, have never sufficed for curious human minds; we like to interfere and see what happens. Chapters 10 to 13 will consider ways of changing brains experimentally: the tools of manipulation used by today's researchers. Chapter 10 sets the scene by describing how meddling with brains has proved its worth, despite its considerable controversies. The rich field of neurogenetics (Chapters 12 and 13) is the main focus of attention these days, but older, electrical technologies are also continuing to prove their worth in the struggle to control how neurons behave, as discussed in Chapter 11.

The final chapters round up the book's major themes and explore implications of the brain supremacy. They outline some possible futures for this remarkable new phase in human understanding, some good, some not so desirable. I will be asking what we can do, now, to bring about the best outcomes while avoiding the nightmare scenarios. And I will even be invoking two ancient deities, from the era often hailed as originating science, albeit only to supply a metaphor for modern research.

That is for the future. In the next chapter, I put the brain supremacy in perspective and look at what modern brain research has done for us.

2

The Many Powers of Science

Science is what made us what we are today, and is our best chance for tomorrow!

(Jon Butterworth, physicist)

Once upon a time human beings were at the mercy of predators and the ferocity of nature. Then they discovered society and superstition and learned that teamwork could protect them from natural threats. They grew to depend on—and started oppressing—each other. Then they discovered science, a paradigm of cooperative enterprise. Ever since that breakthrough, the ills inflicted by both nature and civilisation have on the whole been slowly diminishing.

It's a caricature, of course. Science is often extolled as a way to escape from superstition, but it's more a bedmate than a usurper. Years of science education may have made some impact on human irrationality, but traditional ways of thinking still hold considerable sway even among the science-trained.[1] A paper in the journal *Cognition*, for example, asked US college students, most of whom had studied physics at either college or high school, to work out the trajectories followed by moving objects.[2] Only a quarter of the 44 students got close to the correct answers, which the study's authors interpret as suggesting that people's 'naïve' beliefs about the world are overlaid, rather than replaced, by scientific training. Reason is a hard habit to acquire, especially when its lessons are as counterintuitive as scientific knowledge can be, and older instincts easily reassert themselves.

A social transformation

As for the idea of progress towards perfection, it's a myth, though a popular one. In practice, human societies have developed fitfully and unevenly, with reverses and even extinctions. The twentieth century, our most civilized and scientifically adept to date, provides an extreme example: alongside the many advances in quality of life, a staggering 262 million civilians are thought to have been killed in conflict. That's civilians, note; soldiers are extra.[3] Imagine yourself travelling back in time to 1900, to tell a startled Edwardian gentleman that within a century so very many people—in his time, about one in seven of the entire world's population—would die in wars without even having enlisted. One hopes the next hundred years will have a better record, since a seventh of the population in the year 2000 is over 870 million people (nearly three times the entire current total of Americans).[4] That's an inconceivable amount of death and suffering. The choices we and our leaders make will help determine whether it can be avoided.

Caricatures grow from grains of truth, and the progress caricature is no exception. For the world's luckier citizens, life has undoubtedly improved thanks to the changes wrought by science and technology. This is so often said in these fast-changing days that it's easy to nod and move on, but considering just how great the transformation has been even in the last 100 years reminds us that this truism has depth. The brain supremacy will trigger further massive transformations, so gauging how far we have come already may offer a sense of what's ahead.

Here's a brief reminder of how things used to be. It comes from a memoir of working-class life in an English city, early in the twentieth century:

Every day was washing day. We used to have a big concrete bowl built in the wall and a fire was lit under it to boil all our clothes. We all had to help in those days. Boys had to make the fire, get the coal in, chop firewood. Girls used to iron, hang washing out. I was always given the job of scraping the ash from underneath the boiler as no one could get under easy like me. I must have only been about 9 years old then. We only had one cold water tap, and all the water for baths was in the boiler, or kettles on the fire. Friday night was bath night. We used to have a big tin bath and two of us at a time got in it by the fire. But when we got older we had to have it more private, or go to a public baths.

Baths once a week; clothes washed by hand; hot water by lighting a fire, not flicking a switch. Public baths, and yes, an outside privy. This isn't ancient Rome, but relatively modern England: the writer, Edith Crosby, was born in Liverpool in 1909. What a contrast with our luxurious, computer-dependent lives today—in England and other rich nations—where heat and power arrive as and when required and washing is done by a machine.

Edith was my grandmother. As childhoods go, hers was tough. Manual labour was what awaited this early twentieth-century young-ster and most of my ancestors before her. Her father died when she was five years old, her mother seven years later. By then her three younger brothers had already been sent to an orphanage; after their mother's death the younger girls were also put into care. Edith was too old for an orphanage, so like many working-class girls of her time she went into service, doing the housework of wealthier people, coping with what we would call overwork, bullying and sexual harassment. She escaped into marriage, raised a family, survived the Blitz and cancer, and witnessed the dawn of the Age of Computing—though to my knowledge she never touched a personal computer and would have been bemused by the worldwide web. She died in 1998. A long span, during which life became both easier and far more complicated.

And what a risky life it was, compared with my good fortune. In the concerns over obesity, depression and so on we forget how much more life we have been granted. My grandmother, passing her 88th birthday, was unusual. Life expectancy for girls born at the beginning of the twentieth century was just 49 years, for boys 45. (Of the ten Crosby children, six exceeded these expectations.) For twenty-first century kids like my niece Beth and nephew James the figure is 80 years for girls and 75 years for boys. That's a phenomenal advance: all those extra years to work with (and pay for). If we fall ill, living in Britain, we're treated by the National Health Service. There was no such help when a stroke confined Edith's mother to bed (at home, not in hospital), nor when Edith's older sister Caroline died in infancy of whooping cough.[5]

In work too, career options for women opened up magnificently during the twentieth century. My grandmother was a housemaid, then a housewife. I have a PhD in neuroscience. By the time Beth Taylor is starting her career she may have a job that I'll find hard to understand.

We face threats my grandmother never knew, and it's easy to be absorbed by the miseries of our own era. Yet things could be worse, and for most of the humans who have ever lived they were. In quality as well as quantity, in health and work and in the home, life in the West, especially for women, has changed from slavish drudgery to unprecedented freedom. My niece's life chances, set against those of her great-grandmother, are undeniably, incomparably better.

The power to change the world

Where did this transformation come from? The standard, though inevitably oversimplified, narrative is that modern scientific thinking took shape in the Western world in the seventeenth and eighteenth centuries, initially among clubs of wealthy, bright young men, as part of a great ferment of industrialization, exploration and colonization, religious change and a growing openness to new ideas. We associate such thinking with ideals and principles characteristic of a very specific period in human history, the Enlightenment: among them, reverence for truth, free and open discourse, the idea of human rights, and democracy. The ideals weren't new, but a confluence of external factors—the invention of printing, the Protestant Reformation, competition between small European states, and so on—brought them together in unusual prominence during this one tiny slice of humanity's lifespan.[6]

Whatever the exact trajectory, the result stands apparent in a world where science is increasingly international, spreading its benefits beyond the richest nations.[7] The physical sciences have given us unprecedented mastery of our environments. Physics and chemistry did not achieve their current eminence by virtue of their ability to bore generations of schoolchildren into submission. They give us power; we can see the evidence all around us. From globe-spanning communications to the exploration of the distant universe, from the micromanipulation of matter to sophisticated techniques of energy production, this ability to shape the world has revolutionized politics, work and society. War made famous the atomic bomb, but our lives have arguably been more deeply changed by developments in electronics, which have revolutionized the nature of work and communication. Recent reports promise truly astonishing prospects for the coming decades: real-life invisibility cloaks, augmented reality interfaces powered by your body movements, intelligent houses, fridges and cars to keep you safe and healthy, and a future of machine-wrapped, long-living individuals swimming in a sea of information. That's providing you're born in one of Earth's better neighbourhoods, where disease, war or poverty don't stymie your chances of gaining such luxuries.

As science proved its worth, and governments saw good reasons for funding it, the rate of production became phenomenal: over a million peer-reviewed articles are published every year, and growing.[8] The vastness of even one scientific discipline has long exceeded any single person's capacity to comprehend it, and the quantity of money, people and time consumed in scientific research has mushroomed like the proverbial cloud. And as our control of nature and the environment has improved, the world-shaping sciences are beginning to make good on a promise they have always offered, that one day we'll have the skills to reshape not just the world, but us. The futurologist Michio Kaku argues that we have had the quantum revolution, the computing revolution is ongoing, and we are just beginning to get to grips with the revolution in biotechnology which has come from unravelling DNA.[9] That third and most challenging of changes is helping to push our understanding of ourselves into realms where human nature can be tested as never before. The brain supremacy is underway.

High-value science

With neuroscience, as elsewhere, it's easy to be blasé and shrug off how much has already been achieved. In the past two decades, however, brain research has grown dramatically, transforming a subfield of human physiology into a science in its own right, complete with feuds, frameworks, fringe hypotheses and subdisciplines. The change has been driven by the natural momentum of research and by increasing cultural recognition that brain research is useful to all sorts of people, from advertisers to weapons makers.

Indeed, the influence of brain research reaches far beyond medicine, psychiatry and neuroscience, important as they are. Part of that influence is economic: keeping scientists in jobs. This is not to be discounted. Neuroscience-related industries, from making electrodes to building imaging machines, provide a lot of employment. Likewise for those areas of psychology, economics, art, and culture interested in brains. Likewise for a great deal of academic research and associated bureaucracy.

In 2007, the US Society for Neuroscience (SfN) says that American funding for bioscience research 'created and supported more than 350,000 jobs, generating wages in excess of $18 billion. The average annual salary was $52,000, nearly 25 percent higher than the national average.'[10] Discussing monies provided by the National Institutes of Health (NIH), which doles out US government resources to researchers, the SfN adds that, 'Every dollar of NIH funding generated more than twice as much in state economic output: an overall investment of $22.84 billion from NIH generated a total of $50.53 billion in new state business, taking the form of increased output of goods and services.' In Britain, combined state funding for the Biotechnology and Biological Sciences Research Council and the Medical Research Council has been, on average, almost £600 million per year of late (for the ten years until 2007).[11] Being a bioscientist, in raw financial terms, is good for the economy as well as for the scientist.[12] Bioscience includes neuroscience, and until the global financial crisis in 2008 neuroscience was doing well, helped by the proliferation of expensive imaging scanners in UK hospitals and research centres.[13]

The biggest contributions to brain research have undoubtedly come from technological advances. Neuroimaging techniques such as fMRI (functional magnetic resonance imaging), CT (computer tomography) and PET (positron emission tomography) are familiar to many people because they are used in hospitals. These and other ways of working with the brain have helped us understand much more about its function, as we shall see in later chapters.[14] Yet the images they give us are only glimpses of the array of methods now committed to cracking open the human brain. Better techniques for analysing EEG (electroencephalography) recordings; clever methods of manipulating genes in living neurons using light (optogenetics) or chemicals (immunocytochemistry); stronger magnets for fMRI; improved statistics for more accurate analysis, etc. To call this discipline fast-moving is to understate the case.

New methods have also done much for those with damaged brains. Neurosurgery, for example, is no longer butchery, but precise and skilful manipulation causing minimal unnecessary damage. People are more likely to survive a brain tumour, stroke or car crash with their faculties reasonably unimpaired. Patients incapacitated by severe depression or Parkinson's disease have been given back their lives, at least for a while, by deep brain stimulation, and some of the degenerative disorders which were once among the ugliest of death sentences can now be controlled for months or years.

Gene therapy for neurological syndromes may also finally be starting to deliver. For example, a recent case study treating the condition X-linked adrenoleukodystrophy, though tiny and demanding further research, was encouraging enough to make it into *Science* magazine.[15] The disorder, caused by problems in a gene on the X-chromosome which result in the lack of a single protein, is horrible: affecting brain cell function (among other things), it leads to walking problems, incontinence, weakness and eventual wheelchair dependence, with some patients also facing sensory and mental impairment, paralysis and early death. The scientific hypothesis that fixing a faulty gene may help is no mere intellectual exercise, but an urgent hunt for answers, underpinned by sufferers' desperation.

That better neuroscience can be a life-or-death issue is clearly shown by a recent use of neuroimaging on people thought to be in persistent vegetative states—the kind of damage that prompts court cases over whether medical support should be withdrawn. A few such patients have shown signs of consciousness—apparently answering questions about their family correctly, for instance—by systematically changing their brain activity to signal 'yes' or 'no', albeit while imprisoned in unresponsive bodies.[16] Suddenly the practice of allowing such individuals to starve to death looks less like leaving a personless body to run down and more like awful if unwitting torture. Doing brain research matters.

Furthermore, as we learn more about the neurological and genetic basis of many disorders formerly seen as psychiatric—schizophrenia, for instance—there are hopes that the most severe of mental illnesses may be, if not resolved, at least better understood and managed. There has been much discussion of the limits of psychiatry (particularly its biomedical branches) in recent years, so it is worth noting that not all psychiatric treatments fail. For these improvements, and for many more, brain research has earned our gratitude.

Neuroscience has extracted the brain from a pre-scientific world of spirits and souls, seeking to unravel how the complexity of this most baffling of organs makes it both robust and delicate, resilient under a huge range of stimuli, yet vulnerable to many genetic and environmental disruptions.[17] Today's researchers acknowledge a very peculiar claim, in historical terms: that the brain, more than any other organ, gives life to the mental worlds we value so highly. Mind is to brain rather as climate is to planet Earth. Both thoughts and weather, personality and atmospheric patterns, are intricately woven from the interplay of physical forces.

Brains are harder to model than weather systems, and the problems of understanding brain function and dysfunction are more difficult than those of grasping climate change. The challenge is increased when you take the brain out of its theoretical vat and immerse it in a body and a world. Yet we cannot infer, given the record to date, that this complexity will always be impenetrable. Brains are amenable to being understood, bit by bit, in health and disease, as two centuries of research effort has shown. Understanding brain function now seems less an impossible dream, more a feasible goal.

Of healers, scientists and engineers

The default assumption at present is that most of this activity is being done for the good of humankind. The rapid progress towards the brain supremacy benefits from the close association of neuroscience with medicine, the healing art. Few people argue that seeking cures for brain diseases like Alzheimer's is a bad thing to do (though some might say the money would be better spent on fighting infections which kill the very young). As the World Medical Association declared in 1975, 'The physician's fundamental role is to alleviate the distress of his or her fellow human beings, and no motive, whether personal, collective or political, shall prevail against this higher purpose'.[18] Throughout the book I will return to this key theme of justification: how brain researchers account for their activity to others. In my view such accounts fall into one of three categories: clinical, analysis, or enhancement.

We start with the medical motive: the urge to heal. Clinical research, with its aim of treating or preventing brain disorders, is a major driver of neuroscience and psychology. Very many things can go wrong with an organ so complex. The terrors which dysfunctions of our nervous system can induce, however, are different from those which accompany, say, a diagnosis of heart disease, horribly debilitating though heart disease can be. Brain problems can seem especially cruel: slowly destroying a person's self, making them paranoid and aggressive with their loved ones, imprisoning them in their body, taking away all dignity and independence. Unsurprisingly, the clinical urge to ease suffering and find a cure for hideous illnesses like Alzheimer's, Parkinson's and motor neuron disease has always been strong in neuroscience.

Neuroscientists, however, are not always doctors. Many do not have medical training, and their ethics are those of research more than medicine. Healing is good, of course, but for brain researchers the prime directive is to understand, to seek knowledge. The model is Faust, not Hippocrates; the aim is analysis. Clinical and analytic studies are intertwined, since the pathologies that afflict the human brain have taught us much about its function. Yet the analytic desire to understand that function in healthy individuals goes beyond medical motives to purely scientific ones: wanting to see how things work by taking them apart, whether virtually—by way of neuroimaging—or literally. In later chapters, we shall see how this immensely successful reductionist approach, breaking brains down into their components, has both driven and been driven by new technology—and where that technology is taking us.

Clinical approaches to neuroscience regard the brain as a deeply tangled mystery in which one or more of the coils has been twisted out of shape. Analytic approaches see it as a thing of beauty and wonder, and a fascinating challenge. As well as these two, there is a third, less complimentary way of regarding the brain: as a kludge in urgent need of re-engineering.[19] This is the enhancement approach, which has already given us pills for better concentration, and which promises much more. Enhancement says we can improve on evolution, and neural enhancement offers the ultimate in self-fashioning: changing brains to bring an actual human being closer to some ideal.

If the urge to enhance us is given free rein, and fulfils its promises, what could the world of the brain supremacy look like later this century? No one knows, but we can make an educated guess at some extreme scenarios by assuming that two sets of technologies will become available.

The first, already well underway, will allow the sampling of human brain activity in real time, creating computer-stored records of brain function which can be linked to particular mental states. As we shall discover, what is measured by ways of seeing the brain varies widely, so the recording technologies will capture, in digital format, multiple aspects of neural function as well as of subjective experience. Since 'multiple aspects of neural function as well as of subjective experience' is too long to bear repeating, I will refer instead to digitized neural experience (DNE), to emphasize the bond between subjective experience and the neural activity which is its physical basis.[20] DNE recording will allow the interpretation of brain states to be done in real time in the clinic, perhaps even in the home and on the move. Better treatment of mental illness should result. Mind-reading will also become a genuine possibility, of which more in the next chapter.

The second set of technologies, DNE programming, will allow a DNE recording from one brain to be mapped onto the neural circuits of another, or transferred back into the same brain, by temporarily resetting the states of neural circuits. This may involve electromagnetic stimulation (as is already being done more crudely; see Chapter 11), or physical, chemical, or genetic changes to the neural machinery. Successors to Hollywood and YouTube may begin by remixing existing DNE recordings to create artificial experiences. Initially, these will be crude, cumbersome and expensive—and DNE recordings from people may continue to carry a market premium—but as the brain's repertoire is better understood these mind movies will become more realistic. Eventually, DNE programming will provide the ability to alter individual circuits temporarily or permanently, at the levels of synapses, genes and molecules.

In theory there is no reason we know of to prevent future scientists from being able to reprogram any neural circuit or release any neurotransmitter they choose in the animals they genetically design. And if in animals, perhaps one day in humans? Researchers have already programmed memories into fruit flies, controlled the movements of tiny worms, and triggered dopamine release in the brains of rats.[21] In itself this is extraordinary work, raising the prospect that we may be able to use animals as living robots, doing tasks we cannot or do not want to do ourselves. (The military implications alone are startling.[22]) Controlling animals, however, is only a step on the path towards refashioning human beings. This is the end goal, the ultimate dream of personal remaking, in which any unwanted aspect of the self, from bad memories to an awkward gait, can be adjusted to match the individual's desires.

There are two reasons for setting out the science fiction. The first is that changes in ethical and cultural attitudes can take years to develop, while research is advancing at a fast and quickening pace. The ethical dilemmas raised by the brain supremacy are often familiar: for example, concerns about brain-enhancing drugs map onto other forms of performance-boosting, like cheating in elite sports. Yet its scientific accomplishments, which make human selves the target to be altered, break new ground, and the ethical discussions may not keep up.[23] We can make new people by combining reproductive technologies with traditional biology; we can change them slowly, crudely, and with difficulty; we can destroy them in an easy instant. But no other current method than destruction guarantees control of human beings: not love, education, bribery, or empowerment; not even cruelty, slavery, and fear. If any neurotech could make even the vaguest stab at such control, however imprecise and dangerous, do you trust your species not to use it?

The second reason for highlighting the extreme ideals of DNE recording and programming is that these ideals, however unlikely they may seem at present, are already driving brilliant and hard-working people to produce intermediate technologies: techniques for changing human brains without a proper understanding of the details. We have already had some of those, at considerable cost; notorious examples from the childhood of neuroscience include depatterning and prefrontal psychosurgery.[24] They remind us that side-effects can take a while to become visible, that patients can be driven into the clinic by social pressures as well as by medical needs, and that treatments are also subject to such pressures. (Lobotomy offered relief to the families of difficult patients, just as ritalin today calms troublesome children.) That is especially the case when treatments—or enhancements—affect the brain, mind, and self.

The next chapter looks at one of the most profound enhancements promised by the brain supremacy: mind-reading.

3

Could We Read Minds?

If you have something that you don't want anyone to know, maybe you shouldn't be doing it in the first place.

(Eric Schmidt, CEO of Google)

In Chapter 2, I discussed three motives driving neuroscience research: the clinician's urge to heal, the analyst's urge to understand, and the engineer's urge to improve. Understanding and repairing the brain have always gone along with wanting to improve it, and proponents of human enhancement have eagerly anticipated the brain supremacy. Could brain techniques like neuroimaging be used to extend or transcend natural human capacities, for instance by allowing us more direct access to other minds? Could learning, problem-solving and social interactions be transformed?

Most of us are already skilled mind-readers, using facial expression, tone of voice, body language, and our own experience to infer what the people we interact with are thinking and feeling. Yet these markers are proxies of our inner states, 'accessories accepted in lieu of the internal character', as Charles Dickens called them.[1] As victims of con artists learn to their dismay, our beliefs about other minds are sometimes incorrect. Neuroimaging offers the hope that we could bypass the need to infer mental content from external cues. This is the superpower of practical telepathy: detecting and decoding minds at source.

Back in my graduate days I remember hearing fMRI dismissed as 'brain geography', prettily descriptive but doing little for real understanding. Since then PET, fMRI and their descendants have become an immensely fruitful set of research tools, and the literature they create has burgeoned.[2] Journal articles reporting on fMRI studies now cover everything from sensory differences to psychological biases, courage to empathy, reward processing to print processing—and more.[3] Brain imaging techniques have proved their inventive worth.

In the past year or so, some truly remarkable claims have been made for neuroimaging. Here are some examples:

By using [...] functional MRI, we decoded activity across the population of neurons in the human medial temporal lobe while participants navigated in a virtual reality environment. Remarkably, we could accurately predict the position of an individual within this environment solely from the pattern of activity in his hippocampus.[4]

Traces of individual rich episodic memories are detectable and distinguishable solely from the pattern of fMRI BOLD signals across voxels in the human hippocampus [voxels are 3D pixels, the units of the grid into which brain scans are segmented for analysis].[5]

This article [...] demonstrates how a resulting theory of noun representation can be used to identify simple thoughts through their fMRI patterns.[6]

These [...] models make it possible to identify, from a large set of completely novel natural images, which specific image was seen by an observer. [...] Our results suggest that it may soon be possible to reconstruct a picture of a person's visual experience from measurements of brain activity alone.[7]

So scientists can already do a form of DNE recording. It seems that they can decode where you are and what you're looking at, what memory you're reliving and even what you're thinking. Has the brain supremacy achieved so much already? As we shall see in the following chapters, IMCOTT. At present these startling claims are strictly limited, because it really is more complicated than that. However, there seems no reason why they may not be brought to apply more generally in the very near future. What then might be the consequences of such a technology?

Practical telepathy

At first glance, a world in which mind-reading became available not just to researchers or governments but to anyone who wanted it may look like a place full of promise. Lovers could know, at last, if their partners truly cared for them. Friends could detect betrayals before they happened. Banks, the police and governments could catch more fraudsters. Psychiatry, counselling, welfare and the criminal justice system could be transformed. Lies and cheating would fall out of favour, at least in face-to-face relationships, and honesty would find itself fashionable.

Practical telepathy would force us to be more open with ourselves and others. Like the CEO of Google quoted at the start of this chapter, many people link openness with virtue. If this is the case, opening minds to other people's scrutiny should result in general moral improvement. Imagine government officials, sales personnel, the media and leaders everywhere being put under pressure to say only what they actually believed. Imagine the impact on consumerism and employment, family and friends, if everyone had access to portable, perhaps even concealable, brain-scanning technology.

The consequences of enhancing human capacities to detect mental activity vary depending on what you are detecting, and how. There is a difference between current overt neuroimaging techniques and potential covert technologies. The latter's availability will depend on whether sciences as yet undeveloped, such as nanotechnology and room-temperature superconductivity, can make brain monitoring equipment sufficiently cheap and portable.[8] If nanomachines, perhaps in the form of proteins encoded in synthetic genes, could be designed to emit a signal when certain neurotransmitter molecules were released in certain brain areas, and if the artificial DNA could be administered in food, drink, or as an aerosol, a person thus infected might never know that their privacy had been lost. Until that is possible, computational power and statistical analysis will be used to increase the sensitivity of monitoring technology. The ability to record electromagnetic 'brain waves' at a greater distance from the skull, with less interference from other electromagnetic radiation, would be a considerable asset, for example.

On whom will these technologies be used, and when? Enemy soldiers? Suspect or criminal individuals? Celebrities or holders of public office? Anyone of interest to the media, or the government? If electromagnetic fields are being recorded, is there anything to prevent such recordings being made of more than one brain at a time? Perhaps methods could be developed to monitor groups—looking for signals as to whether a crowd of demonstrators is likely to turn violent, for example—or even entire populations, finally putting electromagnetic flesh, however crudely, on that most elusive of notions, public opinion.

Another important distinction is between techniques presenting their results in real time and those using later, off-line data analysis. In either case, will the information flow one way from participant to researcher, or will it be fed back to the brain that sourced it?—as a method of clinical treatment, for example. How the results are presented, who gains access to the data, and how much training the recipients will need to understand them, also need to be considered, as for any research study.

What exactly would a mind-reader read?

Overt or covert technology, offering immediate or delayed results and targeting individuals or groups: the possibilities are already remarkable. There is, however, a further question: what aspect of brain function will be measured?

One form of mind-reading could involve detecting the contents of a person's consciousness. Here the potential benefits for human creativity are immense. I personally long for a system which could translate my sometimes vivid dreams directly into pictures and videos, since my drawing skills are abysmal. Skilled artists too would surely enjoy the ability to transfer their mental images directly to a screen; likewise for composers, film directors, novelists, web designers, programmers and other creators.[9] So to any scientists working on brain downloading, please hurry up.

These techniques could be used in many domains. Entertainment, education, medicine and psychiatry, and criminal justice are only the more obvious possibilities. We may be able, one day, to make our own DNE records, to share or program our dreams, to learn new skills direct from the minds of experts, or to communicate with loved ones purely by thinking. If the technology can be miniaturized and the computing power made available, real-time recording of brain function could become a routine aspect of everyday life, perhaps even continuously so. Thus applied, it could prove an unparalleled aid to diagnosis, or even prevention, of mental distress. It could change definitions of what counts as unacceptable mental activity, allowing individuals to be treated for thoughts, fantasies or memories they—or others—find disturbing even when a doctor would say that there was no clinical problem. And it could solve one of the biggest problems in medicine by establishing a baseline for normal function against which the clinical symptoms could be compared.

Intention reading

The concept of reading intentions is of very great interest in criminal justice and forensic psychiatry. Thoughts alone are insufficient here. If Edmund sits quietly at his desk, dreaming about how an axe through the skull would improve a tiresome colleague, he is doing no more actual harm than a worker who spends company time on Facebook. However rapt his fantasies may be, they do not hurt anyone as long as he keeps them to himself and doesn't either mention or perform the fatal craniotomy. There may come a time when George Orwell's thought crime is seriously proposed as legislation, but for now a man's imagination is still his own backyard. If intention-reading technology became available, it would have to be able to tell the difference between violent fantasy and the moment when Edmund snaps and looks around for the nearest sharp implement.

Identifying the urge to commit a dangerous action before the action takes place is not as easy as it may sound. In monkeys, scientists can already detect intentions for simple movements like gaze-shifting, where the direction in which the eyes are going to move can be inferred from the activity of neurons in specific regions of cortex.[10] Researchers have also successfully suppressed aggression in male mice, using optogenetics to stimulate part of the hypothalamus.[11] Monkeys and mice, of course, are not human beings, nor is moving your eyes the same as beating someone up. The process of teasing out the neural pathways underlying human violent behaviour is as yet incomplete. Nonetheless, these studies are intriguing hints of what may be possible in the not too distant future.

If detecting violent intentions could be done, especially if it were coupled with mechanisms for preventing such behaviour, it could render prisons virtually redundant, replacing them with clinics where anyone identified as an offender is fitted with the monitoring technology. However, such methods are likely to be used before concerns about their efficacy and ethics have been thoroughly ironed out, by governments struggling with the problems of predicting violence, dealing with addiction and minimizing antisocial behaviour. Thinking about them well in advance is therefore worthwhile. Since in practice any such system will probably begin as a tool for controlling violent killers, respect for their human rights may well be minimal; yet what starts with managing a murderer may spread to anyone judged habitually violent, and then to the only potentially violent. We should be wary of establishing the principle that anyone, even a criminal, should be banned from intending violence, as opposed to actually committing it. The idea that, if you have something that you don't want anyone to know then maybe you shouldn't be *thinking* it in the first place, is something not even the lords of cyberspace have yet suggested.

Researchers have already noted the ethical conundrum posed by being able to predict undesirable outcomes, like violence, partially but not absolutely. Various factors are known to correlate with a greater likelihood of violent behaviour. Some are social (e.g. gang membership, participating in a war, living in a culture which heavily emphasizes honour, living in a dangerous neighbourhood). Some are personal (e.g. a history of violence, childhood physical abuse, lack of early supervision), and some are bio-markers (e.g. being male, being young, perhaps having certain genes or physiological traits).[12] Unfortunately, knowing that your next-door neighbour is a shady character with a troubled background and a savage temper does not give you the means to predict his next explosion.

This inability to apply predictions to individuals is a general feature of scientific explanations, especially in the behavioural sciences, because they depend on statistical analyses of how groups of people—sometimes very small groups—behave under certain more-or-less realistic conditions. Analysing collective behaviour deliberately glosses over the personal idiosyncrasies that make individual actions so difficult to predict. Scientific theories and hypotheses in brain research are thus framed in statistical terms about groups, not persons. They express probabilities rather than certainties and generalities rather than specifics.

Because it would be unethical to deliberately induce violence in a community, or an individual, for research purposes, many studies of harmful behaviour also express correlations rather than causal links. Saying that people with more risk factors have a higher probability of committing violent acts means that, if you took a large sample of people with risk factors and another sample of people without, you would likely find that the high-risk group was more violent. It does not mean that everyone who has the risk factors will be violent, because correlational studies do not tell us that having risk factors causes a person to be violent.

Intention-reading technology, however, would be a step beyond risk factor research. One need not say, 'This person has the kind of profile that violent people have, so let's lock them up/tag them/monitor them just in case', thereby risking the injustice of locking up an innocent citizen. Instead, neuroimaging would be used to identify the neural patterns activated when a person is just about to commit a violent act, and combined with monitoring of the environment to assess whether it was safe for them to do so. Of course, the person might then exercise remarkable self-control ... but if he or she didn't, a system to detect the outgoing motor command and intervene in some preventative fashion is not beyond the wit of scientists. As noted earlier, ethical concerns would remain with such a system, but realistically, progress in ethics is like progress in science—one step at a time—only slower.

Emotion reading

Another possibility is that future techniques will be able to detect moods, emotions, desires, and dislikes more accurately than can skilled human perceivers. Since the capacity to assess other people's feelings is extremely useful and widely variable, the benefits of this kind of enhancement could be considerable, in principle bringing all of us up to the standard of highly empathic, emotionally literate people. Work is already under way on multiple techniques to improve emotional understanding for people deficient in it because they have autism. Some are chemical (e.g. using the hormone oxytocin, applied as a nasal spray), but neuroimaging is also playing a part.[13] For example, fMRI is being used to detect differences in brain activity in autistic people.[14]

Finding a robust and repeatable physical difference, a 'bio-marker', is the first step towards achieving the analytic goal of understanding why autism involves such devastating problems with social interactions. Eventually, the hope is that researchers can devise a treatment to achieve the clinical goal of normal function—and perhaps, thereafter, the enhancement goal of making us all more adept at reading each others' hearts and minds.

Greater access to emotional states, in the sense of more accurate detection, would not necessarily imply more empathic togetherness.

Empathy appears to be dependent on contextual features and on whether or not the person's cognitive resources are already drained or distracted.[15] One important aspect of the context is similarity: empathy for other people's emotions, and their pain, is more likely to be evoked by people like us. If a person sees a friend or partner in pain, they will probably try to help relieve the pain, and they may feel the pain themselves to some extent—it works better in women, apparently.[16] If, however, they judge that the pain is deserved punishment, because for example the sufferer previously acted unfairly, empathy can be reduced—at least in men.[17] If the sufferer is classed as an enemy, empathy may also be lessened; in some cases, the observed suffering may even become rewarding.[18] Then there are the cases where empathy leads to so much distress in the empathizer that they can't bear the pain and react by retreating, denying the suffering, or feeling active hostility to the sufferer who is unwittingly hurting them. Better recognition of other people's feelings through technology, therefore, will not automatically produce better ways of dealing with them.

Furthermore, similarity is not a yes/no distinction but a complex gradient between 'like' and 'unlike'. How similar to myself I judge you to be depends on what aspects of your appearance, behaviour, and personality I happen to value or notice as I make the judgement. That in turn can be affected by what else is going on in my environment. If, for example, I express my delight in classical music, and you adore Mozart, then you may feel we're more similar than my obvious revulsion at your political opinions might have led you to believe. Empathy between people can change extremely rapidly depending on the circumstances. The emotional contagion through which we pick up another person's moods, via subtle changes in body language, prosody, facial expression, and so on, can also be very fast, and these changes are often largely subconscious. Using neuroimaging technology to, in effect, bring them to consciousness might assist people to regulate their own responses.

There is, however, a danger: too much information might lead to overload, stressing people into reverting to stereotyped behaviours.

I have argued previously that the brain can be seen as an effort-minimization device, with conscious perception serving as a marker of effort.[19] This is why learning a skill is initially very much a conscious activity, with awareness diminishing as the skill becomes habitual. Conscious processing of information from neuroimaging technology is likely therefore to be far more effortful than the brain's usual social processing, rendered habitual by many years' experience, which typically occurs below the threshold of consciousness. Compared with what brains achieve, as a matter of course, during a simple social interaction, our conscious processing capacities are woefully restricted. Adding to their burdens will have to be carefully done.

Perhaps the prospect of monitoring other people's emotions in real time is too ambitious. Apart from anything else, not every human being is interested in other human beings' feelings. Surely a major motivation for pursuing wealth and status is the desire to escape the bondage of having to care about what other people feel. Of those among us who are interested in emotions, some are altruistic, but many have instrumental motives: marketing, political leverage, or other forms of manipulation. Is it wise to provide them with yet another tool?

Thought-reading

This brings us back to the traditional form of practical telepathy: as 'silent speech' or thought-reading. Here again the implications of making such powers available are almost unimaginable. Politics, for example, could be transformed, with voting performed via mentally activated computers, and candidates assessed on the basis of the visceral responses they inspire in voter focus groups. Advertising and marketing are already looking to neuroscience; think what they could gain from these techniques. Diplomacy would have to change; so would government, the media, and even science itself. Indeed, it is difficult to think of any area of society that would not be affected, should this child of the brain supremacy be born.

Classic science fiction portrayals of telepathy tend to regard it as a gift (though it may be a curse as well). It is often a marker of superiority and/or the next evolutionary step awaiting human beings: one thinks of the many instances in *Star Trek*, the 'group minds' of telepathic children in John Wyndham's *The Midwich Cuckoos* and *The Chrysalids*, and so on.[20] These stories suggest that, as with many powers, mind-reading is dangerous when unequally distributed, but can also be a positive force for social harmony. If practical telepathy of this kind does become available, therefore, much will depend on who gets it and when.

Devilry lurks as ever in the details so smoothly passed over when merely uttering the word 'telepathy'. Imagine a device—portable or perhaps implanted—that can deliver real-time thought streams: DNE data extracted from other brains, smoothed and remapped onto your cortex. At last, the gift to see ourselves as others really see us. (Be careful what you wish for.) But how will it work? Surely reception and transmission would not be switched on by default—imagine the noise—so we can imagine a focused system with settings appropriate for the circumstances. A 'lecturer' setting, offering one-to-many broadcasting, could transform teaching, politics, and the media, for instance. Requiring consent to 'sync' with someone else and pick up their transmissions would be the equivalent of opting in to data-sharing—and no doubt as easy for governments to override when, for example, chasing a suspected terrorist. Search technologies would allow the system to tune into certain DNE patterns and ignore others, allowing automated analysis to scan the population for 'dangerous' thoughts.

Selecting your choice of partner would be crucial. Enticing as the thought of spying on other people's mental lives may be, there are few Prousts out there whose cranial worlds would be worth raiding. If my head, and the blogosphere, are anything to go by, most of the neural chatter would be inane. Ow-it-hurts, yum-chocolate, must-wash-up, stop-it-do-some-work: we'd need some mechanism to filter out the junk from our transmissions. Who knows, the result might be a gigantic mental clean-up and admirably better internal self-regulation.

A side effect might be that spoken language becomes associated with lower financial and educational status, as is already happening for internet abstinence.[21] Speech and its support systems might even eventually atrophy from lack of use. Another unintended consequence might be that people withdraw still further from face-to-face interaction—where they risk being scanned—in favour of safer, more controllable, virtual connectivity.[22]

The quagmire of ethics

Mind-reading makes the ethical issues already raised by recent developments in social media, such as tailoring adverts to a person's profile and location, seem minor, especially if it becomes possible to apply the technology covertly. Yet it raises many of the same concerns, so we can regard public reaction to social media as a trial run for more distant products of the brain supremacy. I have already mentioned a major anxiety: mental privacy, given the many gaps between thought and behaviour. This is especially problematic when the technology intersects with power differentials in our unequal society. The powerful are likely to have more access, earlier, both to mind-reading and mind-protecting technologies.

Another concern is to do with control and ownership. Whose would the DNE data gathered by mind-reading technologies be? Who could exploit it for gain? If you took a photograph of a person in the street, you might view that photograph as yours, but would that be equally true if you took a brain scan?[23] What if your government scanned you, either without consent or with consent gained by some form of pressure, like making a scan mandatory for certain jobs, benefits or tax concessions? Would you be happy for that information to be held at all, given governments' lamentable history of incompetence when it comes to data security? Would you be happy for it to be passed to all sorts of third parties, in the name of greater efficiency? Or would you want the ability to opt out and delete the data?

A third concern is mission creep. Government allows the invasion of its citizens' privacy for specific reasons, like suspected criminality. Mind-reading scans, however, might well be vulnerable to reanalysis for reasons never used to justify the original study. Some kinds of scans might also provide information irrelevant to the purpose of the scan but hugely important to the individual scanned, such as the discovery of a brain tumour. This could be extremely damaging for individuals if a scan taken for one purpose (e.g. to vet a candidate, by an employer) was then reanalysed for another (e.g. to look for disease, by an insurance agent). Clinical neuroimaging technologies have procedures in place for this eventuality, but if mind-reading is to become available to people beyond the current specialized user base we need to think carefully about who has access, and what training if any they receive.

As brain scanning technologies become able to detect not just blatant disease but more subtle changes, the ethical problems they carry become more acute. Some are familiar from other contexts, like genetics: what if a scan shows up the first small signs of an incurable neurodegenerative disorder? Some, however, are peculiar to the brain, and down to the emphasis we humans place on certain aspects of brain function—the ones we call beliefs and desires. Here's an example: imagine you've applied for a job as a schoolteacher. You reluctantly agreed to the routine brain scan, and are horrified to be told that the machine detected the presence of inappropriate thoughts about children.[24] Not only do you fail to get the job, you risk being stigmatized, losing access to your own family, and being forcibly detained for 'rehabilitation'. The problem? You were so nervous that you found yourself wondering if you could ever have felt a sexual urge towards a child. Anxiously reviewing your past encounters with children, you involuntarily remembered an uncomfortable teenage experience of sex. The machine correctly detected anxiety, thoughts of sex and memories of being with children, but the interpretation was dangerously wrong.

Paedophilia, most people agree, is an evil, its status reflected in law. When it comes to those beliefs and desires disliked by many but not (yet) made illegal, the possibilities evoked by practical telepathy start to look very worrying indeed. If, kept awake yet again by my noisy neighbours, I dream of them dropping abruptly and quietly dead, I don't want that wicked thought made public, with names and dates attached. Especially not if it earns me an antisocial thought order, or whatever equivalent future governments use to crush their less-than-perfect citizens into shape.

People whose sex lives include unconventional—but entirely theoretical—components may likewise want to keep their fantasies to themselves. So may anyone whose criticisms of those in power, if openly stated, might cause them problems. The gap between thought and action allows space for human agency: self-control, the understanding that fantasy and reality are distinct, and the acceptance, essential to maturity, that not all desires can or should be gratified. Remove that gap, and one consequence will be that human beings become more infantilized, less able to control their own behaviour, and more tolerant of external controls like social pressure and state power.

Any form of social control, once applied, is far easier to extend than to roll back. Society, talk of free speech notwithstanding, is already extremely conformist. I've lost track of the number of times I've come across someone saying, 'It may be true, but you just can't say things like that!' Thought-reading, potentially so good for social openness, could be catastrophic for personal liberty. Research scientists may be currently barred by ethical constraints from doing the kinds of studies which would directly threaten that liberty, but ethical climates change—as we are already seeing with ideas about privacy since the arrival of social networking. Even if research restrictions are maintained, streams of progress which find their way blocked by ethics are apt to be diverted into other channels, such as those offered by military research or some private enterprise, where the moral constraints are looser. If ever there were a 'dual-use' technology, offering both benefits and dangers, mind-reading is surely it.

These examples involve potential harms to individuals. There are other cases, however, which do not cause obvious harm but which may nonetheless make us feel uncomfortable about the benefits of ultimate openness. Here is an actual instance, from a conference where neuroimaging results were presented prior to publication. The fMRI experiment involved showing religious and non-religious people pictures of women. The 'experimental' picture had religious meaning; the 'control' picture looked similar but had artistic rather than religious value. The results were as expected apart from one religious gentleman, whose brain had responded more intensely to the control image. When the researchers enquired, he confessed that he had thought the lady in the picture rather attractive. So they slipped that information into the presentation. Cue amusement from presenter and audience.

The data were anonymous, and the participant who gave up his time, unpaid, for science is most unlikely ever to know he's been laughed at, so where's the harm? Again, we have a pre-existing analogy: those noble people who donate their bodies for medical research will never know if students make rude remarks about their corpses (in the past trainee medics did a lot worse than that, but I'm assuming prank control is stricter these days). Since no harm is done, does it matter if the students, or the researchers, are less than respectful of their volunteers? Or is harm not the only consideration here? My instinctive reaction was that the laughter wronged that unknown man and demeaned the gigglers, though they caused no harm. What do you think?

Do we need privacy?

We are, for now, still private people. To take evolutionary psychology seriously implies that having a private self was either advantageous or, at the very least, not problematic for our ancestors. Why might that be? The standard model proposes that limited resources—food, shelter, good-quality mates, etc.—force organisms and the genes they carry to compete in what Charles Darwin called the struggle for existence.[25]

The struggle for existence inevitably follows from the high geometrical ratio of increase which is common to all organic beings. [...] More individuals are born than can possibly survive. A grain in the balance will determine which individual shall live and which shall die,—which variety or species shall increase in number, and which shall decrease, or finally become extinct.

To survive in a changeable world for long enough to reproduce it is a great help to be able to predict at least some of the changes. In social species like ours, many of the most important and potentially danger-ous variables are other individuals, especially competitors. Skill in understanding why they act as they do, and in predicting what they will do next, remains an advantage; people with autism, who seem to have difficulty with this, often struggle to function well in society. For our ancestors, even a slightly better-than-average gift for second-guess-ing others may have been enough of a grain in the balance to tip our species onto a trajectory where theory-of-mind skills were favoured by selection.

Developing better prediction, however, is only one side of the evolutionary arms race, because if your rivals can predict your behav-iour as well as you can theirs, where's the advantage? That sets up another selection pressure: less predictable individuals may be better, over time, at exploiting resources. In a social species, however, trust between members of the same group is so crucial that behavioural extremes are necessarily constrained. A little mystery may procure the impression of charisma—a useful asset—but excessive unpredictability makes you seem unreliable, mentally disturbed and possibly danger-ous. That reputation may get you kicked out of the group, with catastrophic results for you and your genes.

Being able to keep some beliefs and desires hidden, however, allows you to exploit resources without necessarily telling the group about them: to cheat and free-ride, now and again, when you feel you won't get caught. It also gives you a social currency: by strategically revealing hidden parts of your self, and reciprocating when others do so, you can build trust. These benefits require a private self. As we have acquired cultures, symbolic thinking, religions, philosophies, and ideologies, our private selves have grown accordingly to encompass abstract beliefs and ideals. Yet they remain firmly grounded in our individual and separate bodies, which is why, when our privacy is invaded, we feel not only angry and afraid but violated, ashamed, and humiliated.

Be wary, therefore, of those who call for greater openness, especially when they are more powerful than you. Asking, 'Cui bono?' may not necessarily produce the answer, 'Mihi!'.[26] Opening up your private self can be beneficial when trying to build trust, but in competitive conditions it makes you more easily exploited. Encouraging openness among the powerful—among whom I include the media—is no bad thing. Demanding it of the less powerful, especially when it is not reciprocated, may not benefit them and could worsen their lack of control.

If we do ever find ourselves faced with practical telepathy, arguments like the old canard, 'Why worry if you've nothing to hide?', will undoubtedly be produced, as they have been for every invasion of privacy from the Domesday Book to the CCTV camera. They are bad arguments, using social pressure to disguise the coercion involved. We have private selves for good reason. Openness is in itself neither good nor evil, so anyone wishing to extend it must make their case and show us they can be trusted. We may live in a world of technological prowess, but we are still creatures guided by ancient reciprocities. If you ask for a piece of my self, you must show me that you are fit to take care of it.

Will employers, partners or governments demand access to our minds as a sign of trust? Will the media espouse open access as the must-have accessory? Will market researchers and politicians clamour for access to data which gives new insight into voters and consumers? Should we expect the offence of cognitive rape—non-consensual scanning—to be added to the statute book? And will the technologies be sold as entertainment, therapy, surveillance, or essential survival kit in the brave new world?

The problem is not immediate. Mind-reading technologies, whatever the hyperbole may suggest, will not imminently be joining the arsenal of methods ·available to governments and companies who wish to render us more predictable. IMCOTT; as we shall see, there is much more work to be done. Nonetheless, such technologies as DNE recording are possible. The rate of development in science is so rapid, and rapidly accelerating, that every day seems to bring a new trophy hauled from the realms of science fiction into the pages of a journal. We barely raise an eyebrow at achievements which would have had people gasping even a mere few decades ago. Mind-reading is just another notch on science's bedpost.

Except that it isn't. This is a trophy capable of transforming not only our relations with other people (as the internet is doing), not only our quality of life (as the car has done), but our innermost selves: what it is to be an individual human being. It may well be with us before we are ready for it. Between now and then we will undoubtedly hear much about the blessings it could bring us; this chapter has presented only a few. But we also need to look closely at what we may be giving up.

4

Bring on the Designer Minds?

I want to argue that far from being merely permissible, we have a moral obligation or moral reason to enhance ourselves and our children. Indeed, we have the same kind of obligation as we have to treat and prevent disease. Not only can we enhance, we should enhance

(Julian Savulescu, philosopher)

Human enhancement is nothing new. We see it attempted every day, with varying success, in schools, evening classes and training courses. We do it ourselves when we drink coffee to stay awake or accept a glass of wine to ease us into a party mood. Some students take ritalin to help them concentrate, some workers take modafinil to stay awake.[1] Many people read self-help books. Dissatisfaction with one's present state of being is heightened by unrealistic comparisons—the fabulous creatures who stalk the halls of media and fashion set ruthlessly high standards—but these modern gods and goddesses did not invent our desire to be other than we are.

Drugs, legal or otherwise; counselling to learn from the wisdom of others; formal education and training—the details vary, but the methods have been tried for centuries. The brain supremacy, however, promises far more effective techniques of self-transformation than these haphazard behavioural and pharmacological approaches. Firstly, it offers to show us how they change the brain, allowing us to make both pills and behaviours more effective, with fewer side-effects and—importantly—faster and easier results. Secondly, it emphasizes the role of social and environmental triggers in making us who we are, allowing us to notice and alter influences that previously escaped us. Finally, we are already acquiring tools for direct manipulation of the brain by electromagnetic, surgical, or genetic tools. These are steps towards the goal of DNE programming: the ability to alter our neural function precisely, in real time, and on demand.

The dream of enhancement

As with mind-reading, a lot depends on what we propose to change. Much of the attention to date has been on cognitive enhancement: improving long-term and short-term memory, attention, self-control, and other faculties conducive to the exercise of reason, using drugs, electrical stimulation, and so on.[2] Advocates for cognitive enhancement, who often come across as wanting to remake the rest of us in their rational image, argue that we have been modifying ourselves for generations, so why worry? As Julian Savulescu, Director of the Uehiro Centre for Practical Ethics at Oxford University, puts it:

> In general, we accept environmental interventions to improve our children. Education, diet, and training are all used to make our children better people and increase their opportunities in life. We train children to be well behaved, co-operative, and intelligent. Indeed, researchers are looking at ways to make the environment more stimulating for young children to maximize their intellectual development. But in the study of the rat model of Huntington's Disease, the stimulating environment acted to change the brain structure of the rats. The drug Prozac acted in just the same way. These environmental manipulations do not act mysteriously. They alter our biology.[3]

We tend to think of our bodies as machines, taking in inputs from the environment: sights and sounds, food, drink, drugs, and so on. Before machines were so much a part of our lives a common metaphor was the idea of the body as a vessel into which experiences poured, a fleshy container of the human essence. Influential though these ways of thinking remain, they are misleading, because we envisage machines (and vessels) as having a solid structure unchanged by their inputs (or contents). The instincts that human enhancement is 'playing God' or 'unnatural', in a way that sending a child to university isn't, seem to be based on this distinction between inputs—which it is acceptable to change—and a structure which ought to be left alone.

The organic growths we inhabit, however, change their structure all the time. Genes are expressed, new cells grown, others killed off. Education changes not just the inputs we receive but the pathways in our brains along which those inputs run. Why, Savulescu is asking, should the concept of changing our brains be considered any different? Except of course that if we can change those pathways directly, and more precisely, we may be able to learn things better and faster. We trust education more, but that is because we have used this tool for longer. As we get used to brain stimulation, or consuming artificial DNA, or whatever techniques become widely available, we will come to trust them too.

The brain supremacy will offer many opportunities for such acclimatization. Already, electromagnetic stimulation is being explored to boost learning, increase creativity, and treat disorders from tinnitus to depression.[4] As we will see in later chapters, both invasive and non-invasive techniques for manipulating electrical or magnetic fields are available. Chemical manipulation of brain function is also becoming rapidly more exquisite, able to target specific genes, proteins, lipids, and ion channels: the building blocks of neuronal activity. Since greater precision should mean fewer side-effects, these technical refinements are surely to be welcomed.

I am not sure, incidentally, that the prospect of human genetic manipulation is as utterly unacceptable as many commentators seem to think. The furore over genetically modified food in European countries may seem an obvious counterexample, but there are better ways to handle how such controversial issues are presented. (Science communication, like marketing, is a learned skill improved by paying attention to the audience.) It is also remarkable what human beings will do to keep up with the Joneses, and offering gene manipulation as just another form of self-improvement could find enough takers to trigger social competition, as cognitive enhancing drugs are already doing. As it becomes more widely understood that all sorts of things change gene function, all the time, the contrast will be not between leaving our bodies as inviolate temples and mucking about with our DNA, but between mucking about inefficiently and haphazardly, or with precision and all the care of good science. Of course, like any other new treatment this one will have to overcome the technology hump: the problem of how to ensure product safety when people are willing to take up tested products but chary of being guinea pigs for new ones. Nonetheless, my guess—and it is no more than that—is that the potentially enormous rewards will offer powerful incentives to push research over the hump.

Oh brave new world

If the possibilities opened up by being able to read minds leave one gasping, those suggested by the new biotechnologies are frankly dizzying. What the brain supremacy promises is a godlike power, not over the world, but over ourselves and others. Children could be born free of the tendency to depression, old age no longer tainted by cognitive decline. Knowledge could be instilled far more quickly than it is today, anxieties much more efficiently soothed, bad habits altered. Fine-tuning desires, finessing motor skills, bringing awkward beliefs into line, all could become routine manipulations, part of the regular medical review that keeps your mind as healthy as your biotech-enhanced body.

Here are a tiny few of the potential consequences. Firstly, maintaining personal relationships may become easier, as couples learn more about what makes for good compatibility—at the level of neural circuits—and problems can be fixed by DNE reprogramming. If you did have a row, and something unpleasant was said which you can't stop remembering, you can have it erased, like any other trauma. If you and your partner find your sex life ebbing, no need to fret, just have your reward systems retuned. No doubt when you first committed to each other you underwent mutual adjustment to make sure each found the other supremely gorgeous. If your partner's fantasies weren't exactly yours, perhaps you had yourself modified to share them, as a demonstration of your love and commitment.

DNE recording may also be extremely useful. If your child has nightmares, and you can afford the equipment, you can monitor their dreams and better address their anxieties. Couples may like to peruse each other's dreams, creative types to keep a file of theirs. Maybe dreaming could even become an interactive experience for two or more connected brains to share—and, with DNE programming, to develop as they prefer. These facilities and others may enable us to dissolve many of the misunderstandings, and find ways around many of the problems, that currently make being with others such weari- some work at times. Perhaps our descendants will look back on early twenty-first century family dysfunctions much as we look back on slavery: with astonishment that such horrors were ever tolerated.

Work, education, and entertainment may also be transformed by DNE technologies, not least as learning and fun become merged in the single category of 'experience'. If you are ever bored, you can download adventures more enthralling than any videogame; and new industries will be needed to supply them. If you don't like your work and can't easily change occupation—perhaps your genetic profile put paid to your hopes of being a top celebrity—you can have yourself tweaked so the daily grind no longer bothers you. If you want to know what it feels like to conduct an orchestra, read Aramaic, win a boxing match, work as a supermodel, smell a rare orchid, taste the world's most expensive wine, or walk on another planet, you can pay your money and take your choice.[5]

No doubt, if the free market's ideological grip on humankind lasts long enough, there will also be provision for nastier tastes. Those who would like to know how it feels to sleep with a supermodel—or a dog, or a very young child—can fork out and find out. If their tastes run to throwing kittens on fires, to dog-fights or badger-baiting, those too may be satisfied. Likewise anyone who has ever wondered what it is like to die by the guillotine or to be a suicide bomber, to be part of a rampaging mob or to kill a woman slowly and sexually. Fantasies of murder, paedophilia, and so on will thus be available to anyone who wants them—as many do—without real harm ever needing to be done. From war crimes to car crashes, unpleasant but strongly exciting experiences have always attracted a clientele. Adding new technology does not change that.

Except that the fruits of the brain supremacy could make it possible to change the brains of those with unacceptable desires, suppressing the behaviours which fulfil them or even the desires themselves. If and when these technologies materialize they will thus carry with them some interesting moral implications. Violent and sexual fantasies, both of which are very common, have long been considered both private space and part of the way a person is, part of the fate doled out by genes, environment, and experience.[6] The power to adjust them, however, moves them from private to public and from uncontrollable fate to controllable features of an ever-more-malleable self, which means that the person must take responsibility for them. 'I can't help it, it's just the way I am' will lose its force as justification, as will defences which mention compulsive desires or even mental illness.

Anyone who needs violence in their lives—or anything else despised by public opinion, whether actual or imaginary—will then face a choice. They can take the virtual experience, on the understanding that any real crime they commit will earn them severe penalties—which may include being made to feel the emotions of victims of violence, as restorative justice goes neural. Alternatively, they can undergo adjustment to cure them of their dangerous predilections. Would we feel more lenient towards the fantasists if their aberrant urges could be satisfied without damaging a single child, or would we insist that they be cured? Would they themselves be happy in a virtual world, if the thrills it provided were intense enough? Or are there limitations to John Stuart Mill's liberal principle that what matters is the harm being done, because certain behaviours are wrong whether the victim is real or virtual?

The beginning and end of life could also be transformed. Parents could exercise more conscious choice over the psychological traits and disease susceptibilities of their children (it may be that if you want a genius you have to accept a greater risk of mood imbalances). If you want your baby to grow up adventurous or musical, don't forget to mention it to the reprotechnicians; you may have to pay a little more. Intelligence, concentration, excellent memory, and an instinctive liking for fruit and vegetables come as standard. Your genes have barred you from certain occupations, but Junior should have more choice, and both of you should stay mentally fit into your second century. When the sad time comes for end-of-life care, your brain will receive continuous DNE programming to ensure that reality feels pleasant, whatever your physical condition at the time. And when your medical team can do no more, that same manipulation will make death an easy transition, like going to sleep.

Enhancements are go?

Enhancements are often said to require separate justifications, compared with treatments, since one restores adequate function while the other goes beyond normal. Normal, however, is a slippery construct, even without the moral overtones it easily acquires. There are plenty of women of normal body weight who long to be thinner, perhaps because they are influenced by media, rather than medical, definitions of what is normal. If a new diet pill could make them thinner, easily and without side-effects, they would presumably be happier, so providing the pill is surely a good thing. 'What matters is human well-being, not only treatment and prevention of disease,' as Savulescu says.[7] The fact that the women's current unhappiness does not meet clinical standards for mental disorder is neither here nor there; if science can enhance them, science is obliged to do so—providing we can afford it, of course.

Similarly for intelligence, memory, and other features of interest to the cognitive enhancers.[8] These are, like well-being, good things in themselves, and they are also linked to other goods. Intelligence, for example, has been associated with creativity, more liberal, pro-democratic attitudes, higher socioeconomic status, better physical fitness, and longer and healthier lifespans; it has even been suggested that smarter men have better quality sperm.[9] What's not to like about having more of these benefits?—assuming, of course, that the association with life's good things remains when we artificially boost intelligence.[10] Proponents of enhancement have further argued that boosting cognition will benefit both individuals and societies as a whole, and that such benefits are urgently needed given the complexity of the social and environmental problems we currently face.

That argument has several components which need scrutiny. One is the claim that enhancing attention, memory, and so on will improve our ability to think and/or make us better at solving complex problems. Is this the case? A better memory would have been a distinct advantage in the eras of Homer or Cicero, but these days we have high-capacity memory storage devices to assist us, so enhancing memory would be most useful not for itself but if it boosted other cognitive powers. It is not clear, however, that this is the case, at least for healthy adults.[11] Improving the cognitive building blocks may be more relevant to early development, and/or passing exams, but of course applying these techniques to children brings its own issues. Even in adults, safety concerns are far from trivial, because in a system as complicated as a brain, the law of unintended consequences has all the more capacity to wreak havoc.

Another doubtful claim is that boosting individual cognition will benefit societies as a whole. In principle, perhaps, but in practice enhancement technologies, and any benefits which flow from having enhanced workers, are likely to be distributed unequally, thereby widening the already gaping chasm between fortunate citizens and the impoverished rest. Proponents of enhancement, who tend to be Western academics, understandably want to improve the abilities of others as well as their own, but it is not clear how widely that charity extends. To their own students, and to rival professors? To competitor countries? Worldwide? Yet how effective would it be, even if the funds could be allocated, to make enhancement available to students who lack teachers, books, computers, and other necessities, in a world where some children are not even able—or allowed—to go to school?

It is also difficult to see how cognitive enhancement can be considered in isolation, as an individual benefit for which individuals should be held responsible, especially when children are involved. In practice, if something were to go wrong—say if an enhancer given to toddlers turned out to make them more violent teenagers—the state would have to pick up the pieces, whether in dealing with the extra crimes or funding research to try and redress the problem. In other words, the individual gets the lion's share of benefits, while society must underwrite the risks.

In our competitive world, there is also a fear that making enhancing agents so readily available will put pressure on people to take them in order to keep up. If the enhancers turn out to be bad for us—and the jury is still out on that one—then this indirect coercion is a legitimate concern. But what if the side-effects are minimal? Some commentators, such as the psychologist Vince Cakic, argue that if taking an enhancer is as safe as reading a book or going to college, then some people's reluctance to do so can be considered irrelevant as a reason for banning the use of enhancers by others. 'Although indirect coercion would imaginably be an unpleasant experience in those who feel it,' Cakic concedes, 'the expectation that one restrain their actions for fear that it may evoke feelings of coercion in others is not a particularly cogent reason for prohibiting these actions'.[12] If lots of people join a social network like Facebook, the cultural expectation becomes 'You are on Facebook'; but the existence of people who feel pressured to join and don't want to is not a 'cogent reason' for banning the use of Facebook.

Nonetheless, despite the term 'cogent reason' these are moral judge-ments (and logging on to Facebook is not the same as taking an enhancing drug). They balance the harm of interfering with personal liberty against a sense of social pressure for which Cakic appears to have little empathy; others might feel differently. Elisions of reason and morality are common in discussions of enhancement. This can be a problem, since academics claim their authority as experts on the basis of rationality, not moral superiority.

There is a further, more basic objection to the argument in favour of cognitive enhancement. Given the likely inequalities in the distribution of these goods, it is possible that, although better cognition may be a good thing for an individual, cognitive enhancement may not be a good thing for society as a whole. If it were to be used in the clinical sense of bringing less able thinkers up to the standard of the most adept, then it could be of huge benefit, but history and economics tell us that this will not happen. Instead, to use the biblical phrase, 'For whosoever hath, to him shall be given, and he shall have more abundance'.[13]

This prospect has troubled many advocates of enhancement, who are well aware that modern technology has already increased our cognitive capabilities. It has greatly speeded up our access to know-ledge for anyone who can query a search engine; it allows more efficient sharing and visualization of information; and its swelling powers to store, sort and interrogate data make humankind immensely more adept than it was even a few decades ago—let alone in the early years of the twentieth century, when my grandmother, then nine years old, was busy scraping ash from under a boiler. This cognitive boost has in recent years been accompanied by a decline in active warfare, which might suggest that enhancement does indeed provide social benefits. Unfortunately, IMCOTT. As the 2010 report from the internationally renowned peace research think tank SIPRI states: 'The decline and stabilization in the overall number of armed conflicts contrasts with a slow but steady increase in overall global crime levels in recent years, as well as a lack of any discernible decline in global, regional and subregional levels of criminal violence.'[14]

So far, the cognitive enhancements provided by technology have not provided that much of a dividend for one of the world's great problems, interpersonal violence. Would further improvements help? Julian Savulescu has his doubts:

> Technological advance and consequent exponential growth in cognitive power means that even rare evil individuals can act with catastrophic effect. The advance of science makes biological, nuclear and other weapons of mass destruction easier and easier to fabricate and, thus, increases the probability that they will come into the hands of small terrorist groups and deranged individuals. Cognitive enhancement by means of drugs, implants and biological (including genetic) interventions could thus accelerate the advance of science, or its application, and so increase the risk of the development or misuse of weapons of mass destruction. We argue that this is a reason which speaks against the desirability of cognitive enhancement, and the consequent speedier growth of knowledge, if it is not accompanied by an extensive moral enhancement of humankind.[15]

We fear Dr Strangelove. Intelligence without wisdom, the man who thinks that 'I can do this' equals 'I should do it', the terrifying hubris of science gone haywire. Even a philosophy professor, that most rational of creatures, finds the idea alarming; so should the rest of us panic? Perhaps, though probably not any more than we are already frightened by the idea of terrorists using a nuclear weapon, a possibility few of us can do anything about.

With cognitive enhancement, however, we do still have the power to change the future of the brain supremacy. We can demand to know how our governments—and our military researchers—are studying the topic and regulating others who do the same. We can attend scientific talks on enhancement, vote in surveys, email scientific societies, and do much else besides to make our views known. None of this need take unfeasible amounts of time or effort. Being a citizen interested in science is easier today than it has ever been, yet a European survey in 2010 reported that nine out of ten of us rarely or never go to public science events.[16]

No one can accurately predict how the brain supremacy will develop. I have highlighted some possibilities; there are no doubt many others. The fear of a new Dr Strangelove may well be outweighed by the many benefits that widespread cognitive enhancement could eventually confer. On the other hand, it may be that the last thing this overburdened world of ours requires is yet more clever, technical intelligence. Rather, it requires a redirection of motivation along more moral lines, and an increase in wisdom, whatever that may be. Later I will consider how wisdom could help us, and indeed what wisdom has to do with science. First, however, what about Savulescu's suggestion of moral enhancement? Could it help?

Beyond cognition

> The beliefs currently rattling around in the heads of human beings
> are some of the most potent forces on earth
>
> (Sam Harris, psychologist)

Cognitive neuroscience and moral psychology have become close companions lately. The prefrontal cortex has long been identified as important in moral judgement, but it does not act alone. Research has also implicated areas of parietal, insular, and cingulate cortex, together with subcortical structures like the amygdala and hippocampus.[17] Morality does not appear to have its own unique module, but to draw upon networks involved in non-moral reasoning and social cognition (much work has been done on theory of mind, for example). The role of emotional processing has also been highlighted in recent work, notably with respect to the emotion of disgust, which seems to have a much more powerful influence on moral judgements than we might like to believe.[18]

How morality is best deconstructed is a matter for ongoing debate. Joshua Greene has argued for a model in which cortical reasoning battles for control with subcortical emotion.[19] Jonathan Haidt prefers a five-factor model of moral foundations, in which concerns about harming and caring, respect for authority, fairness, loyalty to others, and anxieties about symbolic or physical purity vary across both people and situations.[20] Then there is the 'universal moral grammar' school, exemplified by Marc Hauser's controversial book *Moral Minds*, which argues that morality, like language, has a basic structure, found in all cultures, on which local variation is overlaid.[21] What all these approaches, and many others, have in common is that they accept the analytic strategy, seeking to parse morality into its components.

Some of those components we think of as cognitive: the ability to reason, understand language, decide between two alternative actions without forgetting one of them, and so on. Theory of mind, the ability to imagine what others are thinking, is sometimes called cognitive empathy to distinguish it from the feeling-your-pain kind. Other components are emotional—empathy, disgust, the outrage one feels at unfairness or betrayal of trust—or aspects of character, like sociability, optimism, or trustfulness. In principle, any of these could be manipulated. It has been suggested, for example, that applications of the hormone oxytocin stimulate empathy and so could be used to boost social affability and in resolving conflicts.[22] Alas, more recent research suggests that the so-called cuddle hormone is only effective for people who might be prepared to consider cuddling each other in the first place; enemies are not included in the love-in.[23] Even if empathy can be enhanced between hostile groups, excessive empathy can lead to mental distress and consequent hostility. It can be hard to tell whether callousness is innate, or acquired protection.[24]

Moral enhancement will thus need to be done with considerable care, since the chance of unintended consequences is high. Perhaps a means of suppressing disgust would be effective, or a way of reducing anxiety in those who feel threatened by stimulating their sense of control or manipulating their stress responses—but one would not want too little disgust, or too much self-esteem. An additional challenge is that some of the crucial brain areas are difficult to access with current non-invasive technologies: the amygdala lies under the temporal lobes, the insula buried deep in folds of brain. Moral processes are also tricky to study in animals, which is another reason why this field of neuroscience has not progressed as quickly as some others.

The rapid progress currently being made, however, will not necessarily address concerns over enhancement, whether moral or cognitive. One such worry is more of an instinct than an argument, but none the less powerful for that. It is often expressed as unease about scientists 'playing God' or 'interfering with Nature', and like many of our most emphatic moral judgements it draws on disgust. But it also relies on a concept foundational to the biological sciences: the notion of homeostasis. The idea is that within a cell, an organism, or a group there are balanced states and states of imbalance, and that the system at any level tends to promote the maintenance of balance. One can push so far, within a limited range, and the system will self-correct. Push harder, and it will either become maladaptive—as in chronic stress—or veer into collapse. The instinct frets that, by meddling with human nature, scientists will push too far and do more harm than good. Whether this concern is valid, I do not know; neither does any scientist. As yet we understand very little about brains' constraints and their tolerance of artificial changes to their systems, since such changes have never before been possible.[25]

There are challenges to enhancement, both moral and cognitive, which I do not have the space to consider here. One, though, demands inclusion. It queries not only specific technologies, not even the idea of enhancement, but the notion that this kind of approach could solve the world's most pressing difficulties. Is what we need more intelligence, better memory, more empathy, or a stronger sense of fairness? Are these the most efficient targets for future brain manipulation? Or is the idea of an easy technical fix itself part of the problem?

Beyond enhancement

After all, it is standard to describe the problems we face as 'complex', but are they? Climate change, biodiversity loss, pollution, water and energy security, even migration, conflict, the arms trade and social inequality…one might argue that at base, despite their fearsome intricacies, these share one simple cause: too many people consuming too much. Every day, it is estimated, about 156,000 of us die and 384,000 are born—nearly two and a half times as many.[26] The astounding growth rate would be less alarming if all of those already on the planet consumed only as much as its most restrained members, but that is not the case. Instead the poor seek to emulate the richest, who have contributed the most to the damaging effects of fulfilling all those individual desires. Using up resources too quickly, creating too much toxic waste, too insistent on the differences between us, and far too prone to settle those differences by killing each other, we have plenty of urgent items on the global agenda.

These problems are simple in the sense that they are easy to state and have traditionally been solved by simple methods, namely, migration or war. (Political uses of mass killing and genocide were not developed by sadists for their pleasure, but because these strategies are effective; the dead leave any wealth they have behind and consume only those resources required to dispose of them, which for enemies can be minimal.) The reason that we find ourselves in such difficulties today is that the simple solutions no longer work. We cannot yet migrate to other planets. Nor do today's wars, risky and costly though they are, kill enough human beings to counterbalance our rapid rate of increase; not even the worst diseases can do that. We are coming up against our natural limits, and we cannot or will not control our numbers (what species ever did?). Instead we look to science and technology to help.[27]

And help they do in many ways beyond the scope of this book, from new types of contraception to methods of more efficient energy extraction. Yet these do not solve the underlying problems of our human plenitude, which are problems of will—that is, moral and political, not technological. Furthermore, we already know what needs to be done. Cutting back on consumption, incentivizing greener business practices, and abandoning the fetish of economic growth. Using taxation to forge closer links between the damage caused and the people who cause it so that people who choose to harm the environment actually pay the real costs of doing so. Reducing inequality through redistribution, improving the lot of the world's poorest and insisting on better social status and education, especially for women. And—with the help of brain research—encouraging attitude change to make the rest happen.

Politicians, environmentalists, and other commentators have urged us to embrace all these approaches and more, in the hope of building a better, fairer, and ultimately less destructive society. For myself, rereading the list I've just written, it is all too easy to see why we long for the technofix, the sticking plaster of science. Doing things the more natural way, the hard way, is just too hard. Vested interests, indifference, ignorance, downright inertia...the array of obstacles makes the task seem impossible. Scientists tell us we need to change our behaviour quickly, but even gradual change may be beyond our selfish, fragmented, conservative institutions.

What we need is to be able to change what people care about, because when they care enough, they can work wonders. Highly motivated humans can build cathedrals, set up great companies, or organize immense outpourings of kindness and charity. They can work themselves to death or sacrifice their lives for others. They can start campaigns which change the bad habits of corporations or even governments. These enterprises succeed when they work with human nature, but we have not always found it possible to do that; hence the big problems. In the era of the brain supremacy, however, we may be able to change human nature itself: the ultimate technofix.

Attempts to make better people, from cults to communism, have a long and unsuccessful history. Could a neurotech approach be different? To answer that question we must ask another: how realistic are the visions set out here? The path to the brain supremacy has begun, but how far along the path to end-game technologies like DNE recording and programming have we come already, and how far are we likely to get? Perhaps the extreme scenarios extrapolated here are in fact impossible. Or perhaps they are underestimates, and by 2050 we will have reached 'The Singularity', the moment when, as postulated by futurists like Vernor Vinge and Ray Kurzweil, machine intelligence exceeds the human kind and all bets are off.[28] All the facts we have to go on, when trying to guess what the brain supremacy will bring, are limited to past and present research. But if we can also understand brain research methods, we can better extrapolate to what soon may be.

To think about the future, in other words, we need to take the plunge into neuroscience, and ask what its methods can teach us here and now.

5

Seeing the Brain
through Many Eyes

Every adult should have a base of scientific understanding about how
the world works. But understanding the process through which
scientific knowledge develops is equally critical

(Bruce Alberts, former president of the US National Academy of Sciences)

Neurotech—the methods and machines of brain research—must
surely be one of the most underappreciated marvels in science.
These technologies have given us unprecedented power to understand
the puzzles of being human. Just because the machines are not as big as
the Large Hadron Collider does not mean they are any less interesting.
Far from it: they are fascinating demonstrations of scientific creativity
and craft. Without some familiarity with the tools, moreover, it's hard
to make sense of the glittering contents on display in the house of
brain research.

Neuroscience draws on sciences from organic chemistry to quantum
mechanics as well as on knowledge of brain cells and blood vessels.
Interdisciplinary research is part of its fabric, necessarily, since a single
way of seeing cannot grasp an organ this complicated. Brains are difficult,
and neuroscientists need all the help they can get from other research
fields. In the following chapters, therefore, I will be exploring the subatomic and quantum worlds as well as the world of neurons. Physics,
chemistry, and biology were traditionally taught as separate domains,
but that is increasingly unsustainable, especially for neuroscience.

Brain research is an excellent way to learn science, but it encourages a more pick-and-mix approach.

Tracing the logic of neurotech machines is an excellent way to see how scientific thinking, faced with very tough problems, draws on deep principles to come up with smart solutions. For neuroscience the biggest problems are these. How can we look inside a living human brain without damaging it or murdering its owner? And how do we manipulate it without damaging it more than we absolutely have to?

The hunger to understand, control, heal, and even improve how our brains work is the hunger to understand and control ourselves and others. Neuroscience has developed a fine array of tools to assist us in that quest: ways of seeing the brain, and ways of changing it. The following chapters will look at examples of both. First, however, it will help to know more about the central enigma of the brain supremacy: that fatty pudding stuffed between our ears.

We begin with a very old tool indeed: the knife.

Reach for the knife

At first sight it doesn't seem beautiful (see Plate 2). The pale, swollen shape, crisscrossed with blood vessels brown with age and preservative, is not unlike a cauliflower with the leaves stripped off. The anatomist who fished it out of storage places it gently into my gloved hands. The core of a person, once; now this baffling lump. In the awe-inspiring surroundings of Oxford University's anatomy department, with its matchless displays of immortalized human innards, I and my tutorial partner are getting our first ever lesson in human brain dissection. We cut carefully, as if through a priceless cheese, splitting the amazing thing into left and right halves. Then—being students—we christen one Mary, one Hermione, and begin our exploration.

Appearances can be misleading. Brains possess extraordinary beauty, as the images in this chapter demonstrate.[1] Their cells are gorgeous, their structures and networks gloriously intricate, their functions astoundingly complex, and the management of all these parts remarkably efficient. Intellectually as well as visually they are marvels. They are also mysteries, despite all the advances in research and computing. Each of us carries a treasure we cannot hope to replicate or replace.

And yet a brain by itself looks cumbersome, awkward, out of place if not actively unpleasant. Its colour and texture remind one of porridge or cheese, depending on whether the organ has been preserved. It's wreathed in grimy blood vessels. And when it's alive it's pulsing and swimming in goo: the cerebrospinal fluid essential for nourishment.[2] When I see a naked brain I feel the awe with which other people speak of their holy places, but I can understand why others might be repelled. Like many other pale and squamous things, brains rarely see daylight; their natural habitat is darkness. There is a sad ugliness about them exposed and out of context; they belong in living heads.

Where then do we get those beautiful images? From the methods we use to investigate the brain, dead or alive. Raw vision alone is nowhere near enough to reveal its depths, so we have sharpened our vision with ever more sophisticated machines, like the neuroimaging scanners now capable of watching living brains in their natural environments. Later, I'll be saying more about that remarkable capacity, but brain research began long before neuroimaging. It began with vision. And with a nice sharp knife.

Learning to talk about brains

Humans are visual creatures. Even in writing or mathematics, many of our tricks of understanding use visual language and visual imagination. And despite our long acquaintance with writing and maths, we still rate pictures highly: flooding our world with them, paying huge sums for some of them, deeming them worth at least a thousand words. Certain pictures become iconic, like certain personalities, and that is as true for scientific images as for the *Mona Lisa*. We recognize and respect the DNA helix, the mushroom cloud, the brain scan—albeit with different flavours of admiration.

Images, descriptions and medical treatments of brains date back centuries. In the West until the Renaissance, however, knowledge of brain anatomy was largely based on sporadic case studies, work in other primates, and the studies of the Greek doctor Galen.[3] Knowledge of brain function was also vague: some people even thought of the brain as like a radiator, useful for cooling the blood.[4] Aristotle and Galen, who downplayed the brain's importance, exerted great influence on early European science, though other (Greek and Arab) thinkers challenged their teachings.[5] Also helping to smother innovative European studies were religious objections to cutting up human bodies.[6] Even after the Renaissance shook Europeans' awe of the old Greek masters, it took time both for the horror of anatomy to subside and for technology to develop the tools required (an ongoing project). Western neuroscience is a relatively young field of study. The structure of synapses, for example, was only confirmed in the 1950s, and it is only since then that the discipline has really begun to mature.[7]

Attitudes to dissection—as to scientific research in general—changed in the early modern period, from the sixteenth and seventeenth centuries onward. The curves of the human cerebrum tugged at the pens of scientifically and artistically minded men: Thomas Willis and Christopher Wren; Leonardo da Vinci; the great anatomist Andreas Vesalius (see Figure 2), and others.[8] These pioneers looked more closely at what had seemed a fat white mass, so dully inert that Aristotle thought it couldn't possibly contain human experience, instead assigning that power to the exuberantly beating heart. The men who overthrew the Aristotelian viewpoint reimagined the brain according to the technologies of their day: as an ordered world with numerous realms within, or an engine with distinguishable components. We have done the same ever since, seeing the brain as mechanical or hydraulic, a telegraph or a computer network; but always a mystery.

Among the large-scale structures of the brain an obvious starting point is the cerebral cortex, that mighty, multilayered sheet of cells and fibres which gives the brain its walnut crinkles, crammed into the skull like a crumpled newspaper into an overfull recycling box. Working

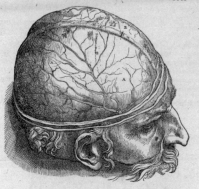

ANDREAE VESALII 605
BRVXELLENSIS, DE HVMANI CORPO-
RIS FABRICA LIBER SEPTIMVS, CEREBRO ANI-
malis facultatis sedi & sensuum organis dedicatus, & mox in initio omnes
propemodum ipsius figuras, uti & duo proximè præceden
tes libri, commonstrans.

PRIMA SEPTIMI LIBRI FIGVRA.

PRIMAE FIGVRAE, EIVSDEMQVE CHARACTERVM
INDEX.

PRIMA septimi libri figura humanū caput ita adaptatū exprimit, quemadmodum id
cerebro ostendēdo opportunè à collo & inferiori maxilla dissecātibus liberatur. Præterea tan
tam caluariæ partē orbiculatim serra abstulimus, quanta quoq; omniū quæ in caluariæ cōtinen
tur amplitudine uidendorū gratia, auferri solet. quanta uerò illa sit, liquidò dijudicabis, si septi
mam figurā sexti capitis libri primi examinaueris, quæ hinc ablatā caluariæ partem interna su
perficie exprimit. Quēadmodū itaq; præsens figura sectionis serie cæteras omnes inuicē ordine
succedentes præcedit, ita quoq; illā septimi libri figurarū primā non inopportunè inscribimus,
quæ durā cerebri cōmonstrat membranam adhuc illæsam, neq; aliqua ex parte pertusam, uulne
ratam ue. quamuis interim ipsius membranæ uincula diuulsimus, quæ per capitis suturas ad mem
branam efformandā porriguntur. quæ quod caluariā succingit, περικράνιώ nuncupabitur. atque
cum his fibris pariter uascula sunt effracta, quæ per caluariæ foraminula & suturas deducta,
ipsi duræ membranæ, ac illi qua caluaria succingitur, communes censentur. Cæterum ex duobus
qui figurā ambire conspiciuntur orbibus, humiliorē, cutis & membranæ ipsi subditæ cōstituunt,
elatior autem ipsa est caluaria. Vniuersum uerò hoc orbe complexū, durā cerebri membranam
refert, omnibus characteribus in figura cōspicuis uniuersim semelq; indicatam. at singuli chara
cteres in hunc modum priuatim habent.

A,A   Dextrū duræ cerebri membranæ latus, seu cius mēbranæ pars dextrā cerebri regionē ambit.
B,B   Sinistrum duræ cerebri membranæ latus.
C,C,   C   Tertius duræ membranæ sinus secundū capitis longitudinem exporrectus, & hic nulla ex
Ee 3   parte

FIGURE 2: An image of a human brain, in its anatomical (and literary) context, from Vesalius' *De humani corporis fabrica*, published in 1543.

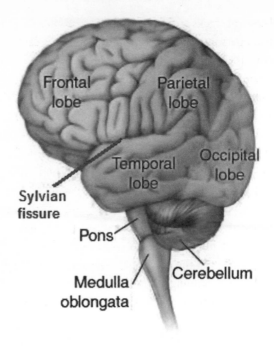

FIGURE 3: The Sylvian fissure.

Figure 3 shows a lateral (sidelong) view of a human brain, with the four major lobes of the cortex indicated. The Sylvian fissure, which runs along the top of the temporal lobe, is also shown, as are three subcortical landmarks, the pons, medulla, and cerebellum.

without modern preservatives, the pioneer anatomists mapped out the cortical territory, starting with landmarks like the Sylvian fissure. It's easy to be unimpressed by the one thing for which Franciscus Sylvius—born 1614, died 1672, Professor of Medicine at Leiden University in between—is normally remembered (unless you are a devotee of gin, which he is said to have invented). To our eyes the Sylvian fissure is hard to overlook, as Figure 3 shows: an abyssal plunge across the middle of each hemisphere, like an earthquake scar seen from space. But the modern gaze has had centuries to adapt, whereas Sylvius was a frontiersman. These days we use his fissure, along with others, to mark off the brain's internal boundaries.

Not all cortical cracks are always obvious. The folds vary greatly with age and from person to person; standard landmarks can be altogether absent.[9] Nonetheless, brains are mostly similar enough to have allowed early neuroanatomists to make gradual sense of the landscape they found beneath the skull. They noted the four neural continents that make up each cortical hemisphere: the occipital, parietal, temporal, and frontal lobes, lying under the bones of the skull at the back (occipital), middle (parietal), sides (temporal) and front (the clue is in the name). They also named the bulges (gyri) and crevasses (sulci) according to their relative positions.[10] The names are often quite sensible, once you get used to them—for instance the occipital and parietal lobes are separated by the parieto-occipital sulcus—but there are a few of what my mother calls traps for heffalumps. The central sulcus is one such: not the obvious gap which splits the left and right cortex, but a fissure running across the brain, dividing front from back. (It's also still occasionally called the Rolandic fissure—but these days only very occasionally.)

Later anatomists like Korbinian Brodmann (1868–1918) and Carl Wernicke (1848–1905) would map the physical territory of the brain's cortex at the level of what we now call cytoarchitectonics: regions distinguishable by differences in the kinds and spatial arrangements of their constituent cells. Wernicke's influence lingers in the term 'Wernicke's area', for a part of the temporal lobe involved in understanding language, while Brodmann's great patchwork quilt of cortex (see Figure 4, Plate 3) is still widely used for mapping the brain.[11] Cytoarchitectonics showed that most of the cortex has six layers, but not all. Areas which get inputs from the senses have a thick fourth layer; those controlling motor outputs have an exceptional fifth layer. Researchers concluded that information arrives at Layer IV and leaves via Layer V. Adding to the torment of future medical students, they further distinguished granular, agranular and dysgranular cortex, archaeo-, paleo- and neocortex, and a host of white matter tracts—the bundles of fibres which connect the 'grey matter' regions of cortex to each other and to subcortical regions.[12]

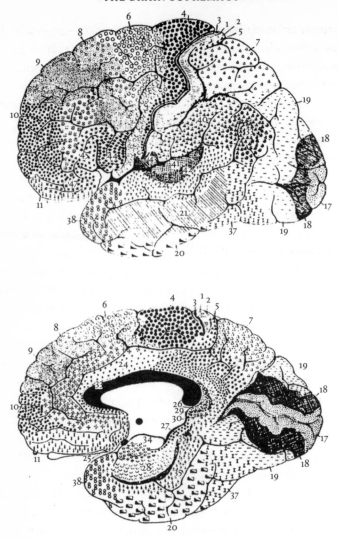

FIGURE 4: Korbinian Brodmann's view of cortex.

The figure shows the original cytoarchitectonic maps of cortex by Korbinian Brodmann. The numbers are assigned to distinct brain regions defined by their cellular structure, which tend to correspond to different functions. For example, Brodmann Area 4 (BA4) is primary motor cortex and has a large number of pyramidal neurons, hefty cells which send signals out through the motor control system (Figure 7 shows an example of a pyramidal neuron). The upper map shows a lateral view of the brain, in which the central sulcus and Sylvian fissure can be seen. The lower map shows a medial view (as if the brain was sliced into left and right halves and the inner face of one half turned to face the viewer). See also Plate 3, for a modern view.

Cortex is far from the whole brain story. Anatomists also traced the cranial nerves which feed the brain data and carry its outputs to the body. And they plunged into the difficult world below stairs, describing subcortical regions such as the hypothalamus, trigger of numerous essential hormones, the neatly ridged cerebellum—literally 'little brain'—which bulges low down at the back of the brain, and the brainstem, which in a living human tapers into the spinal cord.

The brainstem, incidentally, is where most of the information from our bodies flows into the brain, crossing over as it travels so that in general the right side of the body is managed by the left side of your brain, and vice versa. The command signals which underpin your sense of power and free will leave the cerebrum via the brainstem; and much of the routine work of body management—like breathing and the monitoring of blood chemistry and the internal organs—is controlled from this base station. Humans can survive—in a sort of a way—even very severe destruction of their cortex, but damage to the brainstem is another matter.

Another major control centre is the cerebellum, with its deceptively simple structure, which looks more like a computer than do most brain regions. It is thought to be involved, among other things, with regulating movement, posture, and balance. Among many other things. (One neuroscientist I knew was so passionate about the cerebellum that he liked to compare the cortex to a scrunched-up duvet, only there to keep the minibrain warm.) With its close subcortical colleagues, the basal ganglia and thalamus, the cerebellum does a huge amount of work; it is surprising, in animal experiments, just how much keeps going if the cortex is entirely removed.[13] In cases of abnormal human development, where the brain has had time to adapt while it still has the flexibility of youth, it's similarly remarkable how little cortex some people need to function—even though in healthy cases cortex is about four-fifths of the brain.[14]

Anatomizing

As neuroanatomy advanced, many brain parts were named for their appearance. This gave us terms like 'amygdala'—almond-shaped,

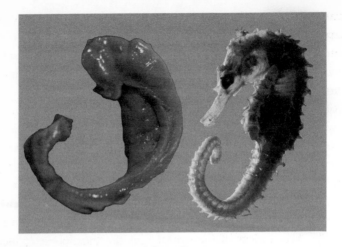

FIGURE 5: The hippocampus and the seahorse.
(Courtesy of Professor Laszlo Seress/Creative Commons licence)

apparently; I've never quite seen the resemblance—and 'insula'—because, tucked deep into the brain, this cortical fold looks like an island cut off from the rest of cortex. Some anatomical terms sound better in Latin, the language in which anatomy was traditionally taught; and they have been kept: an example is the superior colliculus (literally the upper little hill). The word 'cortex' is also from Latin: the bark of a tree.[15] Neuroanatomy can be etymologically tricksy, however, and some names which sound Latin are actually Greek-derived. One example is the 'campus' in hippocampus, which is nothing to do with the Latin word for field. The hippocampus is a subcortical structure heavily involved in memory, which curves around the core of the brain. It was thought to resemble a sea monster (*kampos*) of equine type (*hippos*): a seahorse, in other words (see Figure 5).

The brain's structural divisions indicate functional distinctions, notably teased out by the nineteenth-century and early twentieth-century doctors who gave their names to some brain areas (Broca's area, the island of Reil) and many more diseases (Alzheimer's disease, Friedreich's ataxia, etc).[16] For example, the occipital lobe is primarily

78

occupied with visual processing; the parietal lobe is associated with perceptions of space and of where the body and objects are located; the temporal lobe is linked to hearing and object identification, and the frontal lobe to movement control, planning, and decision-making. As a first approximation; inevitably, IMCOTT.

Complication was also apparent in the naming of parts: the burgeoning jargon of brain anatomy. As well as being called after people, areas could acquire names which reflected their function, such as the primary and secondary somatosensory cortices, which process touch and body perception. They could be named for where they were, like the frontal pole, or the frontal eye fields which help to govern where our gazes point. Today neuroanatomical terms include linguistic gems like the 'bed nucleus of the stria terminalis', 'the pedunculopontine reticular formation', and—a personal favourite—'retrosplenial dysgranular cortex'. Rich variety indeed, but it can be confusing.

If I wanted to tell you about where I took my last holiday, there are many ways of doing so. Some are general: 'Northern Ireland', 'the Antrim coast', 'near the Giant's Causeway'. Others are more specific: 'Portballintrae', 'a lovely little house looking out over the bay', or the exact address or GPS reference.[17] Which description I choose will depend on what I think you need and want to know, as well as on how much I feel like telling you. The same context-dependence is true for naming brain locations, especially in the cortex (see also the legend to Figure 6). For example, you could say 'dorsal prefrontal cortex', 'superior frontal gyrus', 'BA (Brodmann Area) 8', or 'the frontal eye fields' (FEF) to describe the same area; or you could merely say 'towards the top of the frontal lobe'. You could also describe the area in terms of its cytoarchitectonics (layers and cell types), its neurochemistry (frontal areas tend to be dopamine-rich, for example), or the connections it has with other brain regions, should you feel the urge. If you're into neuroimaging, however, you will want more precision, so imagers use a 3D grid reference, as shown in Figure 6 (30 6 60 would put us in the right-hand FEF).[18]

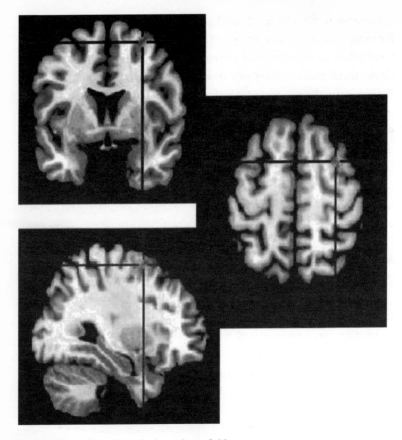

FIGURE 6: Finding the right frontal eye field.

The figure shows three views of the approximate location of the right frontal eye field in the human brain. The black crosshairs target the neuroimaging coordinates [30 6 60]. The upper image shows a vertical section (top of image = top of brain, left of image = left of brain). The middle image shows a horizontal section (top of image = front of brain, left of image = left of brain). The lower image shows a transverse section (top of image = top of brain, left of image = back of brain).

A note on terminology: in the brain (relative to its centre) front and back become **anterior** and **posterior**. Up and down become **dorsal** and **ventral**, or **superior** and **inferior**. The terms for inner and outer also change. Areas nearer the centre of the brain get the label **medial**, while more peripheral areas are **lateral**, from the Latin terms for 'middle' and 'side' respectively. These terms are used, singly or in combination, about the brain as a whole, and also to subdivide brain regions of interest, e.g. dorsolateral prefrontal cortex, posteromedial insula, inferior parietal cortex, and so on. Thus the frontal eye fields' location is anterior, superior, and lateral.

Sometimes 'the FEF' is all you know and all you need to know, but for those who go further, the social nuances are intriguing. Brodmann areas relate to anatomy and provide a useful common currency, so citing them makes you seem more traditional and user-friendly.[19] Referring to the superior frontal gyrus is more old-fashioned, and intimidating: it conveys the impression that you are so expert that you know individual gyri by sight, at once, in any brain. It is also not as helpful, since the anatomical curves can vary from person to person.[20] Mentioning the dorsal PFC suggests you're a systems neuroscientist, focused on function, maybe a computational modelling type or a neuroimager. Talk of the frontal eye fields is definitely functional, emphasizing what the area does, not where it is; someone using this language might be doing behavioural work on animals or humans.[21] Neuroscientists are a disparate collective. Brain research, however, has plenty of room for variety in its practitioners.

Even without social cues, the language of classical neuroanatomy is undoubtedly one of the bigger challenges for novices. For anyone who loves language, however, it offers a cavern of wonders. A lot depends on the teaching. I once watched an Oxford anatomist, over the course of three lectures, reduce a packed house of medical students almost to zero by reciting lists of neuroanatomical structures in a monotone while gazing near-continuously at the floor. (For anyone thinking, 'Told you, science is boring!', I can recall at least one philosophy lecturer who was worse.) Yet though the jargon may have driven generations of students half-demented, it can be as addictive as crosswords or sudoku, because brains aren't pure chaos. Their development, structure and function—and hence the words we use to talk about them—do follow rules. It's just that, as every bureaucrat knows, even a few simple rules can be combined in incredibly complicated ways. And with brains we don't yet understand all the rules.

Ours, however, is a visual age, so perhaps it is fair to say that for brains, as elsewhere, the value of pictures has risen, vis-à-vis words, as the ability to produce better pictures has increased. The brain supremacy will be shaped not only by scientific data, but by the ongoing struggle for public support, and images and their interpretations will be a key weapon in the fight to make people love science, or at least pay for it. Let us turn, therefore, to the pictures served up for our delectation by neuroscience. The best-known of those images today come from neuroimaging, but first there's an older technology to consider: staining.

Colouring the brain

Brain cells are extremely tightly packed. Take a slice out of the brain, and it looks like a layer of whitish cheese with dark smears. Under a microscope innumerable blobs appear: bits and pieces of severed neurons and the glial cells which surround them, with—if you're lucky—a recognizable synapse here and there. The anatomy lecturer I mentioned had slides of such images, bafflingly grey and dusty. Deciphering them as well as noting the names was a challenge too far.

Some of the lecturer's slides must surely have borne some resemblance to the delicate objects you'll see fizzing and sparking in brain documentaries. Neuroscientists associate these pretty skeins of brain-stuff—tracing out cells which seem to be floating in a void—with the Spanish and Italian scientists Ramón y Cajal and Camillo Golgi, true artist-researchers in the tradition of Vesalius and da Vinci. After years of patient work, they discovered chemical processes that would colour only a few neurons, allowing their shapes to stand out from the mass of their fellows (see Figure 7).[22] This breakthrough allowed the structures of individual cells to be understood—squat cell bodies, long axons, clouds of dendrites, synapses and all.[23] That revelation sowed the seeds of the brain supremacy.

Golgi stains, Nissl stains, horseradish peroxidase (HRP) and many other methods of tracing neurons and their connections have taught us an enormous amount about the nervous system. Their underlying principle is that neurons and other brain components fall into distinct categories which can be made visible by using different chemical markers. The consequences have been profound. Chemical delineation

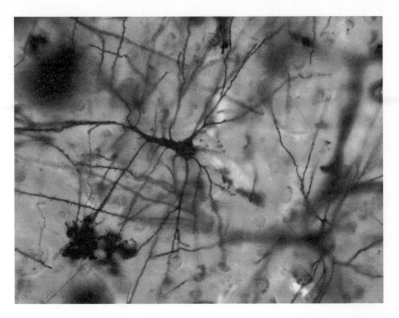

FIGURE 7: A Golgi-stained pyramidal neuron.
The figure shows a cortical pyramidal neuron, stained using the Golgi method to stand out darkly against the pale (originally yellowish) background. The cell body (centre), with its projecting dendrites and axon, is clearly visible. (Reproduced with permission of Bob Jacobs)

of the brain's constituent parts has revealed many types of brain cell, from basket cells to pyramidal neurons to spiny stellate cells and more. It has shown us details of the birth and death of synapses, and of glial cells, nuclei, and fibre bundles; how brains develop; how brain data flow and where.[24] And it continues today, with ever more precision and depth.

The further discovery that some markers, like HRP, could be taken up at one end of a neuron's long protruding axon and transported, within the cell, back to the cell body enabled neuronal circuits to be picked out, telling researchers which regions talk to each other. Do you want to know which parts of the brain send projecting fibres to the orbitofrontal cortex in the rhesus macaque? Prep your monkeys, inject your HRP compound into the orbitofrontal area, give the projecting cells time to suck the HRP back along their axons to their cell bodies, and then fix the brains by soaking them in formaldehyde, which will keep them safe and unchanging until you are ready to see where the HRP has reached.[25]

Of animals and humans

An obvious objection to this experiment will already have occurred to any reader fond of monkeys: fixing brains is fatal to the brain's possessor. Formaldehyde is nasty stuff. Animal research, however, has been invaluable to the development of modern neuroscience. I will have more to say on this topic later; for now, suffice it to say that much of the foundational animal work was carried out decades ago in a different ethical climate. The moral restraints which prevent us tricking, tormenting or slicing open fellow human beings to satisfy our curiosity have forced neuroscientists to infer much of what they know about the brain from studying other species, from zebra fish to mice and rats to primates. It is worth noting that primates are used in very few of the experiments done these days: fewer than 5,000 procedures (on still fewer animals) out of over three and a half million.[26]

Our brains have much in common with those of other organisms. Yet the differences, coupled with the moral restrictions, have fuelled a search for alternative technologies. Post mortem human tissue, meanwhile, has proved a great resource, but the supply is limited and precious, since dissected brains do not reassemble ready for the next student. I am not the only researcher to feel awe upon holding or viewing a human brain, but unfortunately no amount of respect from those who learn by dissection seems able to increase the donation rate—and neuroimaging, marvellous though it is, is no substitute for the act of anatomizing real tissue.

And even dissection, however skilled, is only one way of seeing inside a brain. A lamentably incomplete way, too; the vanished life leaves few readable traces of what it was like to be that individual, the donor. A dead brain, forlorn and naked, jarringly excised from its human apparatus, is a sad and pitiful reminder of past wonders. Whereof it cannot speak, thereof it must be silent—and the silence is vast. To probe that well of ignorance, both science and medicine needed a way of viewing living human brains without inflicting unacceptable damage.

Neuroscience, in its superabundant fashion, has come up with the goods many times over: not just hammers but a well-stocked toolkit. The following chapters will introduce you to three of the most commonly used neuroimaging tools. The first is PET, the second fMRI, and the third MEG (and to understand MEG we will also look at an older cousin, EEG). I have chosen them because they are standard techniques—ones you are likely to meet should you ever need clinical investigation or take part in a science experiment—and because they represent the three main approaches to neuroimaging: measuring the brain's biochemistry, assessing its blood flow, and recording its electromagnetic emissions.

Neurons are multidimensional entities, and to understand them, brain research has drawn on many sciences. In the next decades we may have techniques which use entirely new methods of brain imaging (a way of mapping the number of bits of information transmitted onto neural, biochemical, and genetic circuits would be helpful), but there will also be many which develop from current methods (for example, observing changes in protein levels or gene function within the cell). Understanding our present capacities is thus a necessary starting point. In the next chapter, I will begin with the science of PET scanning: with a chemical view of the brain, and radioactivity.

6

To Physics, With Thanks

We must not forget that when radium was discovered no one knew that it would prove useful in hospitals. The work was one of pure science. And this is a proof that scientific work must not be considered from the point of view of the direct usefulness of it. It must be done for itself, for the beauty of science, and then there is always the chance that a scientific discovery may become like the radium a benefit for humanity

(Marie Curie, chemist and physicist)

In the 1980s brain research received a boost from something happening in another science. Physics was dulling down. The Standard Model was well-established yet obviously incomplete; relativity and quantum mechanics, after years of negotiation, were still not reconciled.[1] Experimental physics was demanding huge investments of time and money, while in some areas of theory, though not all, too many problems seemed dustily uninspiring: what the philosopher Thomas Kuhn termed 'normal science'.[2] String theory was under development, but hadn't yet achieved the recognition needed to pump new life into a discipline feeling its age. Personable TV physicists like Brians Greene and Cox hadn't delighted audiences far beyond their labs; Stephen Hawking's *A Brief History of Time* hadn't yet astounded the publishing world; the Large Hadron Collider was still a twinkle in CERN's collective eye.[3] So when physicists looked for something more interesting, some of them noticed that brain research was not only interesting but difficult, under-researched, and sorely lacking in the paraphernalia with which physicists feel at home: complex equations and big, expensive machines.

They soon put that right. These days neuroimaging scanners are every university's must-have accessory: cheaper than your average cyclotron, but at about a million pounds each, not exactly cheap. As for equations, many articles on the brain still contain distressingly few of those, but work is in progress to rectify that situation. Mathematics is, after all, the language of science, and thus a marker for a discipline's maturity (except when it is used as a private language and token of insider status to ward off the plebs, of course; that kind of tribalism is as clear a sign of immaturity in science as anywhere else). Maths is not, however, the language of science communication, so there will be no equations in this book.

Why I love physics

Here a personal interest ought to be declared. Before I discovered brain research, early twentieth-century physics was my youthful infatuation. In this I am not alone. That revolutionary epoch had huge intellectual charisma, and the science it gave us retains the power to attract and intrigue. How could one not be mesmerized by a discipline replete with concepts like black holes and time travel? With sci-fi machines such as particle accelerators, and studies like the how-can-a-particle-be-just-like-a-wave double-slit experiment? And then there were the personalities—from Arthur Eddington (sweet) and Paul Dirac (strange) to Albert Einstein (far too much of a show-off) and Edward Teller (frankly alarming). Look hard enough, and my teenage self could even find a female role model: Marie Curie, who shared the Nobel prize in physics in 1903 and won the chemistry prize outright in 1911. She is said to have inspired generations of female scientists, and not just because there weren't too many alternatives. (There are other female physicists, but I didn't hear of them in school. And not many reach high levels of recognition: of the 189 individuals who have won a physics Nobel since the prizes began in 1901, only 2 were women.[4])

As for myself, at the tender age of 17 I faced the choice of doing physics, at the excellent, but from where my parents lived extremely distant, university of St Andrews, or physiology and philosophy, at the much more accessible Oxford. Plagued by what psychologists call math anxiety (in my case quite possibly justified), I reluctantly opted for convenience, and biology. I soon learned three useful facts. Firstly, physics was not alone in offering up odd characters. In philosophy, for instance, Gertrude Anscombe and Ludwig Wittgenstein were at least as strange as Teller and Dirac, while in physiology one tutor showed me a slide of an experiment he'd done which required him to stick a hook through his own eye muscle. Secondly, attraction and lasting affection are not the same. Thirdly, and most importantly, humans and their brains are more complicated, more challenging, and more exciting than anything to be found in a hadron collider.

Still, they say you never forget your first love (unless of course a brain disorder destroys your memory), and I owe much to the awe induced by quantum mechanics and relativity. Neuroscience too, especially neuroimaging, owes a gigantic ongoing debt of gratitude to physics and physicists. A clear demonstration of this knowledge transfer can be found in PET scanning, which uses both physics and chemistry to look inside human heads. To see how skulls can be seen through, we need a pinch of radioactive sugar.

PET power

Some neurotech, like EEG and MEG, relies on measuring the brain as it is. Electroencephalography (EEG) attaches electrodes to the skull and records the electrical signals given off by the brain beneath. Magnetoencephalography (MEG), as the name suggests, records magnetic fields arising from brain activity: the other side of the electromagnetic coin in which neurons carry out their transactions. Both techniques, as we shall see, rely on the talent of living cells, including brain cells, for shifting charged particles in and out of themselves. The measuring devices, intimidating though they may appear, are kept safely outside the brain.

Other kinds of neuroimaging add stuff to the person and then assess how the stuff behaves inside the person's brain. PET is one such.[5] These methods are conceptual precursors of one of the most exciting techniques to emerge in recent years, optogenetics, which adds stuff to the brain's genes, providing precise ways of both seeing and changing brains. As our grasp of the biochemical and genetic mechanisms improves, we will be able to design more subtle and specific experiments to elucidate brain function, research which will be crucial to the brain supremacy. Optogenetics, which changes DNA and has many safety issues still to resolve, is currently only used in animals, but what we learn from this, and from other invasive techniques, can be used to improve human neuroimaging—including designing future PET experiments. I explore the potential of optogenetics in Chapter 13.

In PET, the added stuff is a small amount of radioactive 'tracer' injected into the bloodstream: a solution of synthesized molecules whose chemical structure resembles material that the body's cells are used to working with, as part of normal metabolism. (The radioactive dose is very low— about the same as an abdominal X-ray—and PET scans tend not to be used repeatedly on the same person, not least because they are expensive.[6]) There are many possible tracer molecules. One of the most commonly used, and my example here, hijacks the biochemical pathways which process the sugar glucose in the brain. The chemical similarity between the tracer and glucose ensures that the tracer gets treated in the same way by cell processing. Or nearly the same way—and that caveat is crucial. It's a neat technique, and it works like this:

Brain cells gulp fuel like big cars guzzle petrol. Consider how little of your body is actually made up of brain: it's not even the whole of that knob at the top, after all. Adding the tendrils of your nervous system, you're still more liver, by weight, or more intestine, by volume. Yet your brain, about 2% of your overall mass, takes about a fifth of the oxygen you breathe in and about a quarter of the glucose that you eat and drink.[7] Neural consumers are extremely greedy. Or well-paid, depending on your perspective.

Neurons extract glucose from the bloodstream. Once the sugar fuel has moved from the blood to inside the cell, two chemical reactions occur. The first, phosphorylation, adds a 'phosphate group' to each glucose molecule (see Figure 8). If school chemistry is a less distant memory for you than it is for me, you may already have recalled that a phosphate group consists of five atoms tightly bonded: one phosphorus (P) and four oxygens (O). Oxygen carries a double negative electrical charge and phosphorus a positive charge of five, so the charges in this group do not balance out: a phosphate group has a triple negative charge: PO_4^{3-}.

Since glucose itself is electrically balanced, the effect of phosphorylation is to make it electrically negative. This has an effect on the neuron's border control—the cell membrane— similar to what hiding a gun in your hand luggage should do to security at your local airport. Neutral molecules may be allowed to pass, but once negatively charged, the glucose finds its exit barred. Phosphorylation thus keeps lunch on the cellular table, preventing the glucose from drifting out of the cell as easily as it diffused in. The fuel—including the radioactive tracer—is locked into the neurons whose activity the researchers want to measure.

The second chemical reaction, glycolysis, eats the lunch, extracting energy to power the cell by breaking the phosphorylated glucose molecule apart.[8] This chemical change is site-specific: it involves one particular segment of the glucose molecule. The break occurs at a point where one of glucose's six carbon atoms is bound to a negatively charged hydroxyl group (one oxygen plus one hydrogen; see Figures 8 and 9). Herein lies the trick used in PET. By fiddling with that vulnerable hydroxyl, researchers can create a mimic molecule that behaves nearly, but not quite, like glucose in the cell.

The difference is in how quickly the molecules get eaten by glycolysis. Glucose is fine for when a brain needs feeding, but for neuroimaging what you want is a marker which can get into the cells and stay there long enough for you to measure it without being chewed up by cell metabolism. In other words, you want your mimic molecule to undergo

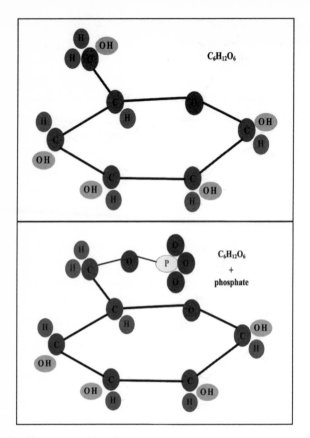

FIGURE 8: Glucose phosphorylation.

The figure shows a model of the glucose molecule before (upper image) and after (lower image) the glucose has been phosphorylated. The backbone of six carbon atoms (C) has chemical bonds with hydrogen (H), oxygen (O), phosphorus (P), and hydroxyl groups (OH⁻). Phosphorylation replaces a hydroxyl group (top left of upper image) with a phosphate group (top of lower image), a molecule made up of one phosphorus and four oxygens.

phosphorylation, so that it accumulates in the cell; but you don't want it broken into bits by glycolysis until after it has served its purpose by being detected. And minimal harm is an ethical requirement, so your tracer mustn't be too toxic and it must break down into something acceptably safe.

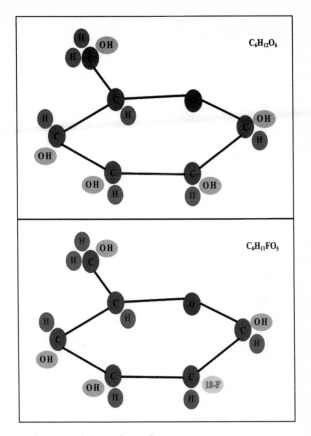

FIGURE 9: Glucose and fluorodeoxyglucose.

The figure shows models of the glucose molecule (upper image) and the radioactive molecule fluorodeoxyglucose (lower image). FDG can substitute for glucose in brain metabolism and can therefore be used as a tracer. The radioactive fluorine-18 (18-F) is shown at bottom right of the lower image.

Tracing a solution

How does PET's way of seeing the brain approach these problems? Its solution is admirably elegant and effective. Change that vulnerable hydroxyl group for something tougher: something with the same negative charge but different enough to delay glycolysis. How about fluorine (see Figure 9)? It's a similar size, and its ion (F^-) has the same electric charge as the hydroxyl ion (OH^-). Take a bow, fluorodeoxyglucose (FDG), chemical formula $C_6H_{11}FO_5$, one of the most frequently used radiotracers. Compared with glucose, $C_6H_{12}O_6$, FDG has added a fluorine (hence fluoro-) and lost an oxygen (hence deoxy-). It's also lost one hydrogen, but they're so common in the brain, as elsewhere, that they don't rate a name change.

However, and this is where the elegance starts to shine through, FDG is made with special fluorine: radioactive fluorine-18. A useful substance, this unstable atom converts itself to stable and harmless oxygen-18 ('heavy oxygen').[9] As F^{18} becomes O^{18} it emits a positron: a tiny particle of antimatter. Finding itself in a brain made of normal matter, the positron doesn't get far—at most a few millimetres—before it meets its deadly opposite-twin, an electron. As science fiction has often enjoyed reminding us, when this happens you get annihilation: an extremely miniscule Big Bang, in which energy is released in the form of high-energy photons, as gamma radiation.

Two shards of light flee the scene of the crime in such perfect synchrony that they arrive at the PET scanner's detectors, on opposite sides of the brain, almost simultaneously, thereby marking themselves out from (almost) all the other photons randomly bumping around in the detector. Not X-rays, but gamma rays mark the spot. Or rather, they draw a line through the brain from which researchers can work out where the spot must be.

There's one last twist in the story which is especially neat. Emitting its positron as F^{18} morphs into O^{18}, F^{18}-fluorodeoxyglucose effectively loses its fluoro- and adds an oxygen, bringing us back to where we came in: glucose. Although the fluorine has been replaced by a heavier form of oxygen than usual, that doesn't snarl up the cell's procedures, so the glucose can be processed as per usual. Back to normal; this form of imaging tidies up after itself. Fairly soon, too: F^{18}-FDG's half-life is around 110 minutes.[10] Visions of participants emerging from experiments with a faint but perceptible glow are tempting but inaccurate: any such halo is one of virtuous satisfaction.

So it's just a question of picking up the gamma rays emitted by the briefly rampaging positrons? Of course not: IMCOTT. All sorts of corrections and processing manoeuvres have to be done. The detectors take time to function, which must be taken into account; some random photons may, by coincidence, appear synchronized; head movements must be adjusted for, and so on. Then a large number of lines through the brain—the paths of the gamma rays—must be converted into a comprehensible map. With appropriate computational wizardry, however, a PET scan can offer a remarkably detailed image of a living brain (see Plate 1 for an example).

PET pros and cons

Invented in the 1970s, PET has been a workhorse of neuroimaging—and clinical medicine—since the 1990s.[11] The term 'workhorse' isn't exactly inspiring, but PET has proved its worth, and there is plenty of exciting research still being done with this technology.[12] One advantage of PET is that it can be combined with other methods, such as MRI, CT scanning, or optical imaging—not just viewing the brain through many eyes, but with more than one gaze at the same time.[13]

Another plus is the variety of radioactive tracer molecules that continue to be used, and developed, in PET. These 'radioligands' can target specific chemical systems, such as serotonin (a neurotransmitter associated with mood) or leptin (a hormone associated with appetite), allowing the behaviour of those systems to be isolated and studied.[14] Just as early anatomists coloured, and thereby picked out, individual neurons, so PET can colour the brain's many chemistries. It can provide invaluable information about molecules used by neurons to communicate, such as the neurotransmitter dopamine. A 2010 study, for example, used PET to show that drinking alcohol causes dopamine release in reward-related areas of the brain, especially the ventral striatum.[15]

That alcohol activates the brain's reward systems is not altogether surprising; that it does so significantly even in young and merely social drinkers suggests one reason why casual intake can lead to problem drinking. Using PET allowed the researchers to estimate how much dopamine was released. Interestingly, they found sex differences: women's reward-related brain activity increased by around two-thirds, men's by double that.[16] This information about changes in a specific brain chemical is not available from other common techniques, like EEG or fMRI. Each way of viewing the brain brings its own unique perspective.

Hammers are widely used, but they have their limitations. What are PET's downsides? One is its spatial resolution: how far an observer can zoom in to the brain's fine details. Emitted positrons, as mentioned earlier, can travel a few millimetres before they meet their doom. At the neuronal scale that's a big distance not to know about: a large neuron may be around five hundredths of a millimetre across. PET pinpoints the neighbourhood, but not the exact address.

There are also limits, built into its machinery, on the scanner's temporal resolution: how quickly it can reflect a change in brain activity. Neurons operate in milliseconds, so PET, with a temporal resolution of seconds or tens of seconds, is not capturing the detail.[17] For clinical purposes (like checking for tumours) the timescale is adequate. But for complex or repetitive experiments, or if you're looking to measure very rapid changes, other neuroimaging tools are better.

Randomness and the physical limits of the technology impose further constraints. No machine, especially one so intricate, can be error-free. (Medieval masons who built cathedrals used to leave deliberate faults uncorrected, albeit somewhere tucked away, because only God is perfect. Scientists now know that the universe has error built in, so science can never be perfect. If some scientists occasionally seem to have forgotten this constraint, that is because they are human as well as scientific, and vulnerable to hubris.) PET is susceptible to all kinds of potential distortions, from variations in individual physiology to human errors of interpretation. In addition, many PET studies have averaged their data over the group of people participating rather than looking at each brain separately. This is a good way to assess normal function, but glosses over individual differences, which can be considerable.

The human side of neuroimaging

As with all neuroimaging, those being scanned can also cause problems in PET, especially if they can't keep still, don't like needles, or if being fed into what looks like a giant washing machine gives them claustrophobia. Behavioural experiments can suffer from too much, or too little, behaviour. Psychologists and neuroscientists, especially those who do experiments with people, soon learn that humans are a disparate and strong-willed bunch, not easily simplified, prone to acting against their rational self-interest, and resistant to rules. Tell them how they're expected to behave and they'll do their best to comply—except when they feel like doing the opposite. They'll interpret your questionnaire in ways you never thought of; they'll misunderstand your inadequate instructions; they'll see things in your stimuli you never imagined, and they're virtually guaranteed to press the one combination of keys which finds a bug in your code and brings your experiment juddering to a halt.

In the fMRI study I discuss in Chapter 14, Rissman et al. (2010), 28 individuals took part in the two experiments, but data from five (18%) had to be excluded 'due to inadequate behavioral performance'.[18] Apparently, 'one participant reported falling asleep for brief intervals throughout the experiment'.[19] You might think this would take some doing, since being fMRI-scanned is like lying next to a pneumatic drill, while PET scans involve an intravenous drip, plus hunger and thirst (fasting in advance is often required). Yet boredom and fatigue can be a problem for any participant, especially the sleep-deprived students who service many of these studies. Scanning experiments can take an hour or more from meet-and-greet to fond farewell, much of which is spent lying flat on a not-entirely-uncomfortable scanner bed. Include behavioural tasks as well, and the time can easily stretch: sessions in the Chapter 14 study were around 3.5 hours. Researchers have a difficult trade-off between packing as much as they can into one session—it's hard to get people to give up enough time for more than one—and keeping their participants alert and awake so that scanning time isn't wasted. As scanning typically costs hundreds of pounds an hour, waste is undesirable.[20]

For PET, supply of the radiotracer (F^{18}-FDG or equivalent) can also be a problem, since it must be made at short notice and near enough to the participant that the radioactivity hasn't decayed too much by the time it's injected. Not everyone has a cyclotron in their back garden, not even neuroscientists or hospitals, and radiotracers aren't cheap. (So if you ever have a PET scan, please make sure you don't miss the appointment.)

PET done for research purposes has a more annoying caveat: gender. As a naïve graduate student, way back when PET research was still quite cool, I volunteered for one of our lab's experiments. The gentleman conducting the research told me women weren't eligible because radioactivity might be bad for future childbearing potential. I must have been having a feisty day, because I enquired why that was his decision, not mine. In vain. I was set to do behavioural tasks instead, which were extremely dull.

Not all PET research studies are male-only, but men undoubtedly dominate the literature, both as producers and experimental subjects— or participants, as they nowadays tend to be called.[21] The change of term reflects concerns about undue scientific authority, as evidenced for instance by Stanley Milgram's notorious experiments on obedience.[22] It takes the volunteers who give up their time for science from 'I will now subject you to this procedure' to 'I hope you will now participate in my experiment', a more tolerable attitude for the guinea pig.[23] The etymology sheds informative light, since the Latin noun *participatio* means a sharing or partaking, while the verb *subicio*, from which 'subject' comes, means to throw under. One term invites you to contribute to an experiment, the other hurls you under its wheels.

Feminist friends have been known to growl that in neuroscience, women are more likely to be subjects than participants. Scientists themselves have noted the distortions which result from sex imbalances in biomedical research and are working to correct them. Comments in 2010 from top science journals indicate that the problem has been regretted, if not yet resolved.[24] It will need to be. Women have much to contribute to the brain supremacy, which to date has been highly male-dominated; its impact will, after all, be felt by both genders. To encourage that contribution, however, we need more female researchers, especially in highly visible 'leadership' roles, as well as female participants. I look forward to seeing a female President of the Royal Society, for example; though as only 5.8% of the current Fellows are women I may have to wait some time.[25] (For science, and especially for science's leaders, male is still the default gender.)

In practice, however, the male–female imbalance has probably not been the prime incentive for seeking alternative neuroimaging methods to PET. More important have been the technique's aggravations—the invasiveness of having a needle stuck in one's arm and a dose of radioactive gunk swilling through one's system—and its blurred vision: the poor resolution in time and in spatial detail. For neuroscience to grow, and for the brain supremacy to approach its dreams of reading off real-time brain data, it needed new ways of seeing faster and better. Let us turn, therefore, to a technology which avoids PET's failings, and to the colourful world of functional magnetic resonance imaging.

7

The Subatomic Chorus

Although not everyone will be a 'brain specialist,' some knowledge about the brain will be considered indispensable for personal and occupational success in the later part of the twenty-first century

(Richard Restak, neuroscientist)

Welcome to the wonderful world of fMRI, the signature technique of modern neuroscience and a major contributor to its increasing presence in our culture. If any technique is the public face of brain research, it's this one. But how does that giant washing machine in the specially designed room enable scientists to watch and interpret a living brain in action?

Understanding fMRI

Don't ask the mainstream media. They operate under different constraints from scientists, and their stories highlight the results of neuroimaging research much more than the methods. Yet what we see depends on what instrument we see with, and without knowing how results have been obtained we cannot judge how seriously to take them. Exciting-looking results can crumble to dust when you look more closely at how they were obtained. Attention-grabbing headlines report new research findings, but the journalist hasn't the time and space to give much context in the article; and the headline-writer certainly doesn't. Take the following examples:

- Neuron Recordings Capture Brain Focus on Josh Brolin (*WIRED Science*).
- Forget Inception, Try Extraction: Dream Recorder is 'Possible' (*TIME* magazine).
- 'Marilyn Monroe' Neuron Aids Mind Control (*Nature News*).[1]

These three headlines are top-ranking science journalism from respectable, widely read sources. They report cutting-edge scientific findings in the language that journalists love to use about science: the language of capture and control, power and possibility. They mention future technologies to excite interest, and cultural references to boost emotional impact and connect with their audience's familiar worlds.[2] All three pieces are from around the same time, which is because they all refer to the same article, a piece in the high-impact scientific journal *Nature*.[3] In terms of providing useful knowledge of neuroscience, however, all three headlines are almost entirely useless. This inadequacy is, of course, intentional. It's how the writers lure you into reading the articles.

These headlines are examples of science-lite, which is as different from actual science as a child's view of being good is from a moral philosopher's—though as with morality you can see the two positions as points on a continuous spectrum of complexity. Science-lite is entertaining, intriguing, bite-size ... and at its lightest, very superficial. (Science is informative, detailed, and lengthy; ultimately more rewarding, I think, though like all the best pleasures in life you have to work at it.) Much mainstream media reporting tells you very little which can help you assess the claims it makes.

So how much do people know about fMRI? In an utterly unscientific survey, I asked a few friends and family, 'What is fMRI and how does it work?' This is what they said:

DAVID, COLERAINE: 'I would probably say fMRI was a way of looking at how the brain functioned, and that it worked in a similar way to X-rays in that a machine was used to scan what was going on inside someone's head.'

GILLIAN, BIRMINGHAM: 'They put you into a big machine and it makes your molecules wobble, and the purpose is to see which bits of your brain are active when you do different things.'

HELEN, GLASGOW: 'I assume it is an imaging scan (I have heard of MRI) but beyond that I am ignorant. I have no idea of how it works but I know it is used in assessing MS patients (I hesitate to use the word 'treating' because I don't think they can really treat it, or that MRI is a treatment for anything). And although one could make numerous suggestions of what the f stands for I actually don't know. Just remembered that MRI uses magnetism.'

ALAN, TELFORD: 'fMRI—really have no idea what f could mean. My guess, without googling, would be 'functional magnetic resonance imaging' which I understand to be a technique for scanning the brain providing an insight into the structures of the brain. Am I anywhere close?'

Not bad! Not quite right, though, and bear in mind that these people know me and have had to put up with my enthusiasm for neuroscience on many occasions. For those who haven't, a deeper understanding of fMRI is an adventure in its own right as well as a way to assess what you read in the media. It's a story of logical steps and ingenious problem-solving, drawing on more than just expertise in brains. Neuroscientists aren't proud; they'll cannibalize other science if it helps. For fMRI, the plunder came from physics, chemistry, and the useful phenomenon of atomic resonance.

Soggy brains

Standard magnetic resonance imaging can be either functional (looking at brain activity) or structural (looking at brain architecture). In either case, it relies on a simple fact: the brain is full of water. H_2O in theory; in practice a looser collective, as water molecules tend to come apart into hydroxyl groups (OH^-) and free-floating hydrogen ions (H^+). Hydrogen, the simplest and most common denizen of the periodic table, is essential for life; it is the third most plentiful element in your body, and were you to be deconstructed into your chemical basics about a tenth of the result would be hydrogen.[4] The behaviour of that tenth is what MRI measures.[5]

A structural MRI scan, the kind you might get in a clinical assessment, uses the fact that different kinds of brain tissue contain different amounts of water to work out what's where—rather like an archaeologist using ground-penetrating radar to see what's soil and what might be the foundation of a temple. It creates an architectural impression of the brain and skull, showing blood vessels, cavities, and brain tissue; muscles, bones, and fat (see Plate 4A).

Functional (f)MRI uses the facts that blood is watery and brains are full of blood to measure changes in the blood supply, and hence what the brain is doing, not how it is built. Blood is where neurons get their petrol: the glucose and oxygen they need to do their work. The ideas behind fMRI are that busy neurons are hungry neurons, that when neurons need more fuel the brain has mechanisms to supply it, and that neurons, unlike people, don't go in for comfort eating. Thus how much blood flows into a brain area is thought to reflect how active the local cells are. In other words, fMRI can be interpreted as measuring neural activity (see Plate 4B).

So fMRI can 'see' blood flow. As science-lite, this is enough explanation, but for curious minds it raises more questions than it answers. How does the 'seeing' work? No one comes out of an fMRI scan with their skull and brain transparent, so how does the scanner peer through the bone and tissue? What aspect of hydrogen's behaviour is being measured? Are the hydrogen ions interfered with, and if so, is that potentially dangerous? To answer such questions, and to understand what lies behind those easy fMRI headlines, we must dig deeper, down into the subatomic world.

Hydrogen atoms consist of one positively charged proton and one negatively charged electron. Hydrogen ions, having mislaid their electron, are simply protons, and their positive charge gives them a 'magnetic moment', as if they were tiny bar magnets. In effect, when an external magnetic field is applied to protons they tilt to align with that field. Just as you can move your bar magnet by bringing another magnet in close, so you can change a proton's angle to the universe.

Order out of chaos

In a typical glass of water—or blood—the directions in which protons are oriented will be fairly random. Apply an external magnetic field, however, and the protons will obey, lining up in the same direction relative to the field. It's a little like what happens when a football crowd starts to sing: hideous to begin with, but soon a tune emerges. Now imagine that one of the spectators in the crowd happens to be the conductor of a top orchestra. If everyone in the stadium sings the same note, he may be able to hear tone-deaf participants (and, if they are nearby, ask them to stop), whereas if everyone is howling any old noise even the best conductor won't have a chance of working out who cannot actually sing. For MRI to work, the proton tune must be similarly clear, so that small deviations can be detected. Thus the first thing you need for an fMRI brain scan is a strong magnetic field (see Table 1) applied across the head in which you are interested.[6]

The second requirement is something that changes the tune: altering the magnetic field as brain activity changes. This is why fMRI measures blood flow. Blood contains haemoglobin, a protein which collects oxygen from the lungs and delivers it to cells which need it to function. Haemoglobin exerts its own magnetic field, and, crucially, as each molecule releases its oxygen its magnetic field changes. Oxygenated blood, in other words, has a different magnetic signature to the deoxygenated blood sent back to the lungs for a refill, so the change when fuel is delivered makes local protons line up differently. That's like altering the note which the football crowd is singing. Just as a skilled conductor can hear when his second sopranos are slightly flat, even when the rest of the choir and orchestra are producing fortissimo, so an fMRI scanner can 'hear' the proton crowd in an active area of cortex through the music made by everything else in the brain.

TABLE 1 Comparison of magnetic fields.

Source of magnetic field	Field strength (in gauss)	Order of magnitude
A typical fMRI scanner	30,000	10^4
A fridge magnet	50	10^1
Earth	0.5	10^{-1}
A microwave oven, close up	0.08	10^{-2}
Background noise from	from 0.001	10^{-3}
electrical equipment (range)	to 0.0001	10^{-4}
A brain	0.00000001	10^{-8}

Table 1 shows levels of magnetic emissions associated with various sources, from the high strengths used in fMRI to the miniscule ripples created by living brains. Magnetic field strengths (second column) are approximate and are given here in gauss (1 tesla = 10,000 gauss). Data are taken from http://www.spaceweather.com/glossary/imf.html. The third column gives the order of magnitude of the field strength for each source, for easy comparison (just take the difference of the superscripts being compared and multiply that number of tens together). For example, the Earth's magnetic field (10^{-1}) is two orders of magnitude weaker than that of a fridge magnet (10^1), or one hundred times weaker.

The third thing you need from fMRI is a way to measure the changes in magnetic field. Because the brain's magnetic signals are extremely small and hard to measure (see Table 1), fMRI scanners do not detect changes in magnetic field strength per se. For that you need a more subtle technology: MEG (of which more soon). Or you could put instruments inside healthy human brains to measure magnetic fields nearer their source, but ethics committees aren't keen on invasive research. Just wait until we have nanomachines and can take internal measurements with a simple injection.[7] Meanwhile researchers make do with less direct methods.

In fMRI they gain their data by cleverly using another physics principle: the 'resonance' of magnetic resonance imaging. Subatomic particles like protons can absorb and emit quanta: packets of energy

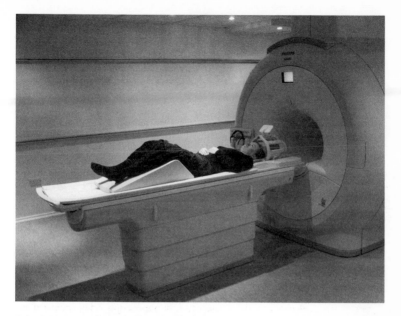

FIGURE 10: A volunteer about to be fMRI-scanned.
(Copyright University of Birmingham 2010)

which we experience as light, heat, sunburn and so on. What these forms of radiation do to us depends on their frequency, and that depends on what's emitting them. Different subatomic entities have different preferences: 'resonant frequencies' at which they will absorb and emit quanta. Applying a magnetic field changes the particles' resonance frequency, and hence the frequency of the quanta.

If an fMRI scanner is like a conductor faced with a noisy football crowd, the magnet's discipline turns the crowd into a choir repeating any note the conductor sings. To give the note, the scanner uses radio pulses, because when protons are lined up in a scanner's strong magnetic field they have a resonant frequency which falls conveniently in the radio part of the electromagnetic spectrum. The scanner's pulse thus adds energy to the brain as the radio waves are absorbed by protons in the water inside a human head. If this sounds alarmingly like what happens in a microwave oven, it isn't, because the pulse of radio waves is very brief, and its frequency is much lower than micro-wave pulses.[8] As soon as the pulse stops, the protons have time to emit radio quanta at exactly the same frequency, so they can get back to their original state. It is these emitted 'echo' pulses which the scanner detects.[9]

The use of resonance is undoubtedly one of MRI's advantages over PET, CT scans, and X-rays. Radio waves beat radioactive liquids and penetrating radiation when it comes to health and safety. As we'll see, the magnet brings its own safety issues, but they are easier to resolve. Participants' physiology—e.g. heart rate—still needs to be monitored while they are in the scanner, but MRI, though noisy, is safer and pleasanter for volunteers and experimenters.

A recent media report described an fMRI 'mind-reading' study by saying that the scanner produced 'distinct patterns that appeared to reflect what the individual was thinking'.[10] You now know that behind that small word 'reflect' lies a very long chain of assumptions. The scanner is detecting radio pulses emitted by hydrogen ions in the brain's blood and tissue. They are interpreted as being correlated with blood flow and hence with neural activity. To jump from there to conclusions about what a particular brain area does, or to decide that some mental phenomenon is real because a bit of the cortex lights up when it is happening, is to take a leap of faith. Yet journalists, and even some scientists, do just that.[11]

IMCOTT! For one thing, the information about where and when the echo pulse arrives at the scanner's detectors must be converted into a map of the brain—a 3D map, not the 2D rendering of the cortical surface you see in neuroanatomical maps like Brodmann's. For another, different brain regions have different proportions of water, fat, and protein, which vary in how quickly they spit out their radio pulses.[12] These time differences offer a way to discriminate between blood vessels, grey matter, and other kinds of brain stuff: the basis of structural fMRI. Scanners can be tuned to 'highlight' particular features, such as blood vessels or the white matter fibre bundles which connect neuron-rich grey matter in cortex and subcortex.[13] That has given rise to a plethora of fMRI-based imaging techniques adept at picking out different bits of the brain. Clinicians and researchers now have a pleasing variety to choose from, depending on their needs: a structural scan if they suspect a tumour, diffusion tensor imaging if they are looking at white matter, arterial spin labelling if they are interested in blood flow, and so on.[14]

What emerges from a neuroimaging scanner, to reiterate, is indirect information, from which we infer conclusions about brain activity. For PET, the item measured is gamma-ray emission following the radio-active decay of atoms incorporated into glucose molecules, which neurons consume for energy. For fMRI, the scanner measures radio pulses emitted from protons manipulated by a magnetic field which changes as blood surrenders its oxygen for neural consumption. For both, an array of detectors provides details not only of what has been measured but where and when. And for both, what is measured is not actual brain cell signalling.[15]

A big advantage of fMRI over PET is that fMRI has better spatial and temporal resolution; it can see finer and faster details. For example, the fastest changes fMRI can detect are now measured in seconds or less, and techniques continue to improve. This is essential if the prospect of DNE recording, able to correlate brain activity with subjective experiences in real time, is to be realized. Moreover, rather than averaging over groups of people, as is common in PET, individuals can be analysed and compared, which gives researchers much more information. And recent developments in fMRI are allowing neuroscientists to understand how the brain works as never before, by looking at the connections which link brain areas through new eyes (see 'fMRI and beyond', below). If anatomists like Sylvius and Brodmann could have understood the work which is going on today, they would have been amazed—and then, I think, indescribably delighted.

Neuroimaging mechanics, and the chain of logic which ties resonating protons to neural activation, are well understood. There are yet more inferences to be added to the chain, however, and they can be rather less reliable.[16] This is a crucial point for the brain supremacy: the methods may be wonderful, but even the best research can be undone by dubious interpretations. To see why, we must look at how MRI data are interpreted. The best way to do that is to explore an example of the process for which all this technology is used: an fMRI experiment.

Inside an experiment

Suppose you are interested in what's going on in the brains of people who hold strong beliefs. Such beliefs often come in sets—belief systems—which can form a powerfully coherent worldview through which an individual makes sense of new information. An extreme case of a belief system would be the kind of paranoid mental illness where everyone else's behaviour, from the glance of a friend to what the TV newsreader says, is read in terms of the patient's conviction that someone is out to get them. Even less clinically severe belief systems, however, can exert huge influence over individuals and groups.[17] You would like to know what it is about belief systems that gives them such power, not least because that might suggest ways of weakening strong beliefs. A treatment for dissolving dogmatism is one of the most potent promises of the brain supremacy, and you hope to contribute towards that goal.

The question of what makes belief systems so strong is too big for one study. As a first step, you would like to investigate brain responses to statements which are part of a belief system, such as a religion. (The research described here was designed, by myself and a colleague, to do just that, though it never got beyond the planning stage.)[18] That is your experimental condition, and you will also need a control condition with which to compare it: statements as similar as possible to your experimental statements except that they are not part of an overall belief system. You decide to use factual statements, which are part of a person's general background knowledge but not of a specific, coherent ideology.

As for participants, you decide to do the experiment on religious people—some of whom may be expected to hold some strong beliefs—as well as on other people who do not profess a faith. This, you hope, will give you a wide range of belief system 'strengths' across all participants, allowing you to see which differences in brain function correlate with differences in belief strength.

Say you have developed a hypothesis that belief systems involve emotion and identity—they matter to people—in a way that other, general beliefs, don't. You've an idea for an experiment, written up in a short proposal; you've got your boss's support, and you may even have persuaded someone to fund your research. What next?

Thinking about experimental design

You know what you want to do. By comparing patterns of brain activity when people read various statements, you can compare your control and experimental conditions: ordinary beliefs (general knowledge) and belief systems (religious statements). If brain regions known to be involved in emotion and identity processing are more active when beliefs are part of a system, as your hypothesis predicts, you will be very happy (if not you will be extremely pensive). In the scanner, therefore, you plan to present your participants with an equal number of religious and factual statements—in lower case for easy reading, and in random order to avoid the effects of fatigue and boredom compromising one condition more than the other. You also need your religious and factual statements to be as similar as possible on word length and suchlike, or else a reviewer may argue that these differences could explain your results.[19]

At this stage, your boss may pick up on a problem. Perhaps religious statements are more attention-grabbing than boring statements of common-sense beliefs, and so easier to remember. Or maybe common-sense statements are so commonsensical that they look rather weird written down, whereas religious statements do not seem so startling. In other words, the level of attention paid to your statements is a relevant variable—it could be an alternative explanation for whatever result you find.

You need to control for (take account of) this possibility. To do so, you plan to give your participants two kinds of tasks. One is to read each statement and press one of two buttons, 'agree' or 'disagree', depending on what the statement means to them. The other is to decide whether each statement is in lower case or mixed case, and press one of the (same) buttons accordingly. This will show you how your participants' brains respond when they are simply looking at and reading belief-statements without interpreting those beliefs as part of a system (because they are too busy deciding on their case). If area X lights up when they are paying attention to the meaning, and also when they are deciding on the sentence's case, then area X is not specifically involved in whatever it is that makes belief systems mean so much to their adherents.

In other words, you have four conditions for your tolerant participants to do. You can give them religious statements (see Table 2, upper row), and ask them to agree or disagree ('attend to meaning'); or you can ask them to indicate the case in which the statement is written ('attend to case'). Ditto for the factual statements (Table 2, lower row). In other words, you have two possible stimuli—experimental and control—and two tasks—meaning or case—which govern the responses to those stimuli. Comparing the four conditions should allow you to isolate the effects of a belief being part of a system.

Now you need to work out how many statements you need to get decent results, come up with some examples which don't make you giggle or raise your boss's eyebrows, and programme a computer to present them in the scanner, making sure the resulting experiment isn't so long that exhaustion sets in. You need to decide how many participants are required to make your experiment statistically acceptable (three friends is not enough), and you must prepare information leaflets to give them and the adverts with which you will recruit them. A more detailed proposal will be necessary too, setting out exactly what you plan to do to how many people, and over what timescale. And of course, this will have to get past an ethics committee.

TABLE 2 Stimuli and tasks for an fMRI experiment.

Stimulus	Task	
	Attend to meaning	**Attend to case**
Religious Statements	There is a spiritual reality in addition to a material reality	ThERre iS a SpiritUAL reaLITY in addition to a mATERIal reality
Factual Statements	There are rainy days in addition to sunny days	ThEre aRe raINy daYs in addITtiOn to suNny days

Table 2 shows the four conditions for an fMRI experiment comparing two kinds of stimuli (Rows: religious versus general knowledge statements) to which there are two possible responses (Columns: attend to the meaning of the statement or attend to which case it is written in). Examples of each condition are given. By contrasting brain activation between two conditions, it is possible to determine which patterns of brain activity are associated with processing a specific feature of the stimulus. For example, to determine which brain areas are involved in processing meaning an analysis would contrast all 'attend to meaning' responses with all 'attend to case' responses. To look at which areas are specifically active when a person ponders a belief which is part of a belief system (religion), the analysis would contrast religious and factual statements. Adding more conditions allows for more precise and detailed contrasts, but makes the experiment long—perhaps too long. It also requires more participants, which is more expensive. Thus any fMRI experiment is a series of trade-offs.

Getting the right people

In addition, you may want to take behavioural measures, to try and make sure that your participants are as similar as possible. You may be explicitly comparing religious and non-religious people, for example, but you want them to differ only on religion, so that you can be more confident that any results you get are due to the religious lot having strong beliefs, not anything else. (Actually your confidence matters less than whether you can convince reviewers when it comes to publication.) As a minimum, you'll want to have every participant rate how much they agree or disagree with the statements before they go into the scanner—just in case your supposedly 'non-religious' participants turn out to be fanatical spiritualists. Apart from anything else, this familiarizes your participants with all the statements, so a reviewer can't argue that the religious statements were more startling than the rest and that's the source of the differences you observed.

Group characteristics are another important issue. Ideally, you want your experimental and control animals to match on at least age, gender, ethnic origin, educational achievement, general intelligence and personality. It's no use saying 'The brains of religious people showed more activation in...' when the only believers you could find were middle-aged, right-wing, introverted nuns and your non-religious participants are liberal middle-class students.

In practice, personality questionnaires and cognitive tests are often expensive to buy and can take a lot of time to administer. And time is limited by what your participants can stand. Before you scan them, moreover, you are ethically bound to explain the experiment to them and allow them enough time for questions, last-minute visits to the loo, and the process of getting settled in the scanner (see Figure 10). Also you need a structural scan of their brain: something onto which you'll map those exciting activation patterns (see Plate 4B).

Another consumer of precious study time is a safety check: taking your participants through a screening questionnaire to make sure they can undergo scanning. This is crucial. Pregnancy, for instance, is an automatic no-no, as is claustrophobia. Likewise metal, which doesn't mix well with strong magnetic fields; some people have piercings in the most extraordinary places. It's important to know whether your volunteer has anything less easily removable—a metal plate in his or her skull, for instance—preferably before you book that pricey scanner session, and certainly before they meet the magnet. (However, over twenty years of fMRI scanning, on millions of people, has not brought up evidence of other health risks.[20])

So you've written up a proposal, designed the experiment, and bought, borrowed or programmed the stimuli you plan to give your participants in the scanner, along with any behavioural measures. You've jumped through the hoops, filled in the forms, and got ethics committee approval, plus the necessary expert references confirming that the project is worth doing. You've checked your local scanner has time available, you've polished a welcoming smile, and you've remembered to make sure that there's cash for participant expenses, as well as for coffee, tea, and biscuits. You have, or someone has, the expertise you need to analyse the data, and you or someone will find the time to write up the experiment for publication. Depending on how many colleagues you are working with, and how much else is on your to-do list, reaching this stage alone can take months. This is why scientific research takes so long.

What next? Experiment! Amid all the standing and waiting, the unorthodox hours, the reassuring of participants who do turn up and the sighing over those who don't, the smiles and thanks even when the person twitched so much during the scan that their data may be worthless...If you can keep your head amid all this, rejoicing is justified. You're finally collecting data: rich, glorious data, the researcher's drug of choice. Now all you need to do is analyse your findings.

Realizing what you've got

A scientific experiment compares a model of some aspect of the world against the world itself. For your fMRI experiment, you will have developed models at different levels of detail. First comes a very high-level, abstract model: your hypothesis about beliefs and belief systems. This is fleshed out during the experimental design, becoming a model of how brains are expected to respond to different kinds of statements. Finally, you have the fMRI model: a precise description of exactly when each stimulus is presented to the participant, noting what kind of stimulus it is, how long it is presented for, and so on.

You know, furthermore, that the brain's blood supply doesn't switch on and off in immediate response to changes in brain activity. Instead it gathers pace over time, peaks, and gradually subsides. You have a mathematical function to model this, the haemodynamic response curve, which describes the fMRI signal's changing reaction to a stimulus over time. Whenever you present a statement, therefore, you can merge your model with the haemodynamic response curve to predict what the fMRI signal would look like in any part of the brain if that part were active. You can consider the whole brain, or select particular regions of interest which you expect to be significantly involved. For any 'voxel'—the cube-shaped basic unit of brain volume used in scanning, which contains around 100,000 neurons—you can predict whether it will be active or inactive when, for example, you show the person a factual statement.[21]

You have a model of how you expect the fMRI signal to behave, in every voxel of your participant's brain, throughout your scanning session. You have the data, which tell you what actually happened. Put them together, and you can use a statistical test to work out how well your model and reality match.

The problem of false positives

Caution is essential. Statistical tests are a staple of brain research, but they can sometimes detect apparently significant results where none exist. In these so-called false positives, random variation—noise in your sample—can create the misleading impression of a significant result. Each brain scan can produce well over 100,000 voxels, and in such a big sample it's hardly surprising that, purely by chance, patterns will emerge. If you tossed a coin 100,000 times, you might get a stretch in which heads comes up again and again, even though the coin is fair. If you were using a statistical technique to detect 'blocks' of heads or tails which might suggest a biased coin, that run of heads might look like a signal that the coin is weighted towards heads, when in fact, over many trials, it turns out not to be. In fMRI you can only rarely have large numbers of trials to check your findings. Except for a few patient, dedicated individuals who come back again and again, there's only so much scanning most people can bear.

Researchers use special statistical techniques to correct for the large numbers of voxels involved in fMRI processing.[22] Uncorrected data can give very odd results, as in the notorious case of the Atlantic salmon. Testing an fMRI scanner to get it ready for people, two US graduate students, bored with the usual procedures, decided to scan something more interesting: a dead fish. Several years later one of them analysed the data and was astonished to find a cluster of significantly active voxels in the fish's brain. Startling evidence of life after death in the marine world? No. The data were uncorrected, and when properly analysed showed no such activation. A neuroimaging journal would reject a paper thus presented—but it's a useful illustration of the problem of false positives.[23]

Looking at beautiful pictures

Even when correction techniques are used, fMRI activation patterns still need to be treated with care.[24] They don't directly show how active a brain area is, any more than an electron's wavefunction at a particular location tells you how much of the electron is to be found at that location. Rather, activation patterns and wavefunctions are both probability maps. The wavefunction tells you how likely you are to find the electron at a given location.[25] The brain map tells you how likely it is that an area's activity was significantly different between whichever two conditions are being compared.

If area X does not 'light up', that doesn't mean X wasn't active. It means the activity was not sufficiently different between the two conditions to pass whatever statistical threshold the researcher has decided is appropriate. In other words, the brightly coloured patterns (see Plate 4B) reflect estimates of how likely it is that, say, the religious-statements/attend-to-meaning activity and the ordinary-statements/attend-to-meaning activity are different. The underlying changes in brain activity are of a few percent at most, but reflecting this in the colour range would make for images so indistinct as to be worthless (see Plate 4C).[26] If area X does light up, it tells you that activity in X may be associated with whatever is different between the task you're interested in and the control task with which you're comparing it. Needless to say, 'may be associated with' is a far cry from 'is the area which does'.

The control condition, in other words, is crucial. Imagine a very simple experiment investigating the effects of red light on the brain. What's the control? Blue light? White light? Darkness? You need to know exactly which variable is being manipulated, since varying wavelength may have different effects from varying whether the light is present or absent. You also, if possible, want to be sure that nothing else has changed except that variable when you switch from the control to the experimental condition. For the experiment comparing beliefs and belief systems, you want to be as sure as you can that there is only one difference between the two conditions: the statements in your experimental condition are part of a system; the control statements are not. But is that the case? Maybe there's something special about religious statements, whether or not they're part of a system of beliefs.

To take account of this possibility, you need another experimental stimulus: statements which are part of a system which isn't religious but which involves the same kind of commitment: a secular ideology. Animal rights activists might be a good population to study, but you'd have to find them, recruit them, and let them inside your buildings. In the Oxford department where I was based as a postdoctoral researcher, the former home of animal research advocates like Colin Blakemore and John Stein, there were plenty of activists around, but scanning them was quite another matter. (I did ask.)

Besides, adding a third stimulus would mean a much longer experiment. This is because you would have to include two extra conditions: attending to the meaning of statements about animal rights, and deciding whether they were mixed or lowercase. That takes your total number of conditions from four to six, and that 50% time increase might make the experiment too long to inflict on volunteers at present, although scanner technology is improving all the time.[27]

In short, when researchers study very high-level processing—phenomena like social judgements, moral intuitions, or beliefs—well-controlled experiments are hard to achieve. This is why so much social neuroscience, fashionable though it currently is, should be taken with a sizeable pinch of salt.

So the next time you read a media piece about fMRI, ask yourself what it is actually telling you. Does it mention anything about who the participants were, or even how many of them there were? Does it tell you what is being compared with what? Does what the text says back up the implications of the headline? Is there a link to a published, peer-reviewed scientific article? And given what you know about the complexities involved in doing these experiments, and the kinds of questions the study appears to be asking, how many pinches of salt are you inclined to take? If the answers which spring to mind are unsatisfactory, you have a fine example of science-lite. Now, however, you also have the framework to deal with it.

fMRI and beyond

As I mentioned earlier, fMRI has burgeoned into a variety of techniques for identifying particular brain features. One is diffusion tensor imaging (DTI), which measures how protons (in the form of water) are moving in the brain. Water molecules are constantly diffusing through brain tissues, spreading from the cerebrospinal fluid (CSF) and blood, passing along the axons of neurons, and so on. DTI can assess the directions of this movement in each voxel of the brain.

In a liquid, diffusion tends to be all over the place; imagine the kind of pattern you'd get if you added a drop of ink to a glass of water. When cell membranes add boundaries, as in a neuron's long thin axon or an artery wall, water molecules move more quickly within the axon or artery—along the tube formed by the membrane—than they do across its perimeter. DTI can use this difference to find bundles of nerve fibres. By highlighting white matter, it gives insight into the brain's internal wiring.

DTI informs us about structural connectivity: the physical links between different areas of the brain. This is vital information, and hard to obtain *in vivo* for humans.[28] If you have a theoretical model which requires strong communication between, say, the amygdala and the hypothalamus, you may have dissected inordinate numbers of rats to demonstrate the existence of vast tracts of axons between these two subcortical regions. Nonetheless, if you wish to extend your model to the human, you need to be sure that the anatomy is similar. Knowing which brain areas are connected was previously assessed, as we saw in Chapter 5, by inserting a tracer chemical into a living brain and then killing it quickly with formaldehyde. Clearly that would face ethical barriers in humans. Thanks to DTI, it is no longer the only way to understand how the living human brain wires up.

There are limitations, naturally. DTI detects large fibre bundles but may miss smaller though still important ones which happen to be aligned at a different angle. Knowing that two areas are physically linked does not tell us which is the sender and which the receiver. Furthermore, the existence of a link only means communication is possible; it doesn't tell you that it actually happens. For that, you need to know about functional connectivity: whether neurons in different regions are using the available infrastructure to send signals to each other.

In an animal brain, this is straightforward: stick an electrode in area A to stimulate it electrically (or by injecting chemicals), and see what if anything happens in area B. In humans, unless they have electrodes implanted for medical reasons, the skull is sacrosanct. Neuroscientists must therefore rely on external interference such as transcranial magnetic stimulation (TMS), which applies a focused magnetic field through the skull. TMS has proved very useful, as we'll see in Chapter 11, but as tools go it really is a hammer, and a sledgehammer at that. So how can functional connectivity be assessed in living, unhammered, unimplanted humans?

This is how researchers have solved the problem. If areas A and B are in communication, that should be reflected in their activity. Think of two people having a conversation in a cafe: the way they speak and gesture is anything but random. While one talks, the other is listening, but also nodding, watching, smiling—a whole set of behaviours which vary according to what the speaker says. In other words, the speaker's activity and the listener's responses may look different, but they are highly correlated. By contrast, the correlation between these behaviours and what the girl behind the counter is doing is low, so one can infer that, although the speaker and listener are causing each other to behave in certain ways, neither is exerting much influence on the girl's behaviour (unless of course she starts eavesdropping).

If brain areas are talking, we should likewise expect their activity to be highly correlated: if A's neurons change their behaviour, B's will likely change too. Using fMRI allows researchers to measure the correlations between brain areas' activity.[29] Even when people are not performing any specific task, their brains are highly active—those daydreams have to come from somewhere. By recording how each area's activity fluctuates over time, it is possible to build a 'functional connectome', a map of how the links between them are used.[30]

One of the problems with many neuroimaging experiments, as noted earlier, is that the weight of the hypotheses they bear is not adequately supported by the experimental design, so that other explanations cannot be ruled out. (The same problem has plagued genetics since the completion of the human genome project in 2003. To read the hype of earlier decades, for instance, you might have thought that major mental illnesses like schizophrenia would have been curable by now.[31] Yet schizophrenia is still wrecking lives, despite all the high-powered genetics and neuroscience applied to it. Perhaps the problem lies partly in our definition of schizophrenia. If the hypotheses are not, in Plato's famous phrase, carving nature at her joints, no amount of technology will do more than temporarily disguise the problem.[32])

One way to escape the problem of poor hypotheses is to reduce their influence by doing what its proponents term 'discovery science': gathering large quantities of data and then investigating patterns in that information without imposing prior hypotheses.[33] (Or, as we used to call it in my day, going on fishing trips.) This can be problematic—banished prior beliefs have a tendency to reappear as unrecognized biases. Yet it illustrates fMRI's continuing fruitfulness and the many ways in which the scanner is transforming research. Functional connectivity studies, DTI and other recent ways of seeing the brain are tremendously exciting developments for neuroscience. Their potential, and that of neuroimaging as a whole, to bypass the barrier of the skull is awe-inspiring.

Nonetheless, fMRI at present remains too slow a technique to capture the quicksilver flows of active neurons. In the next chapter, therefore, we will look at a faster way of seeing the brain, and the exciting potential of electrophysiology.

8

When Currents Flow

I sing the body electric

(Walt Whitman, poet)

Long before PET and fMRI appeared to light up the neuroscene and blind us with science, three older technologies were crucial to laying bare the secrets of the brain. Two have already been discussed: the knife and the anatomist's gift of staining particular cells, fibres, or regions. The third was the electrode. Surgery, dissection, and staining revealed much about brain structure, and something of function too. Yet they were constrained not only by ethics but by practicality, since staining and dissection destroy the brain they aim to analyse. Using surgery to understand brain function is less lethal but still destructive, like trying to understand how a government works by assassinating one senior official at a time. But electrodes do comparatively little damage.

Electrodes able to record the flow of tiny currents in living brains brought modern neuroscience into being around 200 years ago, at a time when the industrial revolution had boosted confidence in man's ability to master nature—even human nature. The development of stimulating microelectrodes able to apply precisely controlled currents or minute amounts of chemicals made electrophysiology a dominant technology in the twentieth century. Central to the brain supremacy's development thus far, it is unlikely to be abandoned in the future; it is far too useful. And its implications have spread well beyond labs and clinics. When the Canadian neurosurgeon Wilder Penfield stimulated the cortex of his epilepsy patients, and evoked not only movements but vivid images, his work came to symbolize a huge and disconcerting change in human self-perception, yanking the ethereal mind down into the all-too-meaty brain. Seventy years after Penfield's book *Epilepsy and Cerebral Localization* made him a science superstar, that wrenching adjustment is far from complete today.[1]

The stream of fire

The topic of this chapter centres on electricity, surely a god for our times. Imagine if some John-Wyndhamesque cataclysm suddenly deprived us of the capacity to trap and channel free-flowing electrons: how life would alter! The world would become astonishingly quiet, and at night spectacularly dark; we would see the stars again. The internet, computers, and many other comforts would cease to function. No mobiles, no email, no muzak, no spam. But also no systems, no helplines, no snug cocoon of state assistance.

If electricity were to vanish altogether, however, we would no longer be able to have any such concerns, for our every cell depends on the movement and separation of electric charge. Eyes and innards, muscles and microglia, bodies and brains need to manipulate ions—charged particles—like sodium and calcium in order to function. That had been known before the early nineteenth century, when it was famously brought to public notice by Mary Shelley. Learning that scientists could make frogs' legs twitch by applying a spark, she commandeered the idea for a novel, updating the Faustian stereotype of the dangerous intellectual in a way which still affects how we see scientists.[2]

> When I was about fifteen years old we had retired to our house near Belrive, when we witnessed a most violent and terrible thunderstorm. It advanced from behind the mountains of Jura; and the thunder burst at

once with frightful loudness from various quarters of the heavens. I remained, while the storm lasted, watching its progress with curiosity and delight. As I stood at the door, on a sudden I beheld a stream of fire issue from an old and beautiful oak which stood about twenty yards from our house; and so soon as the dazzling light vanished the oak had disappeared, and nothing remained but a blasted stump. When we visited it the next morning, we found the tree shattered in a singular manner. It was not splintered by the shock, but entirely reduced to thin ribands of wood. I never beheld anything so utterly destroyed.

(*Frankenstein*, Chapter 2)

Since Shelley's time the destructive power which startled the young Frankenstein has largely—not entirely—been tamed.[3] These days electricity is taken for granted, its basics taught in schools. That is no guarantee, however, that they are remembered, so here is a brief refresher.

It is a truth universally acknowledged, with apologies to another great novelist, that an ion in possession of an electron, must be in want of a partner with whom to bond.[4] Ions, each a positively charged nucleus of protons and neutrons set in a swirl of negatively charged electrons, attract their opposites, seeking quiescence: electrical neutrality. Negative ions like chloride (Cl^-) and phosphate ($PO_4{}^{3-}$), burdened with extra electrons, join up with positive ions like sodium (Na^+) or calcium (Ca^{2+}), which lack electrons. Salt, NaCl, is one everyday result of ionic union, a rapid embrace, as easily dissolved.

Some atoms can hardly wait to shed or acquire electrons. Others, though less unstable, may share their charges with nearby companions without letting go altogether. This joint charge forms tougher covalent bonds, giving many organic chemicals—including many in us—their remarkable robustness.[5]

Molecules such as DNA are not rigid, inactive structures, as the Meccano-style models suggest, but the sites of a constant ebb and flow of electric charge, pulled hither and yon by the play of forces in their minuscule world. Electrons are not the staid little balls of early models, but palpitating, restless surges of energy. They are tugged and shoved by charges in nearby atoms, both in the contorted molecular sculptures of which they are part, and when other entities approach, such as the enzymes which help to untangle DNA for processing. Electron flows power the molecules which control your every function just as they power your computer and the stock markets—and they are key to how brain cells communicate their impulses.

Neurons: cells with potential

Neurons communicate by sending electrical signals along their length to synapses, triggering the release of neurotransmitter molecules into the synaptic gap through which cells converse. The signals are possible because the amount of electrically charged material inside the cell is different from the amount outside, in the extracellular fluid. The difference in charge—or 'potential'—across the cell membrane when the cell isn't doing anything in particular is about 70 millivolts, around 0.03% of what comes out of a UK mains socket. The convention is to write this 'resting potential' as $-70\,\text{mV}$, because the cell interior is more negatively charged than the extracellular fluid.

That difference is not there by chance.[6] Changes in the membrane potential are the cell's signals, and for the fast chat of nerve cells, charges must be shepherded in and out of the cell on a millisecond timescale. Every cell has a multitude of specialized systems which have evolved to provide impressive border control, but neurons are especially skilled players of this game. They can change the potential across their membranes almost instantaneously by moving charged particles from outside to inside, or vice versa. What kind of particles? Most molecules are too big to pass easily through the cell membrane. What are needed are small, loosely bound ions: the migrant workforce of the brain. In neurons, sodium (Na^+), potassium (K^+), calcium (Ca^{2+}), and chloride (Cl^-) ions take major roles in the dance of particles across the cell membrane.

The best-known neuronal signals are the explosive action potentials—also called spikes, signals, firing, nerve impulses or neural activity—which provide the most noticeable currency of brain cell communication. There are others: slower or smaller 'sub-threshold' changes which can make an action potential more or less likely to occur without actually setting one off (more on these in a moment). Only if the membrane potential rises far enough to reach a 'threshold potential' of around −55mV will a spike be triggered.

An action potential happens over a few thousandths of a second, sending an electrical pulse along the neuron's long axon to stimulate the synaptic release of neurotransmitters such as dopamine and serotonin. During a spike the membrane potential rockets up to −30mV or more, as sodium ions flood into the cell, before plunging back down to below −70mV, as potassium ions hastily exit, and finally stabilizing at the −70mV resting potential (see Figure 11).[7] With their brief, on-off

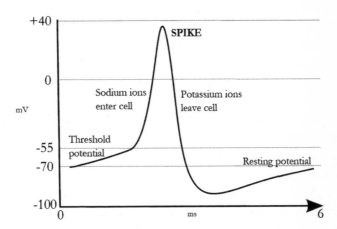

FIGURE 11: The action potential.

The figure represents the progress of an action potential ('spike'). The x-axis shows time, in milliseconds (ms). The y-axis shows the voltage, in millivolts (mV). From the resting potential (−70 mV), the neuron's membrane potential rises to reach the threshold potential (−55 mV), at which point an action potential is triggered as sodium channels in the membrane open and positively charged sodium ions enter the cell. As the membrane potential rises further, potassium channels open in the membrane, and positively-charged potassium ions leave, bringing the voltage back down to stabilise at the resting potential.

nature, action potentials have launched a thousand brain-as-computer metaphors. They translate easily into digital code and computer simulations, are straightforward to record, and hence are likely sources for first attempts at DNE recording and transfer, though the reality of brain electrics is, inevitably, more intricate.

Neurons achieve this swift and masterful control of their electrical potential by opening and closing ion channels: holes in the cell membrane which allow charged material to cross from inside to outside, or vice versa. (IMCOTT: there are also specialized transporter systems, the cell's dumper trucks, which don't wait for stuff to flow in or out but actively shift it.) Some ion channels allow only small particles to cross, such as hydrogen (H^+, protons) or chloride ions. Others are more permissive: for example, there are positive ion channels which admit both sodium and calcium to a neuron's interior. The more charged particles an ion channel can admit, the faster the membrane potential will change when that channel opens, and the more impact it will have on the cell's behaviour. As well as creating action potentials, the influx of ions can trigger all sorts of activity within the cell, including chemical changes which affect the cell's genes and protein-making.

To allow neurons their remarkable flexibility and responsiveness without them descending into anarchy, ion channels are subject to regulation. In many cases they are incorporated into the structure of the receptor molecules which straddle the cell membrane, ready to be opened by neurotransmitters or other molecules which enter the extracellular neighbourhood. An NMDA receptors, for example, contains an ion channel big enough to let in both sodium and calcium ions.[8] It is activated by the close approach of the neurotransmitter glutamate, its ligand ('the thing that binds', from the same Latin root— ligare, to bind—which gives us ligature and ligament).[9]

Once activated, the shape of the receptor protein changes in such a way as to open the channel. Positively charged ions pour into the cell, seeking a new life in a place less oppressively full of positive charges than the extracellular one they're leaving behind. The new life doesn't last long; as the membrane potential soars, it triggers the opening of other channels, the exit of potassium ions and the activation of transporter systems, allowing the cell to rebalance itself. Within a few milliseconds the membrane potential is back at its resting level, ready for the cycle to start again.

Action potentials convulse an entire cell membrane. Place a microelectrode near enough to the neuron and you can detect its firing. In the system I used when doing my MSc research, the spikes could be rendered in audio form as a series of clicks, rat-tat-tatting ever more fiercely, like an out-of-control machine gun, as the microelectrode slid closer to the cell body. Given their pre-eminence it's easy for neuroscience to focus on spikes as the language of brain cells, but spikes are only one form of voltage change.[10] Thinking of neural function only in terms of action potentials is like thinking about cosmology only in terms of stars. Both stars and spikes are undeniably spectacular, but in both cases there's much more going on than the dramatics.

Beyond the action potential

When one of the thousands of synapses through which a cell hears from its neighbours is activated, neurotransmitter molecules spill across the synaptic gap to bond with and activate receptors on the cell's many dendrites—the finger-like extensions with which the cell senses its chemical environment.[11] The activation of receptors affects the electrical balance thereabouts.[12] The result is a small, local signal, sensibly christened the postsynaptic potential, which is either excitatory or inhibitory. It is the overall balance of positive and negative voltage changes from all the cell's synapses, flowing along the neuron's dendrites to its cell body, which determines whether it will fire off an action potential.[13]

(Inevitably the baby potentials bear nicknames: EPSP and IPSP, for excitatory and inhibitory postsynaptic potential. Modern neuroscience articles bear an ever-increasing resemblance to a Scrabble atrocity, with acronyms sprouting like fungi. These linguistic equivalents of barbed wire are, however, a necessary evil in research publications.

Without them things would take too long to say—and there's far too much to read already. The conflations, though ugly, are easier to read than the full-length versions. So EPSP and IPSP it is.)

Changes in electrical potential do not, however, demand that a nearby electrode be poised in order to detect them. There are other ways to read their messages, which is fortunate, since sticking needles into people's brains is currently frowned upon except in dire clinical circumstances (of which more shortly). Movements of electrically charged particles change the electromagnetic fields in their surroundings, and these changes can be detected at a distance. Since the fields pass through solid objects (hence the fuss over mobile phones possibly causing brain cancer), suitable instruments can register the changes even through those very solid objects, our skulls.

Recording the brain's electrical impulses is an old technique, but it forms the basis of many modern 'mind-reading' technologies, including applications which already offer limited powers of thought control, for example to people with spinal injuries. To understand how that can be possible, we must look at an established method of recording the brain's electromagnetic emissions.

EEG

Electroencephalography ('electric-brain-writing') sets one or more electrodes on the scalp, using gel for better contact, to record a person's 'brain waves' (see Figure 12).[14] The first EEG recording, of the dog brain, is attributed to Vladimir Pravdich-Neminsky, in 1913.[15] Since then, EEG has become widely used in research and in the clinic. It is relatively cheap and easy to perform; results are available immediately; it inflicts no worse traumas on the patient than sticky hair and boredom, and it is much quieter and less stressful than fMRI. Most of all, however, EEG is fast and direct. Unlike fMRI, it measures neural activity, not blood flow, and it does so effectively in real time.

(The perfect technique? No, or why would researchers use anything else? Every neuromethod has its flaws, and EEG is no exception. We

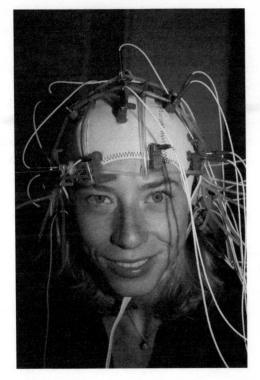

FIGURE 12: An EEG cap. (Daniela Sachsenheimer/ Shutterstock.com)

take our images of the brain through a varied collection of lenses, each blurred or coloured or cracked in a different way. The aim of neuroscience is to combine those imperfect pictures and work towards more accurate ways of seeing.[16])

What kind of neural activity is measured? EEG sheds its amber light on brain function by recording the overall changes in electrical potential produced by the massed activity of cortical neurons.[17] Estimates suggest at least thousands, acting in concert, are required for a detectable signal; examples of such 'brain waves' include the common rhythms labelled alpha, beta, gamma, delta, and theta.[18] This is not the scale required for the fine details of DNE recording, of course.

Technology—and data storage—will have to improve even more than they have since 1913 for that capacity to fall within our grasp.

EEG does not record action potentials either. Most of the signal is made up of EPSPs and IPSPs. Spikes are so brief (lasting only a couple of milliseconds) that the chances of spikes from different neurons overlapping in time—as they would have to in order to make the signal big enough for EEG to notice—are small.[19] EPSPs and IPSPs can be over a hundred times longer: up to a quarter of a second in duration. They are much more likely to overlap, and therefore to merge into a signal large enough to pass through the brain's tough wrappings: the three membranes (the pia, arachnoid, and dura mater, also called the meninges—hence meningitis), the skull, and the more-or-less hairy scalp.

What kind of neurons are measured in EEG? Brains are built with many of their processors on top (the 'grey matter') and much of the wiring tucked away inside as white matter.[20] Cortex, the layer of neuron cell bodies and dendrites which coats the brain's surface, is itself made up of six distinct layers, as noted in Chapter 5. Layer V, which is prominent in motor cortex, contains pyramidal cells which send the brain's instructions to the muscles. These neurons are the major contributors to EEG signals.

Any time you've seen a picture of a neuron, chances are it was a pyramidal cell. They are beauties, with a slender, elongated appearance reminiscent of an Alberto Giacometti sculpture (see Figure 7). Their etiolated form allows plenty of time for voltage changes to be detected, since the currents triggered by EPSPs and IPSPs must flow all the way from the dendrites near the brain's surface to the cell body down in Layer V—where action potentials may or may not spring to life. Furthermore, these cells sit vertically, in row upon row, at right angles to the cortical surface. Electromagnetic fields pulse out from their sources in all three dimensions, but this particular orientation maximizes the signal in one particular direction: from the lines of dendrites out through the skull. The regular layout allows the overlapping electromagnetic 'brain waves' from each neuron to travel in sync—in phase—along the vertical axis, reinforcing each other to build up a signal strong enough for an electroencephalograph to read. Meanwhile waves heading off at other angles tend to interfere—being out of phase—and cancel out.

That at least is the theory. In practice, IMCOTT, because human brains, as many analysts have had cause to regret, do not possess the easy mathematics of a smooth round ball. Far from it. The folds and creases of the human cortex make the EEG signal stronger in some parts of the brain—those nearest to, and set parallel with, the skull.[21] EEG is not the technology one would choose, for instance, to study the insular cortex, which is tucked in a deep fold beneath the temporal lobe. The encephalograph works best for areas like primary motor cortex, where the 'readiness potential' which signals an upcoming movement is easily detectable.

EEG has long been a tool in human–computer interfaces, where motor commands are rerouted from the brain via technology, bypassing the need to move one's muscles. There are many medical applications, including remote surgery, neurofeedback and 'thought-controlled' wheelchairs for people with paralysis. The idea of controlling machines by thought has also extended beyond the clinic to computers, robotics, video games, music-making, and so on.[22] Fantasies about thinking instructions to your fridge remain fantasies at present, but games are already being designed with EEG in mind.

Brain–machine connections could expand human power over the environment into realms where our frail bodies cannot go. From remote surgery to remote mining, from space exploration to investigating the deep oceans, we are already used to extending our self into a distant tool. Wireless technology, once magical, has become mundane. One day, perhaps, we may be able to link directly to each others' minds, rather than needing language, gesture, or neuroimaging as an intermediary. As discussed in Chapter 3, that will be a very interesting moment.

In principle, EEG data from other regions of cortex—like those processing vision or language—can also be used in conjunction with machines. As we better understand the neural codes involved, we should therefore be able to bypass other sensory appendages, like eyes and ears, as well as transcending our motor appendages in favour of a silicon-mediated existence. If this raises in your mind the charming prospect of our species morphing into a conclave of blobs—brains in highly computerized vats—as their bodies become increasingly redundant, bear in mind that interface technology is still at a very early stage. Should you not wish your great-great-grandchildren to be blobs, there is still time to lower the probability of that particular future.[23]

What's wrong with EEG?

Should such a future come upon us, there are reasons to suppose EEG will not be its midwife. One is that brains are more than mere sensorimotor processors, though we sometimes abuse the poor things by treating them as such. A technique which concentrates on the activity of pyramidal cells will inevitably miss other aspects of cortical electromagnetism, since there is much more to brain activity than input and output.

Another problem is the brain's contorted geometry. Not only are deeper areas less accessible to EEG, but signals from all areas are distorted by their passage through the meninges, skull, and scalp in complex ways which depend on individual features like skull thickness. Signals can be detected, moreover, from other sources than brain cells—such as heartbeats or head and eye movements—so these must be taken into account. Also detected, alongside the 'primary' currents which flow within the neurons, are 'secondary' currents flowing in the cerebrospinal fluid outside the cells, which keeps brains healthily damp and acts as a reservoir for ions. This 'extracellular volume', as it is called (brains, like libraries, hold many volumes), is full of charges which can give rise to electrical currents. These secondary 'volume currents' flow in response to the primary currents. They can greatly distort a signal, and taking them into account makes the modelling and interpretation much more difficult. All of which gives EEG a poor spatial resolution, although mathematical techniques can be used to improve it.[24]

The biggest challenge in EEG recording is known as the inverse problem. It is mathematically possible, given a number of electromagnetic field sources, to work out the strength of their combined fields at a particular point in space; this is the forward problem (and it is difficult enough when dealing with brains, because there are so many potential sources). The inverse problem asks the opposite question. Given a cortex full of neurons emitting electromagnetic fields in all directions, many of which are cancelling each other out and some of which are reinforcing each other, where in the brain is the signal you've just recorded actually coming from?

Whether you're a neuroscientist, a driver, or a management consultant, going forward is much the easier move. The inverse problem isn't merely harder, it's mathematically impossible. Identifying a unique source inside the brain from the electromagnetic mush outside just can't be done. I recently met this conundrum in another guise in the house of a friend, the proud owner of 13 vintage clocks, as they all chimed the hour more or less simultaneously. By knowing which clock made which noise and where each one stood, a sound engineer could have predicted the overall racket; but I had no hope of working out which chime rang out from which clock.

The brain presents a similar challenge, except that in the brain each clock can have multiple chimes. Also the clocks are piled in layers, squished and crumpled and at various angles. Oh, and there are around 170 billion clocks.[25] On the plus side, at least you can't normally hear them going off in other people's heads. Until some fool scientists come up with a form of affordable practical telepathy, and some fool government decides every citizen should have it 'to improve social integration', we're safe from that particular version of hell.

Mathematical impossibility, fortunately for researchers, does not mean no practical solutions for the inverse problem. There are technical fixes that constrain the number of possible EEG sources so that, taken together with prior knowledge about where signals should be coming from, it is possible to work out likely origins for the brain waves in question. EEG can also be combined with other technologies. A mathematical solution would be beautiful and a satisfying source of kudos, but the kludges used instead are enough for many clinicians and researchers—as long as very fine detail is not required.

EEG is a widely used, temporally accurate and non-invasive method of brain research. Like all neurotech, it has disadvantages: the spatial resolution isn't great and the inverse problem is a problem. On the other hand EEG setups are cheap and easy to use.[26] So why, when I mention EEG to a neuroimaging colleague, does he groan and roll his eyes? And why have scientists spent gigantic amounts of time and money on developing a far more expensive and difficult technology, MEG, which also measures the brain's electromagnetic fields?

Apart from the fact that MEG is decidedly cool (complex, expensive, and above all still relatively new in neuroscience), and EEG isn't, one of the reasons for disdaining EEG is the flaky uses to which it has sometimes been put. Electromagnetic radiation, like the word 'quantum', tends to bring out the fruitcake fringe, and 'brain waves' are no exception.[27] Applications going far beyond the science are not uncommon in, for example, the use of neurofeedback to treat psychological problems. They give the technique a New Age taint to which many scientists are violently allergic—with reason, since calling someone's work 'flaky' is one of science's most potent and frequent insults. No wonder, then, that websites offering EEG-based 'spiritual technology'— no, I have no idea what that means—and training to enhance your 'human potential' (qué?) are viewed with disfavour by those for whom 'potential' is measured in volts.

You could argue that it isn't fair to blame EEG for attracting weird fry, any more than we blame celebrities for their stalkers. Unfortunately, the tendency to extrapolate beyond the available evidence is a very basic human attribute. Our brains, if they must be summed up in one small sound bite, are prediction machines, continually using evidence to jump to conclusions. Reading some EEG studies, one can forget, among all that detail, that the relation between specific EEG signals and the underlying neural activity is not straightforward. Nor is the brain waves' psychological 'meaning'—the link to subjectivity essential for DNE technology—well understood.[28] Variations in how the electrodes are placed and compared, and the analyses conducted, also contribute to a niggling sense of unreliability in studies using electroencephalographs.

Tracking the brain's grammar

There is another problem with EEG. To illustrate it, I will refer to a 2010 article which uses EEG data to work out which hand movements were being made by study participants while their encephalograms were being recorded. 'Reconstructing three-dimensional hand movements from noninvasive electroencephalographic signals', in the prestigious *Journal of Neuroscience*, attracted a lot of attention, raising as it did the prospect of advancing human–computer interfaces—such as those used in the multi-billion-dollar games industry—beyond the simplistic control of which they are currently capable.[29] EEG was previously thought to be inadequate as a useful guide to how people wave their hands about. However, the study's authors:

> challenge this assumption by continuously decoding three-dimensional (3D) hand velocity from neural data acquired from the scalp with 55-channel EEG during a 3D center-out reaching task. To preserve ecological validity, five subjects self-initiated reaches and self-selected targets.

That is, the participants' brains were monitored as they moved their right hands from a central position to push one of eight buttons in front of them. Ecologically valid tasks are realistic ones, and choosing when and where to move, as these people did, is considered a less artificial situation than being told to do so.

Note that, while this study is recording and analysing data from healthy volunteers, it is not comparing an experimental group with a control group. There is no matching set of five people who, for example, were told how to move their hands. These researchers are after other game: the capacity to predict hand movements from brain waves. The comparison they are making is between how their analysis of the EEG suggests the volunteers were moving, and how they were actually moving. If the two match well, then information about hand movements can be extracted purely from EEG, without a person needing to move their hand at all. That opens the way to more precisely thought-controlled machines, for pleasure, convenience, or life support.

The match between what the researchers measured and what they predicted from their EEG data 'compared reasonably well' to data obtained by sticking electrodes in people's brains. A relief for gamers balking at having implants, no doubt, and a challenge to the default assumption that external recordings of brain activity must always be much poorer-quality than internal ones. For the definition of 'reasonably well' the article cites peak correlations of 0.19, 0.38, and 0.32 for the three dimensions, x, y, and z, in which the movement velocities were measured. Perfection (a correlation of 1) this certainly isn't. There were only five participants and an awful lot of data preprocessing. But hey, I trust the mighty J Neurosci brand. Having said which, wobbly movements make EEGs harder to read, so this technology may not work for people with Parkinson's disease, anxious computerphobes, or anyone keen on drunken gaming sessions. Nonetheless, controlling things fluently by thought without having to stick needles in your brain would be of huge practical benefit.[30]

So what's the problem? Look back at the task description. 'To preserve ecological validity, five subjects self-initiated reaches and self-selected targets.' In other words, they chose to move to one of eight targets. The experimenters knew where the targets were in advance, so they had a good idea of what kinds of signals they were looking for in their EEG data. Decoding hand movements from brain electrical signals is much easier if you start with the assumption that what you are looking for is hand movements—and only a few of all possible hand movements at that, made by a person in a science lab wearing an EEG cap.[31] Ecological validity is relative. Decoding brain signals is a major challenge, and matching EEG patterns to known, restricted outcomes is not equivalent to truly understanding the 'language' of the electroencephalogram.

To see why, consider an analogy from more traditional languages: students learning Mandarin. If you're not a native speaker and haven't tried this fascinating form of self-improvement, imagine you're given a list of characters to learn as follows. (If you know Chinese, this exercise will be a cinch.)

我	I
喜欢	like, prefer
不喜欢	dislike
啤酒	beer
糖	sugar
口味	taste
听见	hear, listen to
喇叭	horn, trumpet
的	possessive particle, 's
声音	sound, noise

You can now decode the Mandarin translation of the sentence: 'I hear the sound of a horn'.

Chinese	我	听见	喇叭	的	声音
Literal English	I	hear	horn	's	sound

Likewise the sentence: 'I dislike the taste of beer'.

Chinese	我	不喜欢	啤酒	口味
Literal English	I	dislike	beer	taste

So here's a test sentence:

Chinese	我	不喜欢	糠	口味

I don't like the taste of sugar, right? Wrong. Look closely, and the fifth character (from the left) is not the one for sugar. 糖 (pronounced 'tang' with a rising tone) means 'sugar'. 糠 (pronounced 'kang' with a level tone) means 'bran', 'husk', or 'chaff', which most people find unappetizing.

If you're an English reader, you're used to 26 letters which on the whole manage to look quite different from each other across a range of fonts. When you learned the Mandarin character for 'sugar' you focused on the features which distinguished it from the other 15 characters you were learning, not on the fine detail of its appearance. If you saw a similar character and assumed it was 'sugar', Mandarin has wrong-footed you. As a fellow-student, I can confirm this is a common experience.

You were led to assume a certain number of characters, and you were pattern-matching the sentence characters against those in the list, when in fact an extra one was needed. An unkind trick to play on a language student, but evolution isn't the kindest of teachers. The brain plays by other rules, and the neural language is one where we're still at the early, pattern-matching stage. There's no grammar book and we're not even sure what are letters and what mere ornamentation. Statistical techniques can help us guess, but many of them also rely on assumptions which may not be correct. And testing all these assumptions is slow work.

Any neuroscientific experiment interprets brain function through the tightly controlled lens of a theoretical model: a particular way of seeing and understanding what is seen. The ideal is a model so thoroughly tested against reality that every other explanation for the difference observed between experiment and control conditions— every possible confounding factor—has been ruled out. If the model has a fixed number of meaningful components (like the 16 Mandarin characters or the choice of movements in the EEG study), then researchers can use statistics to show that their model matches the observed data reasonably well, perhaps better than a range of other models.

Do they test all possible models? No funding would stretch that far. Do they test, or even recognize, all the assumptions underlying their model? No, because they are limited human beings trapped, like all of us, by particular histories and perspectives. Besides, that's the point of laying open one's work to the critical review of other scientists. Critics lack the owner's motivation to defend a precious model, motivation which may blur the gaze of even the best researcher. Peer review and crowdsourcing are far from perfect, but they are the nearest human beings can get to omniscience. Open communication is not merely desirable in research; it is vital.

This is the gigantic challenge facing the science of the brain supremacy. The brain is such a vastly complicated system that the number of its components, never mind their interactions, soars free of the human scale into millions, billions, and trillions: realms more reminiscent of physics or economics. And grasping the components is a mere beginning, just as understanding a foreign language occurs at many levels. A student may recognize every character in a Mandarin sentence while having very little clue as to what it's going on about. Being able to construct new sentences is a further skill, let alone being able to shape them in the way that a native speaker instinctively would. Decoding hand movements from EEG is a neat and potentially very useful achievement. In decoding brains, however, there's much more to do.

And doing it requires better technology. To solve some of EEG's problems, researchers have turned to an alternative way of reading off electromagnetic doings from living heads: magnetoencephalography. It's fast like EEG (much faster than MRI) and it has significant advantages over the older technology. MEG taps the deep and difficult science of quantum mechanics to achieve astonishingly sensitive measurements of brain activity. In the next chapter, therefore, we return to the peculiar quantum world.

9

Neuroscience Goes Quantum

Any sufficiently advanced science is indistinguishable from magic

(Arthur C. Clarke, writer)

Magnetoencephalography does not involve magic. It uses quantum mechanics, which for most of us might as well be sorcery. After all, this branch of physics taps deep forces and works in mysterious ways. It transforms the nature of things, involves spectacular annihilations, creates matter apparently from nowhere. It has its own coven or priesthood—a cadre of specialists who talk in a code opaque to the rest of us. And there's even a cat, the traditional witch's familiar, uncannily rendered by Erwin Schrödinger.[1] The elite are almost all wizards rather than witches, but that has long been the standard model for physics.

Quantum phenomena are notoriously baffling, as its mathematically gifted initiates admit. I'm no priest in that or any sense, but in this chapter I will show you how useful quantum 'magic' can be in a field far distant from its intellectual origins. Some of its applications can be dazzling, and none more so than neuroimaging. We've already seen quantum mechanics used in the fMRI scanner, where energy quanta emitted from subatomic particles are crucial to understanding magnetic resonance. Now we'll see how two other quantum phenomena allowed for the creation of MEG scanners: machines so subtle that they can pick up magnetic fields five billion times weaker than the force which keeps a fridge magnet in place.

Magic magnetic

All neuroimaging machines are remarkable creations. A MEG scanner is a true wonder of the modern world: an elegantly thought-out, precision-engineered transference of quantum subtleties into the realm of the usefully visible. MEG also fills a gap in the neuroimaging toolkit. Faster than fMRI and PET, it is also more direct (measuring neuron activity, not blood flow or radioactive decay), and the signals it reads are less distorted than those of EEG.[2] It needs no strong magnetic fields, the scanner is less claustrophobic than the giant washing machine of fMRI, and unlike PET no injections are necessary.

Magnetic-brain-writing is akin to EEG, measuring the same electro-magnetic fields; but MEG is more precise. It is less affected by the secondary volume currents that form in the brain's extracellular spaces, so the fluctuations it records are more closely related to the processing actually taking place within neurons. It measures magnetic signals, which, though far smaller, are less distorted than electrical ones as they pass through the brain, meninges, skull, and scalp.

If you had been passing my physics classroom during my A-level days, and had glanced curiously in at the solitary student taking the course, you might have observed me apparently practising to be a hitchhiker: right hand extended, the fingers curled, the thumb sticking up. In fact, I was studying electromagnetism, and learning a version of the right-hand rule, a mnemonic variously attributed to John Fleming, James Clerk Maxwell and André-Marie Ampère. Pointing my thumb in the direction of an electrical current, my curled fingers showed the direction of the magnetic field generated around it. The same gesture reminds me that the brain's magnetic fields are at right angles to its electrical fields. MEG, in other words, prefers cortex tilted at angles that EEG isn't so good on (and vice versa).[3]

MEG is as fast as EEG, and at least as reliable: its results can be replicated, over years, even within a single individual. MEG can also offer better spatial resolution than many EEG setups—unless they use electrodes placed directly on or into the brain, and that is normally only done when there is clinical justification.[4] For MEG, the person must recline in a scanner and try to keep still, but the skull stays put and the noise is less alarming than the crunching of an fMRI scanner. Better still, for participants concerned about their appearance, although a MEG scanner looks like something escaped from a hair salon (see Figure 13) it does not, unlike EEG gel, trash your curls.

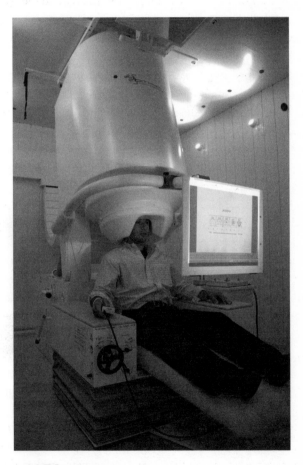

FIGURE 13: A MEG scanner.
(Courtesy of the National Institute of Mental Health, NIH)

MEG can match fMRI on detail—and the costs of a session are similar—while matching EEG on time. And if you must have EEG as well, modern MEG scanners incorporate facilities for collecting EEG data as part of their design, as well as monitoring eye movements, muscle movements, and heart rate. Yet despite its best-of-both-worlds marvels MEG is the Cinderella of neuroimaging. Its sisters fMRI and EEG are well-established, but relatively few researchers or clinicians currently use magnetoencephalography. Why? MEG may seem like exciting new technology, but the key advances were achieved around half a century ago.

Inertia is part of the problem; so is expense.[5] Imagine you own an old car which does what you need as long as you don't ask too much of it. There's no air-conditioning, and you wind down the windows by hand, but you've had it for years and you're used to it. When your neighbour shows off his new high-spec, efficient model, with its fancy electronics, you realize that his lean machine would not only get you up hills without a struggle, it could be immense fun to drive. But the displays make you boggle and the luxury's frankly alarming. And after all, yours cost a fraction of what he paid.

If EEG's an old favourite and MEG's a high-performance hybrid, fMRI scanning is more like driving a truck. It'll get you there, eventually, but your interaction with it is less about the thrilling art of motoring than about trundling along the highway. If you've recently parted with a large sum for your truck, however, and someone offers you a faster vehicle for much the same price, you might well say thanks but no thanks. MRI scanners are now well-established, and MEG facilities are a considerable extra cost.

There is also the intellectual effort required, and this is a considerable barrier. The art of motoring is riskier, and demands more of drivers, than a routine transit from A to B. Likewise new neurotech asks more of its users than older methods. Because fMRI has had more time for the field to develop, and for much of the actual data collection to be automated, the learning curve has become more bearable. It is quite possible to do fMRI experiments without understanding much about fMRI—especially if you choose your collaborators wisely.

MEG, by contrast, currently asks much more from its users in the way of interpretation and understanding, although this is changing (for instance, MEG results are often now presented in a visually comparable way to fMRI data (see Plate 5 for an example).[6] The benefit is that this clarifies what assumptions are being made during analysis, so a researcher knows exactly where he or she stands. The deterrent is that it's more difficult work. Data must be looked at, not just processed automatically by software; decisions about filtering and the choice of sources, how to carve and slice your experimental joint, must be made; time must be taken. MEG researchers talk of 'getting to know your data'—an ideal for all scientists, but one which may not sit well with the pressure to publish.

The workings

Getting to know the data means getting to know the tool which makes the data possible: the magnetoencephalograph, or MEG scanner, in its magnetically shielded room. The shielding is needed to neutralize external magnetic fields, for instance from nearby equipment like the computers required for processing MEG data. Magnetic emissions from machines are many times noisier than the brain's signals (see Table 1).[7] EEG and other electrode recording techniques are also vulnerable to interference from nearby electrical devices—despite its shielding, my MSc electrode setup sometimes picked up the local radio station—but many EEG studies are interested in the brain's big waves, not its subtler distinctions, so interference has been less of a problem. MEG scanners demand expensive wrappings because magnetic fields are so much weaker and harder to detect than electrical ones. Large numbers of neurons firing together produce a signal of around a trillionth of a tesla, which is about 50 million times weaker than the Earth's magnetic field.[8]

The story of how the brain's magnetic signals can be detected at all is an unsung story of modern scientific problem-solving, in which knowledge garnered from quantum physics proved useful in the very different field of brain research. I will set aside details of the data analysis, shielding, and processing to focus instead on an MEG scanner's key component: the magnetism detector.[9] This superb instrument has an unwieldy name—superconducting quantum interference device—but a memorable acronym: SQUID. To see how it works, we must dip a frozen toe into a strange environment indeed: the quantum world at very low temperatures. This is the realm of superconductivity, the first of the mysteries needed to make a MEG scanner.

Into the weird

The problem with measuring the brain's magnetic fields is that you need an extremely sensitive detector. A superconducting metal is a good candidate, because the current flowing through it is in a particular kind of quantum state which is very susceptible to interference (see below), even by the tiny amounts of magnetism emitted by a brain. When interfered with, it 'collapses' to a non-quantum state, a change which can in principle be measured. Unfortunately, taking such a measurement interferes with the superconducting system, ruining the experimental setup before it can yield any data. How were physicists able to work around this obstacle in order to get their supersensitive detectors? To see how they did it, we need to set out from more familiar quantum territory.

One of the best-known quantum mechanics paradoxes is the one dreamed up by Erwin Schrödinger in 1935.[10] In his thought experiment, 'eine Katze' is shut in a box for an hour with a radioactive source. The amount of source is so small that, during the hour, perhaps one of the atoms will decay and emit a particle—or perhaps not.[11] If the particle is emitted before the box is opened, it triggers a hammer to break a flask of cyanide, poisoning Puss. If not, when you open the box you will find Puss alive and well. What state is the cat in while it is in the box?

Only observing the cat can answer that question. Until that observation takes place, in quantum-mechanical terms there exists a wavefunction which describes the probability that the cat is alive and the probability that it is dead. And, at least on some interpretations of quantum mechanics, this is actually how it is inside the box: both potential outcomes—that the particle was emitted and the cat killed, or that there was no decay and the cat survives—co-exist in a 'super-position' of states. At its deepest level reality is fuzzy, probabilistic; it is our gross natures which insist on imposing certainties where the universe offers only a bouquet of possibilities. When we open the box, we convert an uncertain quantum state (cat-alive-with-probabil-ity-X, cat-dead-with-probability-1-minus-X), into an observed non-quantum state in which the wavefunction has a single value (the cat is either alive or dead). If all this strikes you as decidedly peculiar, well, hello and welcome to the club of humans discombobulated by deep physics.

We are not used to probabilistic cats, because generally quantum effects are very small and do not often survive being scaled up to the cat-sized world.[12] For an atomic nucleus or electron, however, although we tend to think of them in terms of tiny spheres, their mathematical descriptions would be in the form of wavefunctions: equations whose outputs, plotted for a range of times and positions in space, would look a bit like what happens to a lake when you chuck in a stone (see Figure 14). As noted earlier, an electron's wavefunction tells us, for a given place and time, how likely it is that the electron will be in that exact spot at that precise time.

All this is a verbal description of a mathematics which appears to work well. Quantum mechanics has been a hugely successful theory. But if you ask a physicist what it 'means'—what's really happening down there in the extremely small—you'll likely get the answer: 'I don't know', or else a heap of equations. Quantum mechanics deals not only in probabilities, but in complex numbers, difficult differential equations, and other mathematical horrors. Over eighty years after Schrodinger came up with his famous 'undulatory theory', it continues to defy attempts to pin down its meaning in any language except that of mathematics. Nonetheless, electron wavefunctions are at the heart of SQUIDs' success as magnetic detectors; so here (without addressing the deepest questions of 'what it means') is my attempt at explaining how quantum mechanics can give us new insights into brain function.

The supersensitive flow

With its subtlety, complexity, and exotic physics, MEG offers a hint of future neurotech, and the remarkable era into which the ascent of neuroscience will bring us. It's an exciting vision, and the study of superconductors is super-cool science. In the case of the metal niobium, one of the materials commonly used in SQUIDs, it's extremely cool—about 9 degrees short of absolute zero (0 kelvin, -273.15°C).[13] When niobium is brought down to this temperature, using liquid helium, it begins to act as a superconductor.[14]

Even at room temperature metals conduct electricity, as coroners, pathologists, and grieving relatives well know. What enables this sometimes lethal characteristic is the metal's atomic structure, in which the atoms arrange themselves in regular, repeating patterns in order to balance the forces between them.[15] When a voltage is applied, it can easily tug outer electrons away from their home atoms, allowing them to flow through the metal as an electric current. Because the metal's structure is so tidy, they can travel for longer without hitting

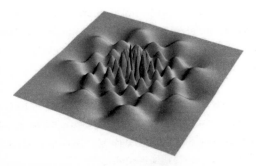

FIGURE 14: An electron wavefunction in a hydrogen atom.
(Courtesy of Benjamin Crowell/Creative Commons licence)

one of its atoms. This is why the electronic tools you and I rely on every day respond when we press the relevant buttons.

Even in a metal, however, an electron can find its path impeded by chemical impurities: atoms out of place. There is also the phenomenon of resistance to weaken the current. Atomic nuclei, as we saw with hydrogen in Chapter 7's discussion of fMRI, readily absorb energy from their surroundings. They also vibrate, shedding energy as they do so. What we experience as warm or cold in a material reflects how actively its atoms are moving within their constraining forces, and atoms, like kids, are more lively when their environment is providing lots of energy. The more agitated the atoms become, the more energy quanta they spit out and the harder it is for electrons to flow smoothly between them without being knocked off course. As an analogy, imagine trying to walk down a crowded street while some of the other pedestrians are busily hurling tennis balls.

Resistance is a wasteful nuisance. Not only is useful energy lost as heat, but the electric current flows less efficiently. Cool things down, however, and the flow is less disturbed. Cool the metal further—much, much further—and the atoms become so sluggish that their vibrations no longer trouble the electrons, which can now flow through the metal without much resistance, except for when they collide with an atom.[16]

At a still lower temperature, something remarkable happens. Not only do atomic vibrations cease to affect electron flow, so do collisions between electrons and atoms.[17] At that point the metal has become a superconductor, a quantum wonder where electrons flow with no resistance at all. It's the equivalent of abolishing friction, so that nothing set moving on a surface would ever grind to a halt of its own accord.[18] If a metal wire is ring-shaped, as in SQUIDs, a super-conducting electron 'wave' will flow continuously around the ring as long as the temperature is kept low—unchanged for years, if nothing interrupts it. This delicate state, so easily interrupted, must be carefully controlled to serve in a MEG scanner.

Despite the modern perception, at least in wealthier countries, of electric current as easily and eternally available, this is not how electricity works at room temperature. The current flowing into your computer has weakened since it was born, costing your supplier money—and therefore you. In a superconductor, that flow would be ageless and intact. No wonder, then, that creating a superconductor which works at room temperature has been described as the holy grail of physics.[19]

The secrets of SQUIDs

How then to manage the electron wave in a superconducting SQUID ring without this touchy, temperamental entity collapsing into the mundane? The answer relies on the second of the quantum mysteries needed to make an MEG scanner: tunnelling.

Under certain conditions, quantum-mechanical entities like electrons display a cavalier disregard not only of common sense but of accepted rules of large-scale physics. Specifically, they can pass through barriers, or jump across gaps, as if there were no obstacle. This, roughly, is because their wavefunctions are spread out in space around and beyond the obstacle. Since an electron's wavefunction at a particular point reflects the probability of the electron being at that point, there is a chance that the electron will be found beyond the obstacle—i.e. on the other side from where one might have expected it. So sometimes it will be found there, as if it had 'tunnelled' through the obstacle. If you see what I mean.

SQUIDs use tunnelling by means of a device called a Josephson junction. This is an extremely thin layer of an insulating material sandwiched between two layers of superconductor. In a common arrangement, two Josephson junctions are inserted into the superconducting SQUID ring on opposite sides. The insulator should break the circuit and collapse the electron wave, but because of tunnelling it doesn't: the electrons simply flow on as if there were no gap. Why then bother inserting the junctions? Because any resistance which does arise across them can be measured. Since the level of resistance changes with variations in the magnetic field passing through the SQUID ring, this is a way to detect such variations.

When the person in the scanner has just received a visual stimulus, for example, the magnetic field near the SQUID will change, just a little. That causes an electrical variation in the SQUID ring. In other words, changes in the brain's magnetic emissions interfere with the SQUID's electron wave, which promptly collapses, raising the resistance across the Josephson junctions.

That resistance is measured by applying an external current, called a bias current, to the SQUID. There is no resistance in the superconducting state, of course, but whenever it collapses, the resistance jumps, causing the external current to fluctuate.[20] It is this fluctuating bias current, recorded from arrays of SQUIDs surrounding the person's head, which is the basic measurement taken by an MEG scanner. Magnetoencephalographs thus do not record absolute values, but changes, in the brain's magnetic fields. They do this in real time and at the quantum scale, a phenomenal accomplishment.

MEG scanners are a marvel of applied physics and a testament to the astonishing resourcefulness of scientific creativity. They are exquisitely sensitive to tiny changes in the brain, and they show how an apparently abstract theory—quantum mechanics—can be used to predict, and then achieve, a remarkable goal in neuroscience research. The only magnetic fields which most of us typically notice are those in everyday magnets, like the ones on a fridge or noticeboard. MEG can pick up fields so minuscule that they are billions of times weaker than this. To match that level of perception, human eyes, which can easily detect a fridge magnet, would have to be keen enough to peer into atoms.

The forward wave

Each neuroimaging technology sees the brain with a different gaze, and each has its pros and cons. MEG is superfast and supersensitive, but difficult. EEG is swift, established, and convenient; fMRI is slower but more fine-grained. Unsurprisingly, a huge amount of effort has gone into bringing these complementary capacities together to focus on a single brain at a single moment.[21] Anything else—like first running one kind of scan and then another on the same person—and problems creep in: fatigue, movements, and all sorts of other potentially confounding differences between the two situations.

Merging EEG and MEG is relatively simple: as noted earlier, EEG is now commonly incorporated into MEG scanners. Merging electrical and magnetic resonance technologies is harder. Participants may wear EEG caps in an fMRI scanner, as long as the equipment has been carefully designed, but the experience is uncomfortable. Worse (from the experimenter's point of view), both signals are degraded by their interaction. An MRI scanner's changing magnetic field mucks up the EEG with artificial signals, which have to be laboriously removed, while the EEG cap distorts the magnetic field in ways which are not easy to take account of in analysis.

MEG and fMRI are even less compatible. Thanks to the high magnetic fields used in fMRI, these two neuroimaging methods are definitely not on speaking terms. You can run one and then the other, but making sure the data match up accurately is a process fraught with error. Yet even this apparently fundamental problem may be resolvable. An ingenious recent suggestion is to use a subset of SQUIDs as MRI detectors in tandem with very small applied magnetic fields (rather than the several tesla used in conventional fMRI), so that MEG can be done at the same time.[22] The MRI provides enough information about location to enable the MRI data—and thus the MEG data—to be matched up to a conventional MRI scan with much higher accuracy than MEG alone.

There is hope, in short, that improvements in neuroimaging technology, and bringing in additional methods such as optical imaging, will help to resolve at least some of the technical difficulties.[23] However the work proceeds—and this will be a fascinating area to watch over the next few years—some form of EEG/MEG will surely be involved, because it supplies the all-important time dimension. Anyone who has ever struggled with voice recognition or video game control will know how infuriating a sluggish response can be. Machines designed to interface with human beings will have to match them—and their neurons—in the temporal domain. This will be increasingly true as the signals those machines are expected to detect become more 'advanced'—not just pre-learned nouns or images or left-versus-right directions for virtual navigation, but the subtle nuances of real-time thought, speech, gesture, and expression. The brain cannot even be crudely controlled, much less comprehended, unless we have a good understanding of brain dynamics.

Two other advances are looming which may well transform that understanding. For reasons of space I will mention them only briefly. The first is wireless technology, which should enable remote access to brain signals—in certain kinds of patients to begin with, and perhaps later in anyone who cares to don the relevant fashionable headwear. That, coupled with the drive to make neuroimaging more portable, is likely to bring it at least partially out of specialist hands, from the lab to the street.[24] Home DNE recording is years off yet, and portability is a vital step on the way.

The second advance is nanotechnology. If we can make our signal-detectors small enough we can abandon the huge machinery that currently anchors neuroimaging to the lab and the hospital, with all the ethical baggage that anchor brings. We may even, one day, be able to insert our scanning technology into a person's breakfast without them realizing, or implant it in children early in life. And if we do so, it will be for admirable reasons: clinical motives, initially; then for research. Later, as society gets used to the idea, we may use DNE technologies increasingly for other ends: like control, or making money.

One of my hopes in writing this book was that it may lead to discussion of these advances before they happen, rather than waiting until powerful tools for brain control are widely available. In technology, 'can create' is often confused with 'should create'; the two are not synonymous. It may not matter when the product is a more efficient car or a healthier sandwich. But better ways of seeing—and controlling—the human brain are in another ethical category, both because they affect us so directly and because of the likelihood that they may be used on people without their consent. Nothing improves a business's, or government's, behaviour like the uncomfortable feeling of critical scrutiny, and advances in brain technology demand such attention more than most scientific developments. Just because the methods may soon allow us to ditch the ethical baggage provided by a research environment is no reason to hand their governance over to the market, the military, or the darker reaches of the state.

Nanotechnology, like electrophysiology, is a bridging power in that it blurs the line between seeing the brain and manipulating it. These two are not, however, the only possibilities for brain control. In the next chapters, turning from ways of seeing to ways of changing the brain, I will consider others, including remarkable techniques from our swelling genetic toolkit. First, however, let us stay on the trail of electrophysiology, which leads us deep into the brain.

10

Poke It and See What Happens

Think occasionally of the suffering of which you spare yourself the sight

(Albert Schweitzer)

One of the remarkable features of human brains is the rapid responsiveness to many external events which makes us such adaptable, accomplished lifeforms. Responsiveness, though, has an alter ego: vulnerability. Our brains can be changed by a quick gin, a sexual touch, or a scented breeze. They can also be affected by more delicate powers: a cutting word, a dream, or a false belief. And a bash on the head, a disease, or a terrible shock can alter a personality for ever.

When interference damages the sensitive substance of the brain it may cause anything from temporary problems or subtle deficits through to loss of function, unconsciousness, or death. Brain damage can leave visible holes, but it often doesn't. The array of possible faults is terrifying, but much of this damage is accidental or collateral. Only rarely do humans deliberately damage brains for clinical reasons. For example, surgical interventions such as lesioning (destroying) a particular area have been used as a treatment for severe cases of Parkinson's disease or epilepsy.[1]

Much more common is planned interference in order to change the brain without (one hopes) doing significant damage, as part of a scientific experiment or clinical assessment. This may involve applying chemicals, or the use of electrical or magnetic stimulation. Such experiments are governed by very strict ethical rules, overseen by ethics committees. Whenever a paper is published, its authors publicly commit to those standards. When they slip, they risk having the article retracted, disciplinary action, or losing their jobs.

More common still, however, is damage deliberately inflicted on the brains of other species. This chapter will take us into the world of invasive research, a darker side of the path to the brain supremacy. The vast majority of this work is done on mice and rats, but other mammals, including primates, are also used. It's the kind of work where blood and brains are on display, where animals die—and sometimes so do patients. Volunteering as a last resort to undergo a new kind of treatment, such as brain surgery, is crucial to how those treatments are developed, but the desperate sufferer is risking damage or death. Animals, of course, are almost all specially bred and do not have the choice.

I will be describing an animal experiment. (If you're squeamish, the animals involved were rats; furthermore, Chapter 12 discusses experiments on mice. Studies using these two species have been central to brain research.) As a meat-eating ex-vivisectionist whose life was saved by scientific medicine, I should make my position clear. I cannot, without hypocrisy, call for a ban on such practices, or condemn the people who do them carefully and well. Unlovely though animal experiments are, and glad though I would be to live in a world without them, I think they remain a necessary evil for the time being.[2] To see why, this chapter will focus on electrophysiology, an elder statesman technique for brain manipulation but one which continues to prove its worth.

Electrophysiology gives real-time access to neuron activity, and implanted electrodes are more sensitive than non-invasive ones. Animals (and patients) are more likely to turn up for the experiment than volunteers are. Because their life history is better known and, for animals, controlled, it's easier to exclude potentially confounding factors. And, crucially, researchers can go beyond merely collecting correlations.[3]

When I was doing my doctorate in the 1990s, neuroimaging was the height of fashion and electrode work had Cinderella status. Today the term 'electrophysiology' sounds very old-fashioned. Yet neuroimaging records signals from a changing brain and leaves the scientists to infer what caused the changes, whereas electrophysiology allows them to cause changes and study the effects. It is also a crucial component of new genetic techniques, as we'll see later, so it will not be left to rust in the neuroscience toolkit any time soon. Sometimes there is no other way to do the experiment than by actively interfering with living brains.

A disadvantage of invasive studies is that results from animals or patients may not necessarily generalize to healthy human brains. Nonetheless, a person fortunate enough to have enjoyed good mental health to date is not a different species from his unluckier fellows. Nor is he altogether unlike the animals killed in laboratories in an effort to save him and others like him from the misery of disorders like Alzheimer's. Research on animals and patients has produced tremendously useful data and considerable benefits. Most of it has been done with far more care for its participants than animals used in other industries receive.

To date, there is no cure for Alzheimer's. Yet to conclude from that sad observation that animal research has been a cruel waste, as some do, is to reveal colossal ignorance. Good science must be slow and careful, adding piece by unpleasantly gathered piece to unravel the gargantuan conundrum of any brain dysfunction. The intricacies of brain systems necessitate the careful and patient untangling of fiendishly complicated webs of cause and effect—in the hope of, eventually, understanding what has gone wrong. Sometimes the clinical implications of a study seem remote, one of very many steps required to unravel how a disease does damage. Moreover, the risks of slipshod work, of not checking potential chemicals thoroughly, are potentially catastrophic in clinical research, as previous medical disasters like thalidomide remind us. To argue from 'there's no cure' to 'there's no worthwhile progress' is simply wrong.

Through the laboratory doors

What is it like to do an animal experiment?

The last time I chopped up an animal for work, rather than for dinner, was years ago now, for a research MSc. The project investigated how particular kinds of receptors for the neurotransmitter glutamate interact in the brain systems which process sensations of touch. Rats are a good model; their somatosensory cortex is well developed, and the whiskers they use to whiffle through the world are more important data sources than vision. To study which receptors were involved in processing whisker stimulation, I recorded neuronal activity while applying a variety of receptor-related substances.

I used to get up about 6 a.m. on experiment days to make my own microelectrodes. It was a fiddly process, and the electrode tips were so infuriatingly delicate that sinking one successfully into the cortex of an anaesthetized rat was always a moment of relief. Those tiny glass tips were essential tools, taking note of nearby electrical activity while allowing me to administer minute amounts of chemicals to the brain I was studying. I was using a sophisticated system with neat automatic recording and analysis facilities, but the basic technique was well-established electrophysiology.

What actually happens in this kind of experiment? Not a lot, to be honest, except at the beginning—when the animal is anaesthetized and prepared for the experiment—and at the end when it is killed. (If animal research is evil, it lacks the glamour of other kinds of wicked-ness.) In my work, there was just enough routine, once the setting-up was over, to keep me from falling asleep in that small, warm, airless room. I gave every one of the rats I killed a name—Fred—but I don't remember talking to them much. No music either, and very few visit-ors. It was dull, prolonged, and sometimes rather peaceful.

My task was to find a cell by moving the electrode in tiny steps, listening for the clicks of a suitable neuron while a small device stroked the unconscious rat's whiskers to stimulate the cortex. After sidling up to the target cell came hours of squirting on chemicals and recording the electrical responses, moving to a fresh cell as required (neurons get tired too). I used glutamate agonists to stimulate cell receptors, antagonists to suppress their activity: tiny doses, applied again and again. Checking equipment and life signals, keeping the rat warm, and thinking; that was how the hours passed. They say science is all about teamwork, but not that project: my experience would have suited a hermit nicely.

That's as long as the hermit didn't object to killing rats with a technique called cardiovascular perfusion, because on a good day—maybe around midnight—I'd round off the experiment by perfusing the rat to preserve the brain for analysis. For readers who aren't squeamish, perfusion involves injecting enough anaesthetic to put the already unaware rat into an irreversible coma, then levering open its rib cage and sticking a large needle full of formalin directly into its heart. This makes it start twitching—just reflex movements, of course, but death throes nonetheless. After the thrashing's stopped the next step is to decapitate the corpse, using scissors, and get the brain out of the skull. I remember that bit very well: the facial skin with the eyes in it sliding all over the place, watching me sardonically as I tweezered off enough bone to remove the brain without damaging it. All in all, not my idea of a good time, ever, let alone 18 hours after crawling out of bed to spend the day in a stuffy, windowless box with only a comatose rodent for company.

For squeamish readers, I agree: perfusion is disgusting. So is cleaning up after a baby with a tummy upset, but it still needs doing. Not to perfuse an animal after an experiment would have seriously weakened the results, since at that time brain sectioning was the only way to check where the electrode had actually been placed. Remember, the rat's experience was limited to being picked up and given an injection; it never knew how it was mutilated. It died, but dying in one's sleep is far less horrific than any one of a number of things both nature and humans commonly do to rats. Disgust often affects our moral judgements—but we are not always right to let it do so.[4]

One of the problems caused by the vociferous and sometimes violent campaign against animal researchers has been that it has made the scientists understandably reluctant to speak publicly about their work. (I thought very hard before writing this chapter.) That prevents a wider discussion about how society would choose to weigh up the differing moral wrongs. When I did my project on rats I don't remember getting much useful guidance on the ethics; my job was to get on with the work. Since my supervisor and I were working in a department where several members vehemently disapproved of animal research (but put up with it because it brought in good money), he may have simply felt too besieged to see long discussions as anything but a threat. I was also warned not to talk about my work outside the department, so it was left to me to weigh up what I was doing against the lives I was ending.

That needs to change. Why should we be afraid of stating in public that yes, we do value our nearest and dearest more than we value a truckload of genetically modified mice? Outside the lab the typical Western response to mice is not to embrace them as fellow beings, but to call the pest control. Animal research is only used on the hardest of problems, but we have no other way to tackle them. Here in Britain we do it well, watch it carefully, and try to do less of it. We also all enjoy its benefits. Our taxes pay for it, and it is entirely consistent and reasonable to say that we need such work to continue even though we don't like it. We don't much like traffic or sewage systems either, but we don't give donations to people who want to destroy them. Instead we ask scientists and politicians to earn their keep by easing congestion, protecting the environment—and reducing the need for animal research.

Things have largely got better

Looking back, the moral issues haven't changed much. We still play God with our fellow creatures. Utilitarianism is a hard habit to break, and for almost all of us human misery outweighs the minimized suffering of experimental animals. What has changed is the experimental setup. A recent 'Perspective' article in *Nature Neuroscience* notes, for example, that 'progress in neural recording techniques has allowed the number of simultaneously recorded neurons to double approximately every 7 years'.[5] With that exponential rise have come massive changes in lab equipment, from data recording and storage to the software used to write up the results. When I cut and pasted photographs into my thesis I used scissors and glue. Those days are gone.

How primitive that distant lab now seems! I could guess what kinds of cells I was investigating, but I'd no idea how close the electrode was to the cell body. I had to wait for histology (the brain-chopping bit) to tell me where the electrode had gone on its travels. Even then I couldn't be precise about how much chemical was reaching which glutamate receptors where, so it was impossible to know the precise source of the electrical responses I recorded.

Today things are astonishingly different. Microscopes, electrodes, labelling techniques for cell identification, and systems for delivering chemicals, not to mention maps of the brain and neuroimaging methods, have all improved so much that brain manipulation is now a precision business. Scientists have specific chemical tools with which they can target receptor subtypes or intracellular enzymes. And they can store gigantic quantities of data from multi-electrode arrays—I used just one microelectrode—in more than one region of the brain at a time, enabling them to understand how neurons interact as never before.

Live-animal research, of course, was only ever part of the picture. Another type of study, still widely used, was the brain slice, extracted and kept alive for long enough to allow for much more precise analysis than a whole brain, at the cost of a more artificial situation. Here too there have been great advances, allowing scientists to exert fantastically precise control over where and when a chemical is applied. They can increasingly see individual proteins and locate receptors on a neuron's surface. An example is the lovely technique of two-photon uncaging, which is related to the optogenetic methods considered in Chapter 13.[6]

Uncaging works as follows. A small extra molecule, a 'caging compound', is attached to a glutamate molecule (or other substance whose effects one wants to study) by chemical bonds. Neurotransmitters and their receptors are often compared to keys and locks. On that analogy caging compounds are like lumps of modelling clay, stuck onto the key to prevent it from opening the lock. The bonds which hold the caging compound to the glutamate are designed to break when a photon of ultraviolet light is absorbed by the caging compound. Until that happens the glutamate cannot activate its receptor. Focus a UV light on the brain slice, however, and the caging compound breaks away, leaving the glutamate free to do its stuff.

UV light can be focused very tightly, 'to a diffraction-limited spot less than a micrometer wide'.[7] The caged glutamate, however, cannot be so precisely delivered. UV photons will therefore activate glutamate in surrounding areas as they travel through the brain tissue to the point where the light is focused, blurring the technique's resolution. (Recall that in cortex, neurons' cell bodies tend to be found in deeper layers.) To sharpen the focus, researchers added a second caging compound to the glutamate. By using two molecules which must both be removed if the glutamate is to become available, researchers can focus two beams of light on a much more tightly restricted region, improving resolution by 57% in the study quoted above.

If brain research on animals has improved, so has the manipulation of human patients. One of the biggest contributors to better brain surgery has been the science of stereotaxy: the development of an accurate system of 3D coordinates for representing any part of the brain. It sounds so simple, but being able to locate some tiny target region, like the focus which triggers epileptic attacks, in a standardized space has allowed neurosurgeons to limit the damage inherent in removing dysfunctional brain matter. Skin and muscle may regrow, but we understand skin and muscle more fully than we understand the brain, and brain damage can wipe out memories or change a person's personality. So minimal destruction is a priority.

When lesions are used to treat patients today, the tools and tech-niques involved are far more precise than in previous decades, and so cause much less collateral damage. An example is the gamma knife: beams of high-intensity radiation which can be focused on target tissue to destroy it with relatively little harm to other cells (unlike an elec-trode, however 'micro', which leaves a trail of damaged neurons in its wake). Radiation brings risks, of course, but it avoids the hazards of bleeding or infection which inevitably accompany traditional surgery in even the most efficient hospitals. We are moving towards being able to treat at least some brain disorders safely and successfully without having to open up the skull.

What have we learned from poke-and-see?

What tool we use to look at the brain shapes how we see it. Modern neuroscience has given us lenses that show us the brain as a pulsing, blood-filled anatomical organ (fMRI), as an evolved set of functions connecting body and world (systems and evolutionary neuroscience), as networks of highly organized biochemical processes (neurochemis-try and genetics), or as an abstract information processor (cognitive and computational neuroscience). The lens of electrophysiology gives us yet another view of the brain: as a ceaseless electromagnetic swirl. Even when supposedly at rest, brains are so vigorously engaged that some areas decrease their activity when the person begins to do a task.[8] We also know that neuronal action potentials are not just 'go' signals, like the on–off switches in a traditional computer. Instead, how spikes vary over time (the frequency of firing) carries useful information: a short burst of high-frequency spikes and a steady, lower-frequency flow can reflect quite distinct features of a stimulus.[9] We know, fur-thermore, that action potentials are not the brain's only signals, nor are neurons the only cells involved in communication.

One of brain research's most difficult challenges will be to stitch the various ways of seeing together. That interdisciplinary work is hard, highlighting conceptual glitches and contradictions as the different views of brain function are brought together, but it is likely to be incredibly productive. Glitches and contradictions fuel advances—and so do new technologies. The merging of methods is already well under way, and it will be fascinating to see how it progresses, steering the brain supremacy towards the goal of a grand unified theory.[10]

One example of how theories arise from methods and bring them closer together is the emergence of the brain network as a unit of analysis in recent years. MEG, EEG, multi-array recordings, and the functional connectivity analyses noted in Chapter 7 have all contributed to the realization that networks are crucial. Thinking of the brain as a kind of cognitive assembly line for converting stimuli into behaviour—a group of anatomical modules, each with its information processing function—is not enough. Overlaid on the anatomical connections are the functional links: the ever-changing electromagnetic discourse of patterns of neural activity flowing through the brain's innumerable paths.

Social psychology studies show that people can mimic each others' behaviour, quite unconsciously, in real time, from the first moment they meet, and that the greater the mimicry, the more empathy they will feel for each other and the more they will feel they have in common.[11] Like people who spend time together, connected neurons also tend to behave more similarly. They too can synchronize their activity, sometimes across vast reaches of the cortical surface. By doing so, the network of connected, similarly firing brain cells creates a pattern which stands out from the crowd: a distinctive signal amongst the cerebral noise. Like coordinated chanting at a public meeting, neural togetherness gets the signal heard in the vast shouting match that is an active brain, giving that particular signal more influence over behaviour.[12]

Moreover, these synchronized neuron networks are defined by the frequency at which their member cells fire, so multiple networks, firing at different frequencies, can use the same anatomical pathways, just as multiplexing allows many telephone or internet communications to use the same physical links. Frequency, in other words, gives brains an additional dimension with which to encode information.[13]

A restaurant menu which described its dishes by texture and appearance would surely disappoint inexperienced guests. Adding information about ingredients would give them a better idea of what the concoction was liable to taste like. Similarly, brains cannot be known by anatomy and chemistry alone; frequency adds flavour. This functional dimension, central to brain complexity, helps to make brain disorders an especially challenging set of problems. Damaged anatomy or disrupted chemistry may not be detectable by any of the ways of seeing described in earlier chapters—and yet there may still be something badly wrong with the brain.

How will the brain supremacy use electromagnetic manipulation to work towards its goal of DNE programming—controlling neural circuits in real time in order to give us the experiences we desire? To imagine that future we need to look at current methods of altering the outputs of brain cells, from both outside and inside the skull. From poking to precision surgery, this is research that goes beyond experiments on animals, into the delicate, dangerous world of human brain change.

11

Poking People

Medicine [is] the only profession that labors incessantly
to destroy the reason for its existence

(James Bryce, politician)

T he previous chapter looked at animal research and its usefulness in
deciphering the brain's electromagnetic emissions. Now we turn to
humans, where research strategies are more limited. The constraints, as
we have seen, have prompted some ingenious solutions to the problem
of how to view a brain you cannot take apart. Approaches to interfering
with such brains have been equally resourceful. In this chapter we
will look at examples of techniques operating through the skull (transcranial stimulation) and from within it (deep brain stimulation).

Poking at a distance: TES and TMS

Modern techniques for manipulating the brain's electromagnetic flows
do not necessarily need to open up the skull. Transcranial electrical and
magnetic stimulation offer non-surgical ways of interfering with brain
activity. By interrupting cortical business as usual and allowing
researchers to see what happens, they provide causal information
about living, presumably healthy brains. They are also being used as
clinical tools, for example in stroke rehabilitation.[1] Moreover, unlike

the traditional 'shock treatment' of electroconvulsive therapy (ECT), they can be focused on a specific area, limiting their side-effects (they don't produce disturbing images of writhing, tightly restrained patients, for one thing).

They are not perfect. Initial attempts at TES poured so much current through the electrodes that it hurt, though in the last ten years newer variants on the method—such as transcranial direct current stimulation (tDCS)—have eased that problem.[2] TMS, meanwhile, can give you a nasty twinge if it catches your neck muscles, and carries a small risk of headaches, fainting, or seizures; tDCS is thought to be safer.[3] Nonetheless both electrical and magnetic stimulation are now ethically acceptable tools for research as well as in the clinic.[4] At-risk participants are screened out by, for example, checking there is no history of epilepsy, just as fMRI safety questionnaires rule out people with claustrophobia.

The electrical stimulation needed to penetrate the skull is not the delicate current I used to squirt chemicals into the brains of rats. It affects much larger areas and requires a lot more current to achieve focal stimulation, since as noted earlier, electric fields, unlike magnetic ones, are greatly perturbed by travelling through skin, bone, and brain.[5] Transcranial magnetic stimulation also uses electrical current, but indirectly, since it relies on electromagnetic induction: a hefty current is passed through a coil, inducing a brief but strong magnetic pulse. This is typically a couple of tesla in strength, comparable with the magnetic fields used in fMRI.[6] It lasts around a millisecond, and in turn induces electrical currents to flow beneath the skull, thereby upsetting neurons in the affected area. Single pulses or repetitive stimulation can be used to excite or inhibit activity. TMS appears able to change brain connections long-term, thereby offering the potential for functionally 'rewiring' faulty networks.[7]

The mechanisms by which brain stimulation achieves these effects are not yet fully understood. But hey, if we waited to understand how our tools worked before employing them the human race would still be relying on lightning strikes for fire. To get around the problem of not completely knowing what they were doing, researchers used a range of TMS frequencies and intensities on sensory and motor systems, where the results of its interference were obvious (for example, muscle twitches when the coil is placed over motor cortex would suggest an excitatory effect of TMS).[8] Once they knew which TMS protocols produced excitation and which shut down activity, they could then apply the technique to 'behaviourally silent' areas of the brain and interfere with the interesting in-between bits, like working memory, mood, and theory of mind.[9] Activity detected in a particular brain region by neuroimaging may reflect neuronal processing related to the task being performed, but it may reflect something else (as the story of the religious gentleman in Chapter 3 showed). By blitzing a specific segment of brain matter, TMS can help establish whether it is necessary for the task to be accomplished.

Standard coils can produce effects over an area of roughly one square centimetre, so TMS's spatial resolution is acceptable, although a pulse still disrupts enormous numbers of neurons. Its temporal resolution is also good: the disruption lasts for under 100 milliseconds. It is easier to use than electrical methods, since the coil doesn't touch the body and no wires need be attached. It also produces more focal stimulation, since TES-evoked currents flow every which way whereas TMS ones tend to flow parallel to the skull.

TMS has its disadvantages, however. It is mostly used for stimulating cortex, since magnetic fields diminish so quickly with distance.[10] In principle it can also be applied to the cerebellum, low down at the back of the head, but in practice its effects on neck muscles can make these experiments very uncomfortable.[11] And the coils are cumbersome and heavy, which makes them awkward for clinical use. Electrical stimulators, such as a cardiac pacemaker or the control unit for deep brain stimulation (more about DBS shortly), can be adapted to allow patients to get on with their lives and regulate their condition without the trouble and expense of frequent visits to a hospital; but TMS coils are larger and less convenient.

The awkwardness is unfortunate, because although the long-term effects of TMS have not yet been studied extensively, the initial research into its clinical usage looks promising.[12] With respect to short-term effects, for instance, TMS has been used as an acute treatment to relieve severe depression and migraine. It has also served to diagnose disorders such as multiple sclerosis and motor neuron disease. Take the case of amyotrophic lateral sclerosis, a type of motor neuron disease also called Lou Gehrig's disease, which slows the rate at which nerve impulses are transmitted through the nervous system. TMS can be used to measure this 'conduction velocity', making it potentially useful in many neurological disorders as a warning of when the nervous system is literally slowing down.[13]

With respect to TES, at high currents it can be an unpleasant experience, but the technique can also be used to create weaker electrical fields which are more diffuse. Instead of stimulating a specific area, these interact with active networks across the brain in such a way that some of the neurons become phase-locked to the stimulating frequency; that is, they start to fire in time to the rhythm of the TES stimulus. The aim is to train the misbehaving neurons into better habits.

Being able to manipulate neural phase-locking has great clinical potential, as shown by recent research into the awful condition of chronic neuropathic pain. Often, after an accident or amputation, a person continues to experience severe discomfort—sometimes agony—long after the physical cause appears to have vanished. Phantom limb pain is an example: the sufferer feels that their amputated limb is hurting, even though that part of the body is gone. Neuroimaging studies suggest that networks of brain areas involved in responding to trauma, collectively known as the 'pain matrix', have changed their activity in these patients. If so, TES or TMS could force that network to fire at a different frequency, at least for a while. TES has been shown to have short-term analgesic effects, and researchers have also begun to use TMS to treat chronic pain.[14]

Probing the labyrinth: deep brain stimulation

Unfortunately for both TES and TMS, not all the brain that matters is to be found in the few centimetres immediately under the skull—the areas most accessible to these techniques. For greater depths, and greater precision, invasive surgery may offer the only means of manipulation at present. Long used in animals, it is done in humans only for clinical reasons—though research is often done in conjunction with the surgery, if patients consent. The trials required to test the medical methods have provided much useful information about how brains work, unobtainable by other techniques.

Developed over decades, deep brain stimulation (DBS) offers hope to patients for whom other measures have failed. It uses a slender electrode through which electrical pulses, driven by an external control unit, can be precisely targeted to specific areas of the brain. This allows stimulation to be switched off and on as desired, giving DBS the advantage of reversibility, unlike older psychosurgical techniques which removed the section of brain seen as problematic.[15] DBS has been used to treat severe neurological and, increasingly, psychiatric conditions: problems as varied as Parkinson's, epilepsy, obsessive-compulsive disorder, Tourette's syndrome, chronic pain, depression, and addiction; it can even be used to reduce high blood pressure.[16] Carefully combined with fMRI, MEG, and/or electrophysiological recording, it can precisely target anatomical or functional pathologies.[17] Lightweight electronic circuitry gives the patient relative freedom and control, and brain surgery does not require a general anaesthetic, so the procedure's physical toll is somewhat lessened.[18]

The procedure itself is rather like what I used to do to rats, except that patients don't need to be sent to sleep with an injection into the stomach muscles (and nor are they cut up afterwards). Local anaesthetic is applied to allow the scalp to be cut and peeled back; it comes away easily. Then one must drill through the skull, pierce the meninges, position the electrode over the brain, and lower away.

In patients, of course, the scale is larger and the process correspondingly more dramatic. Getting through a human skull and dura mater without damaging the brain is quite a challenge, requiring serious elbow grease coupled with extreme care. (Neurosurgeons deserve their salaries for that alone.) As for inserting the electrode, much of the work has been done before the operation, studying the MRI scans and planning exactly where to go and how to get there. Because the electrode is attached to an external control unit—the source of the stimulatory pulses which will (hopefully) change the cells' behaviour—those pulses can be adjusted by the surgical team to best fit the patient's needs.

Anyone who has seen a severely disabled Parkinson's patient before surgery—huddled in a chair, barely able to move—and afterwards, with the pacemaker switched on, walking easily across a room, will rightly be in awe of DBS.[19] For a while, at least, it can give a person back a good deal of their motor function—and their life. Studies of DBS for psychiatric disorders also suggest considerable relief of distressing symptoms and manageable side effects.[20] These are, remember, the most severely afflicted of sufferers.

However, DBS is major surgery. It is not always effective, and how it achieves its near-miraculous changes is not yet fully understood. Much more study is required of target locations such as the subthalamic nucleus (for Parkinson's) and the periventricular gray (for pain). Because these areas are buried far below cortex, they are much less accessible to neuroimaging, so much of what is known about them has come from anatomical studies or electrophysiological work in animals.[21] Also needed is more systematic information on how to set the DBS pulses' frequency, duration, and pattern of delivery so as to make them as effective as possible, while avoiding too much stimulation—which can make the treatment work less well over time.[22]

Nor is it clear how long the benefits of DBS last and to what extent they are masked by negative psychological effects on the patients, many of whom will have had their diseases for years before the surgery. Having a chronic medical condition may initially feel like an unwanted imposition, but as time passes, although it remains a detested burden, the person adjusts to its presence; so its sudden removal can leave unexpected holes in the psyche. Feeling afraid that you can't cope with 'normal' life, worrying about people thinking you're cured when you're only improved, dealing with partners who have got used to caring for you and now have to change their behaviour, and feeling guilty because, after all that time and effort and money, you are still neither healthy nor content, can take the shine off an operation's advantages.[23] DBS is a promising method, but in clinical terms still very much a work in progress.

Probing the future: brain surgery as standard?

I was talking to a colleague about DBS recently. He thinks it could become as common and unremarkable as laser eye surgery. And why not? After all, we're notoriously squeamish about our eyes, and yet, given the chance to do away with glasses or contact lenses, millions of us have gone into a clinic to have bits of our visual organs burned away.[24] DBS is rather more taxing, admittedly, but modern surgical techniques have greatly reduced the physical ordeal.

Besides, science has been telling us for years that we're pure organism, with selves made of synapses and protein-dependent personalities.[25] Technology, meanwhile, has encouraged many people to believe that problems which used to be solved by time-consuming hard work (like acquiring knowledge or controlling weight) might have easier solutions (like cognitive enhancements or short-term diets). Viewing one's body as an adjustable object, a meat machine, leads to the expectation that it can and should be reconfigured according to the fashions of the day—assuming one has the money. Is there really any difference in kind between brain surgery and other body modifications, like getting a tattoo or having your wrinkles botoxed?

Irritatingly for the rich, money to date has been able to do only so much for brain function. Learning, like dieting, must still be lengthy and difficult in order to succeed long-term. But with all sorts of products already on the market to boost your brain power, the under-lying attitude is clear. If the brain is part of the body, technology can in principle fix it, just as a pacemaker or a hip replacement fixes problems in other areas.

The electrical recording and manipulation of human brains now offers possibilities which even a decade ago would have seemed extra-ordinary. In the field of brain–computer interfacing, as noted earlier, work to control machines by thought is well under way. Entertaining though the toys will be, this research is done for the most serious of clinical reasons: to give people kept alive by modern medicine some way of escaping the cage of paralysed bodies. Deprived of the funda-mental power to control our environment which comes with the capacity for movement, and to which we tie so much of our dignity, human beings can suffer intensely whether or not they experience physical pain. If brain interfacing can relieve that anguish even a little, the sooner it becomes widely available the better.

Would you have brain surgery to alleviate a terrible disease like multiple sclerosis? What about another profound disability, the hid-eous black hole of severe depression? Even in the knowledge that brain stimulation may not work, or may only be successful for a while, my guess is that many people would take the risk and have the operation.

What then of milder complaints, especially those complaints which seem to exist only in the minds of the complainers? This is not to downplay the severity of such conditions at all; minds are immensely powerful things. The dismissive attitude of some doctors that 'it's all in the mind' should not be seen as implying the patient's inferiority, but as a defensive admission that some problems are still too hard for doctors to solve. Nonetheless, brain surgery seems a very bloodily physical approach to dealing with these most tangled of mental problems.

Such wariness is justified.[26] DBS alters symptoms, but we are not yet sure how it works and how its mechanisms relate to whatever caused the condition it is treating. Without fully understanding the changes involved, and until sufficiently long-term and large-scale studies have been done, the possibility of unwelcome unintended consequences cannot be set aside. The fantastic promise of brain stimulation techniques cannot yet be wholly fulfilled, even in the clinic. Nonetheless, that promise is crucial to the brain supremacy, and research on such methods continues to advance.

From sickness to health

One day DBS may be extended to healthier individuals. This carries risks, especially when moving from clearly defined organic pathologies like Parkinson's to psychiatric conditions not (yet) associated with specific biomarkers. If evidence for a disorder comes from the patient's self-reports and behaviour, or sometimes other people's complaints about the patient, there may be no obvious tumour, clutch of dead cells, or thinning grey matter to point to as the cause. Studies may show that abnormal activity in a particular network correlates with symptoms of the disorder—as, for example, abnormal signals in the pain matrix have been shown to correlate with neuropathic pain. Are those correlations also causes? For pain it seems so, in that when DBS makes the pain matrix fire in a different pattern the patients report that pain improves. Yet how those signals came to be in the first place is another matter. Nor is it clear what other, perhaps abnormal changes may be triggered by the artificial attempt to make this particular network fire more normally.

The technology-driven change in how we view our bodies and brains has been enormous. Features of physical appearance which were previously part of the fates dealt out at birth have been reclassified as under our control, and therefore our responsibility. It's commonly argued that punishing people for qualities they cannot change is immoral. Once the option of change has been created for us, however, the pressure is on to take it. As more people do, they find it all too easy to condemn those who will not improve their imperfections. As we acquire more power to change the brain, the pressure to self-enhance will start to bite in that domain too, even more than it already does.

I remain unconvinced, incidentally, that this view of our bodies as organic tech is especially new. It may have democratized somewhat in recent decades, and its remit has widened, as medical advances came up with new ways of body shaping and more of us gained the resources to access those facilities. But the desire to bring the actual person closer to some ideal, however misguided, is surely as old as humanity itself. What else is education but an attempt at remodelling that part of the body which sits within the skull, in the hope that the person will fit more comfortably into the world for which school is preparing them? And if science and technology can give us new ways of changing our brains, why not take them on and turn ourselves into better—that is, more socially acceptable—people? No matter that the techniques were designed to heal the sick. If we feel we have something wrong with us, why shouldn't we have it cured, even though others think us healthy? Thus the path from healing to enhancement proceeds by privatizing the definition of dysfunction.

It may soon be possible to improve brain function, cheaply and with few immediate side-effects, in order to relieve not just clinical distress but social imperfection, thereby stepping from neurology and psychiatry to fashion. We humans are exceptionally prone to comparing ourselves with those around us, forming our expectations and changing our behaviour accordingly. (By fashion, I do not mean the true state of public opinion, were such a thing at all coherent, but the individual's interpretation of the social forces exerted by the people he or she happens to encounter—an interpretation distorted by his or her personal anxieties.) If your mind offends you, you may soon be able to adjust it, again provided you can afford to do so. If it causes sufficient offence to other people, of course, they may find the same technologies useful for adjusting you, whatever your opinion on the matter.

The risks inherent in this 'mission creep' of brain treatments, from medicine to psychiatry to lifestyle choice, are already apparent. One example is the psychiatric diagnosis of hypoactive sexual desire disorder (HSDD).[27] A woman whose lack of libido distresses her can apply to the medical profession for this label, and for treatment (e.g. hormone therapy).[28] What if researchers found that deep brain stimulation could enhance a woman's sexual desire? The idea is not unutterably far-fetched; HSDD is already treated with drugs.[29] Were a more drastic treatment available, my guess is there would be takers.

If the treatment worked, some very unhappy women would have their medical needs met and their sex lives improved. It sounds great; but there are thorny caveats. For one thing, if the neuroscience of the near future announces in a confident press release that stimulating area such-and-such relieves HSDD, the technique might pass the required regulatory checks and still do more harm than good. It might have severe side-effects which only become apparent over time; or it might only work for a while, as L-dopa therapy does for Parkinson's. We are not adept at perceiving subtle or long-term consequences before they happen, and to do this for DBS treatment would require expensive research studies, running for years with large numbers of participants.

A second problem is the vagueness of the HSDD syndrome. Women may lack sexual desire and be quite at ease with an asexual lifestyle, so what distinguishes patients is not the lack of lust but their reaction to it as a failure to fulfil their roles as sexual partners. A sensible system would try reducing the weight of expectations which so torment these women, and the stress and fatigue which often afflicts them, before resorting to pills, drills, and electrodes, but human society is not that system, and changing social pressures is not easy.[30]

Making a DBS treatment available would put extra pressure on already unhappy women to risk surgery, while raising expectations it might or might not fulfil—depending on how much of their unhappiness with their low sex drive relates to what they themselves want and how much to what they feel society expects of them. The new advance would also pressurize women whose unwillingness to sleep with partners has more to do with the shortcomings of the partners. In either case, human behaviour is being forced closer to a tightly confining norm, while remaining less than fully understood. Because technofixes offer short-term results, and are easier to change than the social demands on women, they seem more attractive to patients and policy-makers.

Could DBS become as routine a technique as vaccination? It began as a treatment for specific disorders, but why should we not extend its remarkable capacities to prevention? Adjusting brain plasticity, with regular follow-up retunings to keep your neural networks optimal, might one day be part of standard health checks: a mental MOT to go with the physical.

The electrophysiology which gave us DBS is one of the oldest methods for changing the brain, but it is not the only one. Developments in other fields may offer workarounds to treat sick brains without the need for surgery. One obvious example is the burgeoning science of nanotechnology, with its capacity to create what Prince Charles memorably called 'grey goo'.[31] Building tiny devices from atoms and molecules is at a very early stage, but its potential applications for brain research are legion.[32] Getting useful chemicals into the brain, preventing damaging pollution like cigarette smoke from reaching foetuses, and providing maintenance 'nanobots' to clean up dangerous detritus from dying cells are three examples, all of which would be of huge medical benefit (and all of which will rely on animal research and human volunteers for their development).

While we wait for Prince Charles' grey goo to take over the earth, however, there is already a field of research which operates at the level of the very small and which is already laying the foundations for the most ambitious visions of the brain supremacy. Here, in the intracellular domain of ions and lipids, proteins and genes, is some of the most exciting work being done in neuroscience today. As I write, a table of contents has come through from one of the discipline's top journals announcing a special issue on the topic, a sure sign that it is coming of age.[33] That topic is neurogenetics, and it is to this fascinating field of research that I now turn.

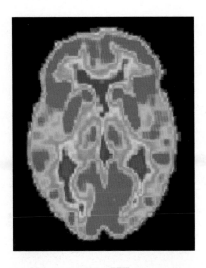

PLATE 1 a PET scan

Plate 1 shows a positron emission tomography scan of a healthy human brain. (The image is courtesy of the Alzheimer's Disease Education and Referral Center, a service of the National Institute on Aging.) Note that despite the scan's beauty and apparently authoritative status as a scientific product, it is impossible to interpret when presented without its research context, as it is here (and as such images are often presented in media reports). For example, the standard colour code uses reds and yellows to indicate areas which are highly active during the PET scan, with greens and blues indicating areas of low activity; but we do not know how active 'red' is compared with 'blue'. The image could also be of a single brain or a composite across a group of volunteers. Moreover, we are not told what task was being done, by whom, using what tracer, and with what control conditions. Even working out which end is which, and whether the brain is being viewed from above or below, can be problematic. Pictures in science communication need to be used with care.

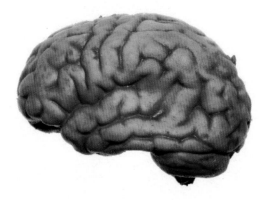

PLATE 2 a naked brain

Plate 2 shows a preserved human brain. The frontal cortex is on the left.
© (mikeledray/Shutterstock.com)

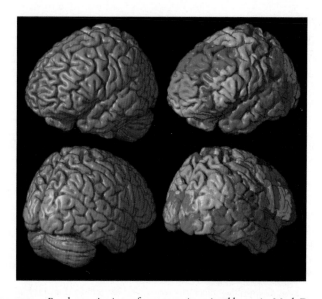

PLATE 3 Brodmann's view of cortex re-imagined by artist Mark Dow

Plate 3 shows lateral 3-D views of human brains from the front (top) and back (bottom). Images on the right show the Brodmann areas in colour. (Image copyright: Mark Dow, available from http://markdow.deviantart.com/art/Brain-Brodmann-43568326.)

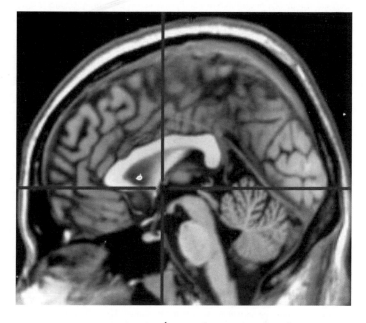

PLATE 4A structural magnetic resonance imaging

strength, flexibility, and success. Certainty is unscientific, and ultimately always self-defeating. Moreover, certainty is not the same as clarity, so doubt need not be perceived as obfuscation, though it often is.

I am not alone in thinking this, incidentally. *EDGE* magazine has recently elicited similar views from 'leading thinkers' (or as the *Guardian* put it, 'Planet's biggest brains', which conjures visions of flippered journalists interviewing whales).[3] Perhaps, therefore, one can hope that change is finally on its way, and that the media's consuming demand for certainty can give ground to a better understanding of science.

Genes means minds?

In the last decade, the science of genetics has been transformed. With the completion of the human genome project in 2003, it became clear that genes alone could not explain the complexity of brain development; there weren't enough of them. Since then, more and more research, with better and faster equipment, suggests that genes themselves are only one component in the convoluted mesh of heritable factors.[4] Epigenetics, of which more in Chapter 13, offers mechanisms whereby environmental factors may affect which genes play an active role (by being 'expressed' as proteins) and which do not.[5] Some of what in the 1990s was dismissed as 'junk' DNA is proving to be far more interesting—and functional, with potential long- and short-range effects on gene expression.[6] And, as we'll see in Chapter 13, even the shape of the DNA coil in a cell is more important than researchers previously realized.[7]

The pathway from DNA to protein, moreover, is far more complex than the model I learned as an undergraduate, in which DNA was transcribed to RNA which was in turn translated to protein.[8] For example, RNA now comes in flavours—such as mRNA, siRNA, lincRNA, and miRNA—which can interfere with each other to prevent genes being expressed.[9] As each additional embellishment is uncovered, the flexibility of control increases, the demands on computing power increase, and the inability of any single scientist to get his or her head around the details becomes ever more apparent. Genetics articles are becoming more like those produced in experimental physics, with many authors and ever more reliance on computer power.

As gene science has developed, brain research using genetic tools has expanded rapidly. I have a first edition of a well-known neuroscience textbook, published in 1996.[10] Its third edition, published in 2006, is half as long again, and, as I write in 2010, is nearly five years out of date. In neuroscience terms, that's an aeon.[11] The latest issues of the current top five monthly neuroscience journals, ranked by impact factor, contain 35 full-length articles, plus letters, commentaries, and so on. Taking only these high-powered sources, and assuming the numbers are typical, that's over 400 articles a year, each of similar density to Richardson-Jones et al. (2010), the publication analysed in this chapter. That's ignoring general science journals, like *Nature*, and high-profile journals which don't publish monthly, like *Neuron* (twice a month) and the *Annual Review of Neuroscience*. It also excludes the many more specialist neuroscience journals. This is far beyond manageable, which is why neuroscience, like physics before it, is fragmenting into subfields whose practitioners know increasingly little about each other's work.

Neuroimaging has undoubtedly contributed to the surge, as have advanced staining, microelectrode, and neurochemical technologies, but the role of genetics has been crucial. In 2009, for the first time, the UK government's Home Office recorded more genetically modified than 'normal' animals—mostly mice—being used in research. Developments in gene manipulation have provided unprecedented opportunities to carry out well-controlled experiments in basic neuroscience, because they allow researchers to manipulate a single variable in half of a sample of animals and use the other half as a control group. A single gene can be prevented from expressing its protein, to create 'knockout' mice, or one can be added to make 'knock-in' mutations, as when jellyfish DNA is used to make animals glow in the dark. Keeping everything else constant, the effects of that single manipulation on living mice, their neural structures and circuits, and their brain development can all be studied. Gene-by-gene, researchers are unravelling the nets of cause and effect which build mouse brains, and thereby helping to understand human brains. Mice are not human, but we need to understand the areas of overlap as well as the differences, and genetically the species have a lot in common.

To illustrate how powerful a method genetic manipulation can be in neuroscience, we'll look at a study which uses the technique to further the understanding of depression. We will see how the scientists thought through the logic of their research, and the remarkable skills and techniques they used to solve problems. To illustrate the extraordinary level of human labour required to make the brain supremacy happen, this chapter discusses the research in sufficient depth to show the immense amount of work which lies behind a single publication. (This is undoubtedly science, not science-lite.)

Reasons to do research

Those of a squeamish disposition, be warned again. Since our governments prevent us from doing these kinds of experiments on <insert your least favourite people>, the article considered here involves some unpleasant things being done to innocent mice. Exposed to bright lights and new environments, forced to go swimming and consume strange brain-altering chemicals, hung by their tails, and of course given Prozac. So far, so murine stag party. Add decapitation and brain extraction, however, and this party ends up being no fun at all for the invitees.

The paper I've chosen as an example is very different, however, from the rat project described in Chapter 10. It is part of a large body of work by a well-established team, and its potential clinical good is clear and distinct: alleviating depression. Research is why these mice existed at all.[12] They are instruments, designed for certain ends. And as ends go, depression, one of the heaviest health burdens of our age, is a high priority. This isn't the lacklustre, 'I-feel-a-bit-down-today' syndrome which everyone gets now and then. It's the genuine black dog, a debilitating disorder which sucks the colour out of life. Numbness, indifference, thoughts of worthlessness, and suicide attempts are well-known symptoms, but there is more to this illness than apathy and low mood. Depression can also involve intense anguish: a feeling of tension, hard to describe, as if the person's self has become intolerably painful. The feelings aren't 'bodily', like those a cut finger would produce; indeed, physical pain can relieve the mental kind somewhat, which is why some depressed people self-harm. Instead, the experience is more like the most excruciating stage of grief. In addition, depression saps energy—the one thing we all need, more than youth or beauty or money or a job, to function successfully as social creatures. It can last for years, wreck relationships, devastate lives, and end them prematurely. In terms of raw agony it is therefore undoubtedly much worse than unexpectedly having your neck broken, which is how the animals in this study were killed.

Enough. Setting aside the cause for which the creatures died, let us proceed to the experiments themselves.

The neuroscience of Prozac

The study I've chosen, Richardson-Jones et al. (2010), is a paper in *Neuron* from the research group led by René Hen at Columbia University (citations are given by first author, not senior author).[13] Its title is '5-HT$_{1A}$ autoreceptor levels determine vulnerability to stress and response to antidepressants'. The article is nicely typical and beautifully illustrates the uses to which genetic technology is being put, as well as being a showcase for skilful scientific thinking. It discusses a set of experiments in mice which aim to help us understand a major clinical concern: the inadequacy of drug treatments for depression. Specifically, the researchers are interested in why antidepressant drugs like fluoxetine (Prozac) take weeks to start exerting their effects, and also why these drugs don't work for everyone.

picked up what we could as we went along—while searching for a tutor who could use the term 'non-medic' without following it with that demoralizing sigh. I was lucky: I found one, and one who could teach, what's more. He did neuroscience, you may not be surprised to learn. But my studies never did include much formal genetics.

Why am I telling you this? For three reasons. The first is that it excuses me from making this chapter a guide to DNA, of which there are plenty already.[1] Given how important genes are to modern neuroscience that would be a justifiable approach, but it's not mine. Instead I will consider genes only instrumentally, as a means for learning more about brains. By showing you some methods and principles, using an actual piece of research, I trust that any necessary facts will slot in along the way.

The second reason is simply to encourage readers who are not geneticists. If I can make sense of a neurogenetics article, so can you (though if you have some other background than science I won't pretend this chapter is going to be easy).

The third reason to undermine my status as an expert is to offer a gentle reminder: the word 'author' need not be inexorably followed by the suffix '-ity'. The link is usually implicit if not explicit in science writing (it tends to become more obvious when a scientist is discussing something outside his area of expertise, like religion). Unfortunately, the problem with authority is that it tends to be taken as certainty. Hypotheses become theories, theories are spoken of as if they are gospel truths, and the risk is greater when science is diluted into science-lite by the pressure to communicate. 'True science teaches us to doubt', as the physiologist Claude Bernard remarked, but doubt doesn't sell well compared with dogmatism.[2]

Dogmatic assertion, however, is a corruption of science, and especially dangerous in the science of the brain. IMCOTT, remember. To be certain is to simplify and distort, to step away from reality, but also to lay yourself open to the threat that some new contradiction will painfully shatter your rigid belief. A scientific hypothesis, by contrast, bends in the wind of change, adjusting to new evidence without, ideally, breaking any egos. Doubt is at the core of science, key to its

12

Chemical Control

Genes means minds

(Anonymous)

'Ah, come in,' said the tutor. 'You're the non-medics, yes?'
Dina and I were final honours students studying for a degree in physiology, psychology and philosophy. 'Er...PPP?'
'Right. So, let me see, you won't have done any biochemistry?'
We shook our heads. Students taking the physiology section of the PPP course studied a number of subjects alongside medical students, but biochemistry wasn't one of them.
'Hmm. Or genetics?' said the tutor, clearly losing hope that this was going to be easy.
'No.' *I could write you an essay on René Descartes,* I didn't add, *but something tells me, sir, you wouldn't welcome one.*
'Right,' said the tutor. And sighed heavily, before proceeding to deliver one of the dullest tutorials either of us had ever experienced.

Authors and experts

Welcome to the University of Oxford in the 1990s, a place where medics, in between drinking, studied biochemistry and genetics among much else. Meanwhile non-people like Dina and myself, drinking rather less,

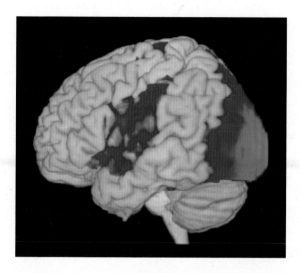

PLATE 5 a MEG scan

Plate 5 this composite image shows a typical MEG scan, collected during a word reading experiment which uses the same tasks and stimuli as the fMRI scan in Plates 4B and 4C, though with 20 different participants. Activity reflects changes in the brain's magnetic signal after stimulus presentation, compared with before presentation. Green indicates more significant activity than blue.

PLATE 4A, B, & C *(see previous page)* structural (A) and functional (B, C) magnetic resonance imaging

Plate 4A: structural magnetic resonance imaging. The image is of a typical structural MRI scan, showing a horizontal section through the brain (at the level of the subthalamic nucleus), in which the encircling skull and outer wrinkles of cortex are clearly visible. The frontal lobes are towards the top of the picture. (Courtesy of John Stein, University of Oxford)

Plate 4B: functional magnetic resonance imaging. The plate shows results from an fMRI scan taken during a word reading task (see the appendix for details). The image is a composite of 20 individuals' data. Areas highly active during the task (as compared with a resting condition) are superimposed in colour on a lateral view of the brain in which the cerebellum and brainstem (lower right), highly active visual cortex (right), and frontal and temporal cortices (towards the left) are clearly visible. On the colour scale used, red is more significant than orange or yellow. The equivalent MEG scan is shown in Plate 5. (Plates 4B, 4C, and 5 are courtesy of Peter Hansen, University of Birmingham, and Piers Cornelissen, University of York)

Plate 4C: fMRI statistics in proportion. This image shows what the fMRI image in Plate 4B would look like if a maximum 5% change in activity was reflected by using only 5% of the colour range. Clearly the colour image is easier for human observers to interpret; yet such clarity can sometimes encourage over-interpretation.

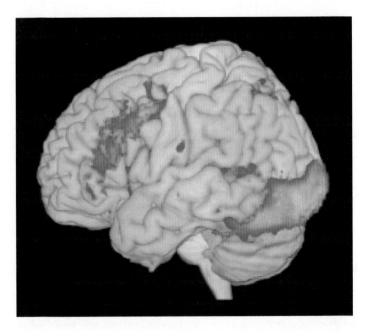

PLATE 4B functional magnetic resonance imaging

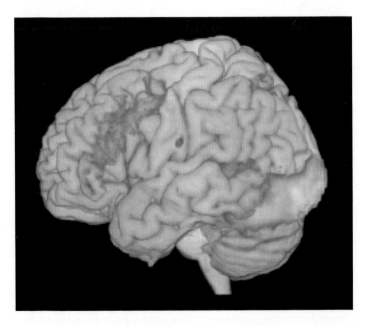

PLATE 4C fMRI statistics in proportion

(for full captions to plates 4A-C, please see overleaf)

This piece of work clearly shows the collaborative, interdisciplinary nature of modern neuroscience. There are 12 authors, and seven more helpers are mentioned in the acknowledgments. They come from departments of pharmacology, psychiatry, neuroscience, anaesthesiology, and radiology, and they work at three different institutions in two different countries: two universities—one American, one French—and a US hospital.

The article cites 65 references: 61 articles, from 38 journals, and four standard textbooks (on mouse neuroanatomy, brain pharmacology, health statistics, and methods for analysing behaviour). The journals referred to cover the ground from general science (*Nature*) through psychology (*Learning and Memory*), psychiatry (*Archives of General Psychiatry*), and genetics (*Genomics*) to neuroscience (*Journal of Neuroscience*) and brain chemistry (*International Journal of Neuropsychopharmacology*)— one citation even ventures as far as *Gastroenterology*. That's a vast amount of information from many sources, funnelled into a single publication. As the type of neuroscience involved—the brain chemistry of mice—is well established, the publications range back in time as far as 1977, though most are from the last decade and nearly half from the last five years.

The ineffectiveness of antidepressants is a big issue. As Richardson-Jones and colleagues comment, 'fewer than half of depressed patients respond to their first drug treatment'.[14] Understanding why this happens is an urgent priority. Better drugs would offer both economic and social benefits: lower costs and less misery for sufferers and their families.

To address the issue, the authors begin, as is traditional, by summarizing previous research: setting out the article's intellectual ancestry. They then present their results, discuss them, and finally, in small print, provide the methods section. This chapter, however, will focus on the small print, because one of the delights of this article is the range of awe-inspiring methods it employs.

The background to the problem

In their introduction, Richardson-Jones and colleagues set the context by discussing the brain neurotransmitter system on which Prozac is thought to act. Low levels of serotonin (aka 5-HT, 5-hydroxytrypta-mine) have been implicated in stress, anxiety, and depression, and common antidepressants like Prozac are selective serotonin reuptake inhibitors (SSRIs).[15] That is, once the 5-HT has been released by neurons into the synapse, SSRIs prevent it from being recycled back into neurons. Since this reuptake process removes serotonin from the synapse, it lowers the chances of a signal being triggered in the recipient neuron. Inhibiting reuptake, on the other hand, keeps synaptic serotonin levels higher (see Figure 15). SSRIs thus lend the sender neuron's 5-HT signal more impact, for longer, raising brain levels of 5-HT and relieving the symptoms of depression.

If the only factor governing serotonin release was how efficient its recycling was, antidepressants would be much more effective. There are, however, other players in the synaptic arena: the 5-HT receptors (see Figure 15). Receptors are proteins embedded in a neuron's surface membrane which change their shape when they come into contact with a neurotransmitter molecule. This process, called activation, triggers a chemical cascade in the cell's interior which affects the chance of that cell producing a signal of its own. Receptors can be either inhibitory (their activation makes the cell less likely to fire) or excitatory (when activated, they increase the chances of the cell firing). Note that one neurotransmitter, like glutamate or serotonin, can activate both inhibitory and excitatory receptors.

There are many kinds of 5-HT receptor. Previous work pinpoints the 5-HT_{1A} subtype as the most relevant to stress, anxiety, and depression, and that is the one investigated by Richardson-Jones and colleagues. I say one, but if only it were so simple. In fact, 5-HT_{1A} receptors come in two categories, autoreceptors and heteroreceptors (see Figure 15). (If God exists, he must have a taste for rococo: in neuroscience there's always another playful curlicue to ornament the complexity already on display.)

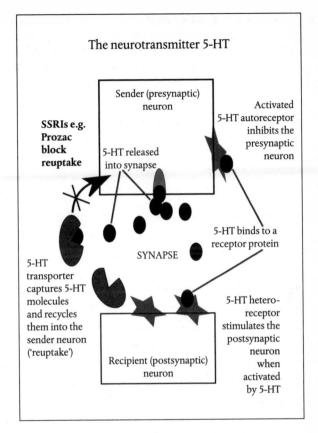

FIGURE 15: The serotonin system.

The figure represents a serotonergic neuron and its connecting synapse with a recipient (postsynaptic) neuron. Dark solid circles represent molecules of the neurotransmitter 5-HT (serotonin) released from the presynaptic neuron into the synaptic cleft. Also present in the cleft are transporter molecules, which recycle 5-HT into the presynaptic neuron. SSRIs like Prozac interfere with this chemical pathway, resulting in more 5-HT in synapses, where it can bind to receptors (shown as grey solid star-shapes). Some of these are postsynaptic heteroreceptors, and their activation makes the postsynaptic neuron more likely to fire. 5-HT molecules also bind to autoreceptors on the presynaptic neuron, and their activation reduces 5-HT release into the synapse (negative feedback).

The first category of 5-HT$_{1A}$ protein is the heteroreceptor. Named from the Greek word for 'other', these are receptors found on the receiving cells which serotonergic neurons stimulate via their synapses. Heteroreceptors modulate their own cell's ongoing electrical activity and release of neurotransmitters. For example, activation of 5-HT$_{1A}$ hetero-receptors in the frontal cortex stimulates the release of dopamine.[16]

The second category of 5-HT$_{1A}$ is the autoreceptor, from the Greek for 'same' or 'self'. These sit on the surface of the sending, serotonergic cell, affecting its release of 5-HT. The 5-HT$_{1A}$ autoreceptors exert negative feedback—they are inhibitory—when they pick up a serotonin molecule, reducing the rate at which more 5-HT will be released. These receptors can therefore control global serotonin levels in the brain. Table 3 sum-marizes the differences between auto- and heteroreceptors.

Serotonin is released by cells in the midbrain, in an area known as the raphe nuclei. Though these serotonergic neurons have their cell bodies plumped down in the brain's depths, they send long filaments on exten-sive expeditions—notably to the hippocampus and prefrontal cortex. The 5-HT is squirted out from the ends of these axons, where it binds to and activates heteroreceptors on other cells. However, it is also released from the cell body and dendrites, where it activates autoreceptors.[17]

Why do you need to know this? Because the distance between cell body and synapse allows researchers to separate out the neuro-transmitter's effects on other neurons—e.g. in the frontal cortex—from what the released 5-HT does to the neurons which release it, down in the raphe (see Figure 16). That is a crucial step, as we shall see.

The problem

Every good science article needs a previous hypothesis to step beyond. Critiquing something dear to someone else is part of the fabric of science, as of academia in general, and this paper is no exception. Its target is a hypothesis presented in a 1998 paper by Pierre Blier and colleagues at McGill University, Montreal.[18] The hypothesis proposes that 5-HT$_{1A}$

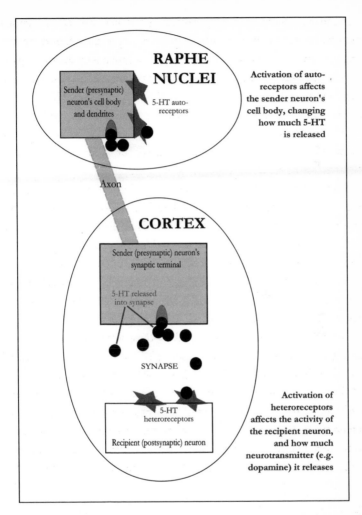

FIGURE 16: A split-level neuron.

The figure represents a serotonergic neuron (shown in the upper image and the top of the lower image) and a connecting synapse (shown in the lower image). Dark solid circles represent molecules of 5-HT, which is released into the synapse, but can also be released from the neuron's cell body. In the cortex, 5-HT molecules bind to heteroreceptors which excite the postsynaptic neuron (lower image). In the raphe, they bind to inhibitory autoreceptors on the presynaptic neuron (upper image).

TABLE 3 5-HT$_{1A}$ auto- and heteroreceptors.

	Autoreceptors	Heteroreceptors
Neural location	Cells sending 5-HT signals (presynaptic)	Cells receiving 5-HT signals (postsynaptic)
Brain location	Raphe nucleus	Hippocampus Prefrontal cortex
Function	Reduces 5-HT release from the sender cell	Facilitates release of neurotransmitter (e.g. dopamine) from the recipient cell
Mechanism	Negative feedback effects	Positive 'feedforward' effects
	(inhibits the sender cell)	(excites the receiving cell)
Range of control	Overall levels of brain 5-HT release	Release of 5-HT in specific areas of the brain
Source gene	*Htr1a*	*Htr1a*

Table 3 compares features of the two kinds of 5-HT$_{1A}$ receptors discussed in Richardson-Jones et al. (2010), namely autoreceptors and heteroreceptors. Note that the brain locations are those discussed in this study; serotonin receptors are also found elsewhere in the brain and body.

autoreceptors are responsible for slowing down people's response to Prozac.

How would that work? As noted above, fluoxetine, the active ingredient in Prozac, blocks serotonin reuptake, making more serotonin available for longer in the synapse. However, that also makes autoreceptors more likely to be activated. Their stimulation tends to shut the serotonergic neurons down, limiting further release of 5-HT. Not a great way to boost brain serotonin levels.

Over time, though, autoreceptors, like other drug consumers, get jaded and tired. They become desensitized, needing more serotonin molecules to get the same response. Gradually, therefore, their blocking of serotonin release becomes less effective. This allows the full impact of the antidepressant's boosting of synaptic 5-HT levels to take effect. Thus runs the Blier hypothesis.

The problem tackled by Richardson-Jones and colleagues is that until now it has not been possible to distinguish the auto- and hetero-receptors, so the Blier hypothesis—that only the former slow the brain's response to Prozac—couldn't be tested. Desensitization of autoreceptors may indeed be the reason why SSRIs like Prozac take so long to benefit some patients, but there could be other explanations. For example, some people might have different numbers of receptors to begin with, because of genetic variation. If so, the Blier hypothesis would need to be reconsidered.

The solution

Richardson-Jones and colleagues needed to achieve two goals. First, they needed a mechanism that would let them switch the gene for the $5-HT_{1A}$ receptor on or off as they pleased, so that they could control levels of the receptors in specific areas of the brain. Next, since the same gene codes for both receptor flavours (auto- and hetero-), they needed a way of distinguishing the two so that each could be manipulated independently. Only then would they be able to test experimentally whether the autoreceptors do indeed provide a key to how SSRI antidepressants work.

Here's how they did it.

Goal 1: a genetic switch

To make a working switch you need three things: the switch mechanism itself, some way of turning it on, and some way of turning it off. To make their genetic switch, the researchers created a type of 'knock-in' mouse—one in which segments of DNA are artificially added to the natural DNA. The type used in this study had two extra components. One was for the switch mechanism itself. The second coded for a protein which, once expressed, acted to turn the switch off.

What about turning it on? Instead of adding yet more DNA, the researchers relied on a curious feature of the switch mechanism: it only works in the presence of an antibiotic. As long as the mice had antibiotic as part of their diet, the switch would be on. Remove the antibiotic, and the off-switching protein would be able to act, preventing the production of more 5-HT$_{1A}$ receptors.

Suppressing receptor production will reduce receptor numbers, because individual receptors aren't permanent features of the synaptic landscape. They are built inside cells to their genes' specifications, then shipped to the surface—the cell membrane, where they can interact with neurotransmitters—rather like books being printed on demand. Unlike the books on my shelves, they do not thereafter stay put until the membrane is full and forces a clear-out. Instead, like a company trying to match supplies to customer demand, the cell is constantly recycling and adjusting, changing receptor numbers depending on the levels of neurotransmitter in the synapse (if many receptors are activated quickly, send more). How many receptors a cell has is not, therefore, set in stone. It changes in response to what is happening around the cell, and so it can be manipulated by ingenious researchers.[19]

The switch mechanism, and how to switch it on

Richardson-Jones and colleagues' target was the 5-HT$_{1A}$ receptor gene, *Htr1a* (following the convention of writing gene names in italic to distinguish them from their protein products). Immediately prior to the code for building the receptor itself lies a section of DNA called a promoter, which gives the signal to a cell's internal systems to start transcribing the DNA to make protein (IMCOTT). Analogously, picture a rail commuter who has learned that when her morning train grinds to a halt for no apparent reason, that's a signal that she is nearly into Birmingham New Street station and it's time to start gathering her things. The promoter tells the cell's DNA-readers that a gene's coming up and transcription should begin.

He who controls promoters controls gene expression, so to build their genetic switch mechanism the researchers inserted a segment of DNA into the promoter DNA sequence for the gene they were interested in manipulating (the *Htr1a* gene). The extra segment is called a tetracycline operator (*tetO* for short) because it is regulated by the antibiotic tetracycline (and by its more stable close cousin doxycycline, which was used in this study). The modified mice were given doxycycline in their food to keep the *tetO* switch on. Since *tetO* does not by itself interfere with receptor-building, the mice's neurons transcribed the *Htr1a* promoter and gene as usual to produce 5-HT$_{1A}$ receptors. (I did warn you; neuroscience's favourite dish is acronym soup.)

Back to the books for another analogy. Pushing two volumes apart on a shelf to slide a third between them does not affect your ability to read them, or turn novels into dictionaries, or do anything else untoward to the rest of the library. Likewise for adding *tetO* to the *Htr1a* promoter's DNA. The adjacent genetic 'book' (the *Htr1a* gene itself) remains as readable as it ever was.

Except not quite; analogy is not identity. In this mouse library the genes, unlike books, have one very peculiar property: *Htr1a* DNA can be transcribed only when there is doxycycline present in the cell. Inserting *tetO* into a promoter is like sliding a book onto a shelf and then discovering that you can't remove the novel next to it—except when the librarian (doxycycline) is in the room, whereupon the novel (*Htr1a*) can easily be pulled off the shelf and read.

How does this work? The answer lies in the second modification made by the researchers, which involves the gene for a protein called tTS.

Switching off the gene

We have seen that Richardson-Jones and colleagues built their antibiotic-dependent genetic switch by adding *tetO* to the DNA of mice and feeding them doxycycline to keep it switched on. What they needed next was some way to turn it off. To achieve this, a second genetic 'knock-in' added the DNA for the off-switching protein, tTS. This tetracycline-

A GENETIC SWITCH

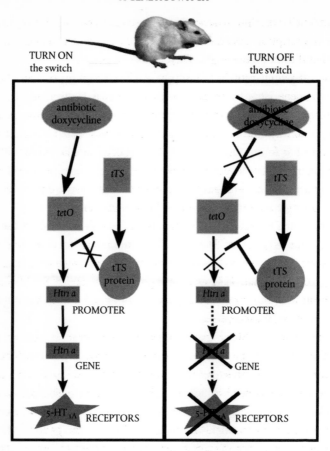

FIGURE 17: Building a modified mouse.

The figure illustrates the 'knock-in' genetic modifications used by Richardson-Jones et al. (2010) to maintain normal production of 5-HT1A receptors in the brains of mice (left panel, control condition) or to reduce receptor production (right panel, experimental condition). Arrows indicate a positive effect, inhibition is shown by a stop line, and an X or dashed arrows indicates that the result or process has been blocked.

The genetic switch mechanism is provided by the *tetO* DNA, which is inserted into the mouse's own DNA. The *tetO* operator controls the promoter of the *Htn1a* gene, which in turn controls the production of 5-HT1A receptors, such that while *tetO* is working normally the *Htn1a* gene can be transcribed and the receptors built. While the mouse is being fed the antibiotic doxycycline, the *tetO* switch is on (left panel). Mice were also given a second modification, the *tTS* gene. This produces the tTS protein, which can switch *tetO* off. However, tTS can only inhibit *tetO* if there is no antibiotic in the animal's food. In the control condition, the antibiotic prevents the tTS protein from inhibiting the *tetO* operator, and receptors are produced as usual. When the mouse is no longer being fed the antibiotic (right panel), the tTS protein is no longer prevented from inhibiting the *tetO* operator, which in turn means that receptor production is inhibited. The researchers can thus use a simple change in an animal's diet to control the production of serotonin receptors in its brain.

dependent Transcriptional Suppressor is so called because it suppresses gene transcription (receptor production) in a manner dependent on whether the antibiotic—here, doxycycline—is present.

The off-switch protein tTS suppresses transcription of the 5-HT_{1A} receptor gene *Htr1a* by binding to *tetO* (the switch mechanism). The transcription enzymes work their way along the DNA coil like trains along a railway, and tTS bars their progress, rather as placing a large concrete block on the line into Birmingham would suppress our commuter's ability to get to work. Note that Richardson-Jones and colleagues did not add the tTS protein itself. They inserted the relevant DNA, giving mice brain cells the ability to make tTS.

How the tTS protein affects the *Htr1a* gene depends on whether doxycycline is present. If it is, tTS can't bind to *tetO* because the antibiotic gets in the way, so *Htr1a* can be read off as usual and the 5-HT_{1A} receptors built. Take away the doxycycline, and tTS will clamp down on *tetO*, blocking transcription of *Htr1a* and switching off production of 5-HT_{1A} receptors.

Doxycycline antibiotic (switching on), tTS protein (switching off), and the *tetO* gene (the switch itself) together provide the mechanism for controlling whether the *Htr1a* genetic novel gets read. Crucially, all the researchers need to do, once they have built their mice, is add or take away the doxycycline from the animals' diet. That simple change in the environment is enough to flick off the genetic switch, determining whether the *Htr1a* gene is transcribed to make 5-HT_{1A} receptors.

This is real genetic engineering: constructing artificial systems, piece by piece, for manipulating cells' production of proteins. It shows how difficult, time-consuming, and careful such work has to be, requiring expensive funding and lengthy training. It also demonstrates what is already possible: precise targeting of just one type of brain receptor in order to change how neurons respond to one particular neurotransmitter, serotonin.

This achievement, however, was only the start for Richardson-Jones and co. They could alter whether 5-HT_{1A} receptors were being made, but recall, the receptor proteins come in two distinct flavours. The scientists now had to work out which was which.

Goal 2: telling auto- and heteroreceptors apart

Tests showed that Richardson-Jones and colleagues had successfully bred a strain of mice with the genetic switch incorporated in their DNA. For the next step, distinguishing autoreceptors from heteroreceptors, they relied on the fact that these two flavours of 5-HT_{1A} receptors are found in different areas of the brain. As noted earlier, the heteroreceptors are located on the surface of cells receiving 5-HT signals. These recipient neurons, which themselves use other neurotransmitters like glutamate and dopamine, are widespread in the brain; for this study, the researchers focused on two areas, the prefrontal cortex and the hippocampus. Autoreceptors, on the other hand, sit on the dendrites and cell bodies of the serotonergic neurons themselves, down in the raphe nucleus.[20]

What is needed, therefore, is a marker of whether a cell is producing 5-HT or not: some feature which serotonergic neurons (in the raphe) have and other (hippocampal and prefrontal) brain cells do not possess.

As it happens, previous research had identified just such a marker: a gene called Pet-1. Richardson-Jones et al. were able to modify this gene also, by linking it to the gene expressing the tTS (off-switch) protein. The result: tTS was produced only when the Pet-1 gene was expressed. The power to turn off the tetO genetic switch was thus only granted to serotonergic neurons in the raphe, since other cells lacked the Pet-1 wherewithal. The mice had neurons with the switch mechanism (tetO) in their hippocampus and cortex as well, and they were eating doxycycline from birth, so the switch was on. When the doxycycline was removed, however, only the raphe 5-HT neurons could flick the off-switch.

It worked a treat. Without doxycycline, the tTS protein switched off 5-HT_{1A} receptor production—but only in the raphe. That meant only the autoreceptors were affected, not the heteroreceptors. Mission accomplished. All the researchers had to do was check that the systems were working and run some tests to see how the mice were affected.

The inevitable IMCOTT

By taking you through the logical steps which the researchers followed, I hope to have illustrated not only how scientists think, but the accomplishments of which modern genetic science is now capable. Now for a cautionary note, lest you should come away with the idea that gene-tweaking has reached such heights of perfection that we can programme animals as easily as we do computers. That is not yet the case. The brain supremacy's dream of DNE programming in humans remains a very distant vision. In this study, the researchers found that autoreceptor levels were reduced by about 30%—a significant difference, but hardly a complete switch-off. In addition, there was evidence of what geneticists call mosaicism: rather than every neuron in the raphe reducing its receptor levels by a third, some of the serotonin neurons seemed to have switched off their receptors altogether, and others not at all. 'The reasons for this mosaicism,' write Richardson-Jones and colleagues, 'are unclear.'[21] In research, remember, unclear is good. Unclear is another mystery to solve, and who knows, perhaps a future grant application.

First build your mouse. Then set up your experimental and control conditions. In this study, the independent variable is dietary doxycycline. It serves as a proxy for the number of 5-HT_{1A} autoreceptors, because its presence or absence governs how many of them are made by raphe neurons. Doxycycline present = normal receptor levels (HIGH, the control condition). Doxycycline absent = low receptor levels (LOW, the experimental condition). By comparing groups of mice fed chow with or without doxycycline, using various tests of serotonin function, anxiety, stress, and depression, the researchers can see how the results of those tests (the dependent variables) are affected by eating antibiotic, or not.[22]

The way these mice are engineered bypasses one of the biggest problems in neuroscience: the effects of development. Subtle changes early on can have such widespread consequences that tracing the causal links back to their origin is practically impossible. The researchers could have simply deleted the *Htr1a* gene, so that no 5-HT$_{1A}$ receptors were produced from conception onward, but that would have made it impossible to tell what effects were due to not having any receptors (now), and what was the result of other mechanisms.[23] For example, the brain might boost production of some other kind of 5-HT receptor to make up for the lack of 5-HT$_{1A}$ types. Brains are like weather systems in that a small change early on—recall that famous butterfly flapping its wings and causing a hurricane elsewhere—can make a profound difference later in all sorts of areas which one might have thought had nothing to do with the original tweak.

Instead of those potential confounds coming into play, the mice are allowed to grow up normally (as long as they are eating doxycycline), and only once they reach adulthood does the genetic switch get flicked—in some of them. This lets the researchers be as sure as possible that any differences in their dependent variables are down to not having enough 5-HT$_{1A}$ receptors up and running, rather than to developmental alterations in the mice themselves.

Having built their experimental animals, the scientists ran a number of tests on them.[24] These fell into two categories: system checks to make sure that the gene manipulations had worked, and tests to see whether the dependent variables had changed. (Remember, this is all part of the necessary background to a single scientific publication.) The system checks were all as expected.[25] What about the dependent variables observed in the experimental and control mice?

The researchers were interested in a number of variables. Some were behavioural: how anxious the mice were, how well they responded to sudden stress, how they reacted to longer-term (chronic) stress, and whether they showed evidence, under stress, of what scientists call behavioural despair. If you're wondering how to spot a despairing mouse, it's one that stays extremely still, as if it has decided the situation is so hopeless, there's no point in struggling any more. Richardson-Jones and colleagues also wanted to know whether changing receptor levels would change the spontaneous activity of the 5-HT neurons. And, of course, they wanted to know how the mice reacted to Prozac.

Testing behaviours

To see how anxious a mouse is, you can place it in a new environment. You can also offer it the choice between exploring a brightly lit area and retreating into nice safe darkness. The researchers did both these things, and noticed no differences between their experimental and control groups. Baseline levels of murine anxiety, in other words, were unaffected by the gene manipulation.

To stress a mouse you can put it by itself in a new environment; its body temperature will rise. LOW (experimental) mice showed a more pronounced hyperthermia than HIGH (control) mice. In other words, the experimental mice showed a bigger acute stress response.

To stress a mouse still further, to the point of despair, you can hang it by its tail or throw it into a bucket of water. To be fair, the water is warm, and 'throw', in a lab, is 'gently place'. Again, the researchers found no differences. LOW mice were no more or less inclined to freeze into immobility when finding themselves suspended or having to swim.

Then the researchers did something else: they retested the mice a day later, on the forced-swim test. They found that the HIGH mice began to give up fairly soon, as normal mice do, but the LOW mice showed more resilience. In other words, these creatures, with fewer autoreceptors, react more to stress but seem better able to cope with it over time.

Is repeated stress the key variable? The next experiment applied what scientists call a mild stressor—gavage—for four weeks, before retesting them on tail-hanging etc. Since gavage involves sticking a tube down their throats once daily, you may query the 'mild'; nonetheless, stress happened. What was the result? The researchers again found no differences on the anxiety tests, and the hyperthermic (acute stress) reaction was also as before. But the HIGH mice were noticeably worse on the tests of behavioural despair than their receptor-deficient cousins. Lowering the levels of 5-HT_{1A} autoreceptors, therefore, seems to lessen the measures of despair (the mouse equivalent of depression), without affecting measures of anxiety.

To see what was going on in the brain, Richardson-Jones and colleagues took electrical recordings from living, anaesthetized mice. They found that serotonergic neurons in the LOW, experimental mice were spontaneously more active, releasing more 5-HT. That was as expected, since 5-HT_{1A} autoreceptors inhibit the neurons in whose membranes they reside. Fewer receptors should therefore mean more active neurons.

So far, so very good. All the researchers had to do now was give the mice Prozac, and run the tests again. And check brain 5-HT levels before and after, using a technique called microdialysis.[26] And administer the Prozac for different lengths of time, to see whether the autoreceptors were involved in the delayed response so characteristic of antidepressant drugs. And try another behavioural test which is specially designed to pick up the effects of long-term antidepressant treatment.

You see why research takes so long and costs so much.[27] The problem with slow science, in a world of fast media, is the gigantic mismatch between the effort of production and the ease of consumption. Consumers see little of how science is produced. (Even most of the people who read the title or abstract of Richardson-Jones et al. (2010) will not have read the full 13-page article.) What consumers do see is plenty of science-lite in the media, from mentions in magazines to TV documentaries, presented in easy-to-read and open-access formats. Add the habitual assumption that 'easy' means 'cheap', and it is no wonder that the effort and expense of science is grossly undervalued. This is a problem when the public has a say in science funding—as for example it does on the 'YouCut' website, set up by the US senator Eric Cantor, where readers can vote to end funding for 'questionable' research grants made by the National Science Foundation.[28]

Richardson-Jones and colleagues did manage to get their study funded. What that study found was that as expected, normal HIGH mice did not immediately change their behaviour on Prozac; but the experimental LOW mice did respond. They were more resilient and less despairing, and they had higher levels of 5-HT in their brains. In other words, a genetic manipulation which lowered the levels of one particular brain protein (the 5-HT_{1A} autoreceptor) on one particular type of brain cell had made Prozac work faster.

The scientists did one last check to make sure that the normal HIGH mice weren't failing to respond because their autoreceptors weren't desensitizing over time for some reason. Perhaps the genetic interference could have somehow changed the receptors' boredom thresholds? It seems not. So the important difference seemed to be that the 5-HT neurons in LOW mice were more spontaneously active, and hence pumping out more serotonin, even before the mice were given Prozac.

Richardson-Jones and colleagues had hypothesized that manipulating autoreceptors in mice could alter how the animals responded to stress, and to antidepressants. The hypothesis was confirmed. LOW mice were more resilient when chronically stressed, and they responded more quickly to Prozac. Richardson-Jones et al. also considered Pierre Blier's hypothesis that autoreceptors delay SSRI action by taking so long to desensitize.[29] Their results suggest that desensitization may not be the main culprit, since their tests implied that the HIGH mice 'displayed desensitized autoreceptors' but did not respond as quickly to Prozac as did the experimental LOW mice, which 'differed only by possessing lower autoreceptor levels before treatment'.[30] They conclude that their findings do not support Blier's hypothesis.

The study grew out of earlier work on this very specialized area of brain chemistry, standing on the shoulders of predecessors like Blier and his colleagues. It built on and tested a specific hypothesis, and its results suggest an alternative explanation.[31] In the same journal issue where it was published, the author of that hypothesis—Blier himself—commented on the research, commending it to public attention, noting its limitations, and offering ideas for future experiments which could help to move the field on still further.[32] This is the working practice of everyday science. It's wonderful stuff.

This particular fragment of everyday science also has important practical implications for us all, since we are all susceptible to depression and many of us will experience it during our lives. The research confirms that genetic differences, in this case variations in the brain levels of certain serotonin receptors, do indeed affect the response to antidepressants. Mice with fewer autoreceptors responded better to pharmacotherapy. This is crucial information if we are ever to conquer the scourge of severe depression. If mice genes play a role in the effects of Prozac, human genes may also matter. That opens up the possibility of distributing antidepressants more efficiently, and beyond that of altering the genes themselves. The potential for improving the human condition—and saving money—is immense.

The human story

Human beings, like these mice, come in two different flavours of 5-HT$_{1A}$ receptor. A recently identified variation in the human *Htr1a* gene causes some people to express higher levels of the 5-HT$_{1A}$ receptor protein (like the HIGH, control mice) compared with others (who more resemble the experimental, autoreceptor-deficient LOW mice). Richardson-Jones and colleagues were attempting to build a mouse model of this human genetic variation.[33] Might this genetic difference be part of the reason why some people do not gain much benefit at first from treatment with antidepressants? If so, genetic testing could identify such patients. Personalized treatments are one of the great hopes of twenty-first-century medicine.

Furthermore, if the crucial difference is indeed in spontaneous activity among serotonergic neurons, rather than in how fast the receptors desensitize, then treatments can be designed accordingly and perhaps targeted at patients with a genetic profile which makes them less responsive to antidepressants.

Plenty of questions remain to be addressed, but another important step has been taken, and researchers now have better tools, thanks to this article, for understanding why some people fare well on Prozac while others are disappointed.

In this chapter, I have used just one of the thousands of papers in neuroscience published in the year 2010 to display the skill and beauty of brain research, as well as the huge effort that goes into creating a single publication. Rather than focusing on genetics as a discipline in its own right, the aim here has been to show you its usefulness as a tool for neuroscientists, enabling them to answer new questions in areas vital for human well-being. Transgenic mice, and to a lesser extent other species, have transformed the study of the brain and continue to do so. We have a long way to go yet until we can alter human genes at will, but in the 60 years since the deciphering of DNA, genetic science has made astonishing progress in identifying genes and controlling them in living animals.

In the next chapter we will look at where the gene path is leading.

13

Tweaking Genes

Let there be light!

(Genesis 1:3)

In the summer of 2005 a remarkable six-page technical report was published in the high-status journal *Nature Neuroscience*. At the time, it seems not to have rated a press release from the journal, nor did it attract much media attention. It was cited, however, by articles in other high-profile journals, and among the research community word spread.[1] A new way of doing brain research was starting to make its presence felt.

These days, so many scientific advances are described as remarkable—if not revolutionary—that one half expects to find it listed in funding agency application forms, under 'impact'. 'Will your research (a) revolutionize the field, (b) get you a TV documentary, (c) reach the international press/blogosphere, (d) achieve a mention in local or specialist media, or (e) add one small piece to a very large jigsaw? Please tick one box only.' Most applications, to be honest, should tick box (e), since most advances are of the incremental, piece-to-jigsaw kind, which is as it should be. Science, among whose ideals are thorough checking and healthy scepticism, has systems which tend to squash young revolutions until they've put on enough weight of evidence. Besides, the sheer quantity of modern scientific research makes it harder for hypotheses to stand out.

Having a higher threshold for accepting new beliefs has its down-sides. Journals and funding agencies pay lip service to innovation but are quite conservative in practice. Interdisciplinary research—a fruitful source of scientific creativity—is an ideal, like virtue, which many espouse but rather fewer achieve. And when a novel hypothesis or method does eventually surmount the barriers there can be a rush to acceptance which sways science fashion at the expense of other, perhaps more useful competitors (as in the case of MRI crowding out the market for MEG, discussed in Chapter 9). Sometimes, however, the new intruder deserves its accolades—such as being crowned 'Method of the Year 2010' by the journal *Nature Methods*.[2] A laurel to put others in the shade. Let us hope a Nobel prize swiftly follows, though opto-genetics hardly needs the extra recognition.

Lighting the brain

Optogenetics is the control of genetically altered neurons by light. One of the attractive features of the method, as often in science, is the mesmeric simplicity of the core idea.[3] By flashing light at suitably modified neurons, their activity can be controlled with astonishing precision, allowing the details of neural circuitry to be teased out with unprecedented accuracy. That precision is spatial—optogenetics can pick out a particular kind of neuron from all its myriad fellows—but an additional selling point is the level of temporal control. Instead of waiting for neurotransmitter molecules to reach and activate their target receptors, or for blood flow in an active area to surge, researchers can have an immediate impact, turning neurons on or off at the same incredibly rapid timescales on which the cells would naturally operate.

The method set out in that *Nature Neuroscience* report, Boyden et al. (2005), was not the first attempt at optogenetics, and indeed that term was used only later. Nonetheless, 'Millisecond-timescale, genetically targeted optical control of neural activity', by a group at Stanford University headed by Karl Deisseroth, established the field, and that lab has dominated it to date. Used together with established methods, such as electrophysiological techniques for measuring neural activity and staining techniques for identifying cells post-mortem, optogenetics looks set to take the understanding of brain circuits to a new level of refinement.

Neurons with light switches

Some organisms, like humans and certain algae, contain cells with specialized receptor proteins which are activated not by a chemical but by light: their ligand is a photon. The human retina has this capacity, which is why we are so good at detecting even small quantities of light. Other organisms which are simpler to manipulate also have such ion channels, and in some cases the relevant genes have been identified. One, found in green algae, codes for a protein called channelrhodopsin-2 (ChR2). Now for the simple and beautiful idea.

Boyden et al. (2005) took the gene for ChR2, built it into a virus, and infected cultured neurons with that virus (see Figure 18). Viruses commandeer cells' internal machinery to reproduce their DNA, and sure enough, the neurons incorporated the virus (including the *ChR2* gene) into their DNA. They began producing the ChR2 protein and shipping it out to their membranes as if it were a normal part of their range of cell membrane receptors. Once settled in the membrane, the protein acted like any other receptor: when activated, it changed its shape. For the ChR2 protein, that opened an ion channel which let sodium and calcium ions into the cell, triggering an action potential. This receptor, however, needed no neurotransmitter as its ligand. All it required was a photon—a flash of blue light.

Neurotransmitters may be more 'natural', in a skull which keeps brain cells in the dark except when that skull is deliberately broken (and yes, that is required for some optogenetics work, depending on the species and experiment). Light, however, is much faster and more precise. Researchers don't have to assume that the neurotransmitter diffused to the point where they wanted it to act, or worry how much of it did something somewhere else which might blur their results.

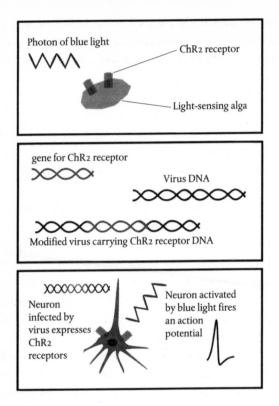

FIGURE 18: Optogenetics.

The figure shows the basic principles of optogenetic methods, using the example of channelrhodopsin-2 (ChR2), a light-sensitive ion channel found in certain algae (top panel). This receptor protein is activated by blue light. Its gene is extracted from the algae and inserted into the DNA of a virus (middle panel). The modified viral DNA is then used to infect neurons, which produce ChR2 receptors and transfer them to the cell membrane (lower panel), where they function as normal, responding to blue light by opening their ion channels and activating the neuron.

They don't have to wait for it to 'wash out' before they can try the next experiment. They don't need complicated drugs, with potential side-effects, to mimic its actions (agonists) or block them (antagonists). They can control individual action potentials with pulses of light, fulfilling, as Boyden et al. remark, 'the long-sought goal of a method for noninvasive, genetically targeted, temporally precise control of neuronal activity, with potential applications ranging from neuroscience to biomedical engineering.' (As already implied, the term 'noninvasive' is relative here; see below.)

The optogenetic mechanism described by Boyden and colleagues offered control over a positive ion channel (one which allowed sodium and calcium ions into the cell) using blue light. Since then, researchers have added, and continue to add, more tools to the kit. Alongside the ability to control positive ion channels (and thereby excite neurons to fire), there are now several 'opsins' for shutting down neural signalling, including a protein responsive to yellow light, another responsive to blue light, and a chloride channel responsive to a range of colours.[4] Groups of neurons can therefore be turned on, or off, depending on which channels they have been modified to possess. Furthermore, by using channels responsive to different colours of light (e.g. blue light to excite the cells, red to inhibit them) researchers can manipulate different neural groups in the same experiment, achieving an extraordinary degree of control over neural circuits.

Optogenetics applications have been extended from cell cultures to living animals (including worms, fruit flies, zebra fish, rodents, and macaques).[5] In mammals, this can be done either by craniotomy—removing a piece of the skull—or by inserting an optical fibre through a smaller hole.[6] This is why the term 'noninvasive', in the quotation from Boyden et al. above, is relative. Flashing lights onto a brain is less damaging to the neural tissue than sticking needles in it, but craniotomy and optical fibres bear risks—of infection, for instance.

To solve the problem altogether, you'd need a light-sensitive protein responsive to longer wavelengths, like infrared, which can pass through a human skull. I'm not aware of this having been done yet, but it may not be long before a suitable 'opsin' is developed.[7] Red-light-responsive varieties are already being used.[8]

Optogenetics has also been used in combination with other methods of brain research like deep brain stimulation, electrical recording of neurons, fMRI, and even the *tetO*/doxycycline approach described in the previous chapter.[9] Scientists have analysed a variety of neurotransmitter systems, from usual suspects like dopamine and glutamate to acetylcholine and orexin.[10] They have also been able to study specific kinds of neurons, such as the fast-firing 'interneurons' which seem to be involved in synchronizing the activity of other cells. Interneurons thereby help to create electrical oscillations: the 'brain waves' formed by millions of neurons firing in rhythmic patterns, which seem to be such important forms of neural mass communication.[11] To be able to tell an interneuron from its fellow cells is thus a step on the long road to making sense of what EEG and MEG reveal.

Optogenetics, in other words, can be used to study different ana- tomical cell types (including glia as well as various kinds of neurons) and different neurochemical cell types (neurons using various neuro- transmitters).[12] It can also explicate the functional networks formed when neurons synchronize their firing. The hope is that one day it will help researchers to understand exactly how these circuits are wired up, and therefore the basis for both normal brain function and such challenging disorders as depression and schizophrenia.[13] Because all known behaviour depends on the electrochemical activity of interlinked cells in the nervous system, the possibilities granted by a technique for carefully distinguishing these cells and their connections are innumerable. Those possibilities have barely begun to be explored.

At present, of course, optogenetics is a technique restricted to other species. It requires the deliberate addition of DNA (via a designed virus) to an organism, and such research is not likely to gain ethics committee approval in the current climate. Climates change, however, and our attitudes to adjusting our genetic material may soften as familiarity breeds less anxiety, just as attitudes to cosmetic surgery have changed in recent decades. Consequently, it is not inconceivable that patients *in extremis* may one day be treated using optogenetics as part of the medical arsenal, especially if this can be done non- invasively.

Beyond DNA

As optogenetics was starting its ascent towards the stratosphere of scientific fame, another hot topic in brain research had already been simmering for a while. Epigenetics, which offers us DNA-plus, attempts to answer many questions about genes, physiology, external circumstances, and how these three fates interweave to make us who we are.[14]

At the core of this burgeoning research field is the increasingly well-supported notion that genes don't just sit in your cells like bored publicists in an office, churning out the same old material until they die or their instructions change. Instead, genes switch on and off depending on circumstances. That means cells make more or less, or none at all, of the proteins they encode—depending on circumstances. Epigenetic effects, furthermore, can extend beyond an individual's existence: the messages which switch genes on and off can pass from parent to child, even on to grandchildren. (Jean-Baptiste Lamarck, you may hold your battered head a little higher.[15]) It now seems that what your mother did in her youth, as well as during her pregnancy, may have tweaked your life chances before you were even born. Likewise for your father's younger days. When environmental activists talk about us having responsibilities to future generations, they usually mean what we're doing to the planet, not to our own and our descendants' bodies.

Epigenetics makes everything much more difficult. Cells can change their protein-making depending on all sorts of factors, from diet to smoking. So much for the common impression that genes line up in rigid order to fix your destiny. Instead, they are less like machines and more like employees on a production line who work with variable efficiency depending on how distracted, hungry, or bored they happen to be. But there's more. We tend to think of our DNA 'genome' as a unique, fixed code; yet DNA can be edited, so your genome can vary in different body tissues.[16] Some bits of DNA can 'jump' about within the overall sequence, like a production line whose workers can move and take their equipment with them. A recent paper in *Nature* shows that brain cells have higher levels of these shifting genetic components than do cells in other organs from the same person.[17] Brains are much more flexible, even in genetic terms, than had been realized.

This explains why we've gained so few rewards, so far, for the large expense of decoding human DNA. Two decades ago there was a great deal of hype about how wondrous the human genome project would be for medicine: 'Potent tool fashioned to probe inherited ills', as a *New York Times* article claimed in 1987.[18] Alas, the anticipated potency was not immediately obvious. As the media and patients waited for cures, geneticists found themselves under growing pressure from the creak and groan of unfulfilled promises and unduly heightened expectations. They had to explain why, having decoded the 'book of life', they weren't producing treatments for innumerable diseases at the rate expected by their audience. The answer was, in essence, IMCOTT. We're working on it; more funds please.

Epigenetics is still young, and its findings need to be treated with caution. Nonetheless, it has one high scientific virtue: it more accurately reflects reality than the simplistic genetic models which preceded it. Fixing a faulty gene may solve some inherited disorders, but for many more the genetic effects seem so intertwined with lifestyle and environment that gene-tweaks alone seem unable to resolve the problems. Instead we must look at how genes are regulated.

Epigenetics research has snowballed lately—even, since 2006, acquiring two dedicated journals.[19] Epigenetic effects have already been identified in adults and during development, in multiple species including humans, in germ cells—eggs and sperm—and in other cells including neurons. Epigenetic mechanisms have been implicated in growth and ageing, memory, mental disorders like post-traumatic stress, and cancer, among other areas.[20] What is already clear is that, in comparison with *The Book of Epigenetics*, the human genome project will look like a leaflet for toddlers. Scientists looked to the genome for answers and found a whole new set of fascinating questions.

This being a common pattern in research, many scientists were always unimpressed by the popular notion that biology was well on its way to being neatly wrapped up. Possibly they recalled the unfortunate Lord Kelvin, who is notorious for saying much the same about physics a few years before relativity and quantum mechanics came along to shred the then-standard worldview.[21] Geneticists always knew that the nature–nurture debate, that ancient distraction, was unhelpful because the two must interact in many subtle ways. After all, a single-celled human embryo copies its DNA as it divides; yet a human being is not an unsightly blob of identical cells. Even allowing for errors in the copying process and the capacity of some genes to regulate others, there must be factors beyond the genes themselves which turn some cells into neurons and others into nasal hair.

Anyone who likes mystery and enjoys having plenty of puzzles still to solve, on the other hand, can rejoice at the discoveries made in the years since the genome was decoded. Those advances have turned the DNA-to-RNA-to-protein story into a rich and intricate epic. A genetically determined world, and the people in it, would be incredibly dull. The world now being uncovered, thanks to technologies driven by the human genome project, is inexpressibly more interesting. That great endeavour is indeed delivering its promise. It's just doing so more slowly, and with more intriguing twists and turns, than we'd expected.

Of course, the motives which drive scientists, who like having problems to solve, are not fully aligned with the longing to heal and improve that is felt by doctors and patients. For them, newly discovered complexity is yet another bar to the goal of preventing suffering from disease. Many of them have had their hopes agonizingly raised that a gene-driven fix, whether gene therapy or a more effective drug, would arrive to make life better for them. Those hopes have not been fulfilled, to date. As *Nature* recently put it, the best is yet to come.[22] Let us hope that when that best is reported, there will be better management of people's expectations.

Simplistic views of rapid, widespread 'gene therapy' did not just torment patients. They risked errors which could have proved worse than the diseases they tried to cure. Incorrect models do not merely lead researchers astray; in the clinic they can have catastrophic consequences. By understanding the limitations of genetic influence, and the mechanisms by which environments conduct each individual's DNA-and-protein symphony, scientists may be able to work out which 'lifestyle factors' do what damage for people with which genes, and how. Therapies, when they eventually emerge, may thus be better adapted to help their patients more, while harming them less.

To invoke 'the environment', 'social factors', or 'lifestyle', however, is to tell human beings that they'll have to do things the hard way. This is not a popular message. Instead of taking a pill, it means working to change behaviour. Ensuring that some desirable but harmful facet of reality—like sugar or alcohol—doesn't connect with the body in dangerous amounts is a good way to ensure that it can't interact with genes in damaging ways. But an injunction to 'go, and sin no more' lacks the cachet of a technological quick fix.

We already know a lot about what in the world is good and bad for us, but that knowledge is notoriously ineffective at reducing the behaviours which lead to illness and death. This is due in part to deliberate obfuscations perpetrated by various lobby groups, in part to human laziness, and in part to our dislike of being told what to do. Talking about lifestyle factors places more responsibility for our defects on us and our choices. After all, how can we be blamed for our genes? (An old attitude, that, but one which will have to change as science brings our DNA increasingly under our control.)

The situation isn't helped by the fact that most health messages are not yet targeted to our genetic makeup and so can seem irrelevant. Some people can eat cake ad lib without putting on weight; others feel as if being in the same room with a sugary snack is enough to make them heavier. If epigenetics can steer its way in public opinion between the crass simplicities of genetic determinism and the equally unhelpful extreme of assigning every fault to a person's environment, it may promote a better understanding of how healthier behaviours can be encouraged.

Epigenetics is carrying the weight of many promises, as yet unfulfilled. It will be central to the brain supremacy, since brains are especially fluid, genetically speaking. Can epigenetics bear the load of so much expectation? To judge that, we need to look more closely.

Regulating genes

Epigenetics is an exciting area to work in—especially in relation to the brain. We're beginning to grasp the many interacting layers of control between DNA and proteins: subtle regulatory mechanisms which complicate the journey from genetic vision to cellular reality. At their core is the concept that DNA has a kind of memory. It can be marked, by events occurring in the cell, in a way that alters how genes are expressed thereafter. Some marks tell the cell to reduce production of that particular protein, others facilitate production. Crucially, the mark can be retained long after the transient event that placed it on the genome, changing the life history of that particular cell.

Epigenetic changes can affect not only ordinary body cells but the germ cells which transfer genes from parent to embryo. What has aroused so much interest in epigenetics, beyond the purely scientific, is that it offers a way of lumbering the next generation not only with one's genes—about which no parent can as yet do much—but perhaps with the unlovely consequences of one's less-than-optimal choices. One thinks of the God of the *Book of Exodus* (20:5), 'visiting the iniquity of the fathers upon the children unto the third and fourth generation'. Could He have included on His already lengthy list of iniquities poor diet, drugs and alcohol, and being severely neglected, starved, stressed, or abused? All of these have been linked to epigenetic effects on offspring.[23] The distinction between 'genetic' disorders and 'lifestyle' diseases, between blaming fate or your parents, and blaming yourself, is less sharp than it might seem. That idea carries enormous implications.

First, however, to epigenetics itself. The quest to tease out the threads of genetic regulation is very much work in progress. Although I could happily take the rest of this book to discuss it, I will resist that temptation and confine us to brief inspections of two epigenetic mechanisms, methylation (for turning genes off) and acetylation (for turning them on).[24] Bear in mind how science revises, rejects, and reinterprets, so any or all of what you read here may need correction at some point. (Such is the common lot of scientists and science writers.) With that caveat, let us proceed.

Deoxyribonucleic acid, the famous stuff of life, is built from a type of sugar called 2-deoxyribose, which links itself into chains using phosphate groups (PO_4^{3-}) as chemical hooks. Phosphorus (P) is often associated with death and danger because of its use in fire-setting and explosives. Yet it is central to human life, not only as a constituent of the fertilizer that grows our foodstuffs but as a key player in every cell.

The long sugar-phosphate chains give DNA its ladder-like structure. Ladders need rungs, though, and these are provided by each sugar binding to a 'base' molecule which crosslinks to another base on a second sugar strand. For DNA, the four bases are adenosine, thymine, guanine, and cytosine: ATGC, the four-letter alphabet of genes.[25] An A on one sugar strand binds to a T on the second, and likewise for G and C, giving us the famous double-stranded helix.

In a living cell, however, DNA does not typically appear as an elegantly twisted ladder. Instead it is curled and clumped around lumps of protein called histones, rather as a mobile phone charger's cable wraps around its plug. This makes for an interesting exercise in 3D geometry, since areas of DNA which are nowhere near each other on the stretched-out helix may come into close proximity when coiled around a histone.[26] Near neighbours can thus affect each other electrically, since the molecules carry electric charges, or by physically blocking access to the DNA, so that the transcription processes which read off a gene to create a protein cannot take place. For such gene expression to happen, the relevant section of DNA must be unwound. The structural arrangement of chromatin—DNA together with its histone support—can thus affect which proteins are made within a cell.

Changing bases

To this tangle epigenetics adds the capacity to mark, and hence modify, stretches of DNA. One mechanism, methylation, interferes with one of the bases, cytosine (C). Adding a methyl group (CH_3) to this molecule to make 5-methyl-cytosine tends to attract gene-silencing proteins, which bind to the methyl group and, like possessive spouses, block other interactions.[27] DNA methylation, therefore, is usually though not inevitably associated with turning genes off. Furthermore, this silencing can be reversed, for example when a 'demethylase' enzyme removes the methyl group.

A second mechanism, histone acetylation, is more associated with increasing gene expression. This process, carried out by enzymes called acetyltransferases, transfers an acetyl group ($COCH_3$) to the histone molecule—as the name acetyltransferase suggests. (When chemists name chemicals, information takes priority over prosody, poetry, or pronounceability. Stereotypes often coalesce around grains of truth, and that includes stereotypes of scientists.)

Back to acetylation. The acetyl group carries a positive charge, so its arrival alters the electrical balance between the histone molecule and the wraparound DNA. The positive charge repels others already present, causing the histone structure to expand. That allows easier access to the DNA for the enzymes which initiate transcription and do the work which turns gene instructions into proteins. Acetylation, like methylation, is reversible, via a mechanism, you will not be surprised to learn, involving enzymes called histone deacetylases.

There are, in short, ways to raise or lower the production of specific proteins, not only in response to the state of other genes, but dependent on what is happening in the organism—and, moreover, to maintain a record of those altered settings, perhaps even through the reproductive process. Some genes, for example, are more or less active depending on which parent they came from, a phenomenon known as imprinting. Interestingly, the relative influence of Mum and Dad appears to change with age (maternal genes contribute more to the developing brain, paternal genes more in adulthood)—at least if you're a mouse. A pair of articles in *Science* in 2010 reported many more imprinted genes than previously thought: well over a thousand in the mouse brain.[28] Other studies suggest roles for epigenetic changes in the effects of early-life environment—e.g. whether a parent smoked or was suffering stress—on an adult's susceptibility to numerous diseases, including allergies and autoimmune conditions, osteoporosis, heart disease, cancer, and mental illnesses.[29]

Known unknowns

In epigenetics, however, the amount known is vastly outweighed by the questions still unanswered. It seems, for instance, that in egg and sperm cells some methylation marks are erased, though not all. Why? Do similar processes affect other forms of epigenetic modification? How long-lasting are the changes, and what exactly are their underlying mechanisms? Why are there several kinds of histones and several kinds of epigenetic changes that affect them; why so many RNAs and interfering enzymes?

Why, in short, is the system so incredibly complicated that you'd wonder how any gene ever got transcribed into a protein, let alone combined with all those other cellular happenings to produce the extraordinarily coincidental you? (Being human is improbable enough; being yourself, here, now is a phenomenal stroke of luck.) How much impact does epigenetic modification really have in adults, as compared to during development, and how much is passed on from parents to children? How is that impact exerted—through effects on neuronal activity, synapse structure and function, neurotransmitter and/or receptor profiles, or what? Can results in other species, like mice, be replicated in humans? And what degree of environmental disturbance is required to do the damage to you—and maybe your offspring?[30] Work proceeds at an accelerating pace, but there is much, much more to do.

An example: the power of parenting

Evidence is beginning to emerge that epigenetic changes may be involved in many psychiatric disturbances where no obvious genetic 'smoking gun' has yet been located. Differences in methylation have already been associated with mental retardation, suicide, schizophrenia, and post-traumatic stress disorder, among others.[31] One promising candidate for study is a gene promoter which regulates production of a type of glucocorticoid receptor called NR3C1.[32] These receptors mediate many of the effects of glucocorticoids like cortisol—'stress hormones'—on the brain.

Cortisol is made in the adrenal glands, above the kidneys, in response to stressful, threatening stimuli. We evolved to fear predators, including other humans, as well as dangers like lightning, falling trees, and landslides, because fearful ancestors were more likely to dodge the peril in time and thus survive to raise a family. These days we are less vulnerable to being eaten, but stress can be triggered by many other stimuli: anything from a speeding car to an aggressive boss.

Cortisol release from the adrenals is prompted by activity in the brain's hypothalamus and in the pituitary gland at its base. When the stimulus is a one-off, this hypothalamic-pituitary-adrenal network (the HPA axis) serves a useful alarm function, preparing the body for the extreme efforts it may have to make in order to survive (leap out of the car's path, deal with the yelling boss). Problems arise when the stress becomes chronic and the HPA axis adapts, producing patterns of abnormal function. HPA axis changes have been implicated in many disorders, from chronic fatigue and depression to severe antisocial behaviour.[33] Constant vigilance wreaks havoc on body and brain.[34]

That havoc is in part transmitted via NR3C1 glucocorticoid receptors. Post-mortem analysis of the brains of people who have died by suicide suggests that the stretch of DNA which regulates production of the receptors, the NR3C1 promoter, appears to be more heavily methylated. That implies lower production of the NR3C1 receptor itself, suggesting that these people's stress responses may have been abnormal—as one might expect, given how they died.[35]

That, however, is not the whole story. Studies in rodents show something both entirely reasonable and quite extraordinary. The NR3C1 promoter in an animal's neurons may be more or less liberally studded with methylation marks depending on how well that animal's mother looked after it when it was a baby. Poor maternal care (in rats and mice absent fathers are the norm) stresses the youngsters. This alters their HPA axis function, leaving them more nervous and inhibited as adults—and it does so in part via epigenetic changes to the NR3C1 promoter.

Abusive parenting by humans is known to have similar effects on their offspring's behaviour and HPA axis.[36] Does it have similar epigenetic features? It seems so. The researchers who analysed the brains of suicide victims (and controls who had died from other causes) looked at two experimental groups: victims who had reported child abuse and those who had not. They found significantly more NR3C1 promoter methylation in the abused victims, suggesting altered HPA axis function—their brains were making fewer glucocorticoid receptors. As the authors remark in a later review, 'The data are consistent with other data from the literature suggesting that suicide has a developmental origin.'[37] This is a neutral statement of a truly terrible conclusion. If these researchers are correct, really bad parenting can do such enormous and long-lasting damage that, years later, it may make grown-up children more likely to kill themselves. Yet there is also hope, because epigenetic changes can potentially be reversed.

Methylated spirits: epigenetics and us

This is where the moral issues really start to rear their carping heads: when epigenetic transmission bridges the generation gap. Take another example: a postulated link between maternal smoking in pregnancy and an increased risk of cognitive and behavioural problems in children.[38] It's one thing for Susie to kill herself slowly with cancer sticks if that's her poison, but what if the causal links between her smoking and baby Josh's inability to focus can be firmly established? Would Josh be justified in suing his mum for his academic failure and consequent loss of earnings? Besides, it may be that Susie's longing for cigarettes is not unconnected with the fact that her mum smoked throughout her pregnancy. Who then is to blame for Josh's problems and Susie's craving for nicotine? This way lies madness—or else original sin—regressing our problems back through our ancestry.

Yet this is not a new concern. As the mention of original sin makes clear, the concepts are familiar. What is changing is the accuracy with which we can apply those concepts. Epigenetics is revealing which aspects of a child's personality and behaviour are most affected by its parents' good or bad behaviours. A good dose of information might help to reduce the heat of the current highly ideological—and often poisonously vitriolic—arguments about parenting styles, which can be extremely stressful for parents. Better definitions of what is harmfully bad behaviour, rather than telling parents what to do, could encourage more state intervention in the worst cases, reduce the interference with other families, and leave most parents reassured that they are doing reasonably well. Clearly stating what damages children and what doesn't might ease the unrealistically high standards society often seems to set its families.[39]

Perhaps I hope for more than human nature can deliver. Yet passions are not always ungovernable, and adding knowledge can, over time, resolve even the most ferocious arguments. In the UK, there were furious complaints when the government made car seatbelts compulsory, but the evidence showed that wearing a seatbelt saved lives. Now the topic is rarely even mentioned. There may be some who still resent having to belt up, but their impact on public conversation—in government and the media—is negligible.

Epigenetics matters for many of the reasons we used to think genetics mattered: not only for the chances it dangles before us of improving the human condition, but for what it may imply about that knotty conundrum. The implications in themselves are of long standing, but they shine the brighter when burnished with a scientific gloss. Some scientists may attempt to avoid the moral and societal consequences of their work, but for the rest of us those are the juicy bits, and such interpretations have surrounded research on epigenetics— and indeed genetics, since long before the discovery of DNA.

Yet whereas genes were traditionally seen as uncontrollable, the fate doled out at conception with which each growing embryo had to make do, it appears that some epigenetic marks can be reversed.[40] Genetic fate is no longer written in immutable chromosomal text—at least, not all of it. The language is biochemical, far more complex, and susceptible to influences over which we can exert control.

This new understanding shifts at least some aspects of 'genes' from the uncontrollable category into the class of things we may be able to work on, a change which cuts both ways. It offers hope, for example, that the negative effects of extremely poor parenting may be amenable to treatment, but it also suggests that such parents—and the society which fails to make good their inadequacies—should be held to greater account for their behaviour. Not only is parenting now a choice, so is parenting badly, and both choices, in our crowded world, have implications beyond the parents and children involved. Parenting, in other words, is increasingly being seen as a public health issue, not a private decision, and very poor parenting as a worse choice than deciding not to become a parent at all.

This is only one of the many implications which are already starting to trouble us as the brain supremacy takes shape. In the next chapter of the book, we return from the world of genes and enzymes—the understanding of which is so crucial to that developing revolution— to the more familiar social world, where brain research will have its most obvious effects on the way we live now.

14

The Problems of Neurotech

Shiny thing make it all better

(*The Daily Mash*)

This book began with a glimpse of an astonishing future: the world of the brain supremacy. We are already entering that remarkable era. Modern neuroscience draws on the massive technological achievements of the physical sciences. They, however, have focused on analysing, manipulating, and improving the environment around us. The science of the brain offers more intriguing capabilities.

As the brain supremacy develops, neuroscience will give us more and more power to monitor and manipulate ourselves—and each other. Ultimately, two kinds of technologies are likely to emerge. DNE recording and programming will allow us to record, transfer, and reprogram aspects of brain function in real time and with high precision. They are the distant goals of the brain supremacy.

I have used the phrase 'digitized neural experience' (DNE) in order to assert the majority view among neuroscientists: that by changing the mind you change the brain, and vice versa.[1] The idea of DNE is also useful, however, because it suggests that DNE recording and programming could be done in ways accessible to the public. Future brain technicians may script their programs not directly in neurochemical codes, but in a high-level language not too far from everyday talk of thoughts, emotions, beliefs, and desires. Just as I see words on my computer screen, not strings of ones and zeros, DNE programmers may work in terms of subjective experience, not neural activity—whether turning up an emotion, weakening a belief, boosting a good intention, or generating an artificial dream.

Neural activity can already be digitized, recorded, and experimentally altered. That does not make the brain a digital computer just waiting for a sufficiently clever programmer. It does not imply that we will shortly be able to simulate a human brain in silicon, or equip ourselves with portable mind-reading devices. And it definitely does not mean that DNE recording and programming technologies are likely to be with us in the next few years. Those who hope one day to download themselves, gaining immortality through electronics, may die disappointed. As I hope the previous chapters have convinced you, IMCOTT. Today's neurotech is phenomenally successful at seeing and manipulating human brains, but it has a long, long way to go.

I have mentioned some of the obstacles specific to each method: the slowness of PET and fMRI; the difficulties posed for EEG and MEG by brain geometry and the inverse problem; the crudity of TES and TMS; the risks of DBS. I have also raised some of the ethical concerns which are likely to preoccupy societies coming to terms with the many changes wrought by the brain supremacy. In this chapter, I will consider a third set of challenges: ones affecting not the specific technologies but the assumptions behind them. These will need to be addressed if the brain supremacy is to fulfil its great potential.

Ecological validity

As the experiments described in this book have shown, a brain research lab is a very unusual environment. Stimuli and tasks are often highly artificial—real life rarely involves such carefully controlled comparisons—so their ecological validity is low.[2] This is particularly true of fMRI, where being scanned requires you to a) sign a consent form, b) answer intrusive questions about whether you are pregnant or have piercings in private places, and c) lie still for ages in a machine which, being shed-sized and noisy, is not exactly inconspicuous. Since the clunky mechanics of neuroimaging techniques, and current ethical constraints, do not let researchers spy on the brain activity of passing strangers, boosting ecological validity will not be easy.[3] Until we achieve considerable shrinkage in the mechanics, neuroimaging by deceit—the kind of study which leaves its subjects as undisturbed as a BBC wildlife camera—will remain a formidable technical challenge, though not an insuperable one.

Spying in real time is also problematic, since many imaging analyses are done hours, days, or weeks after the data have been gathered. This is changing, however, and it may soon be possible to use imaging as a feedback tool. Being able to show a participant images of his or her brain while it is in the scanner would be very useful, not least because the authority carried by such images makes them an effective tool for clinicians trying to alter thinking patterns.[4] ('See that red blob going yellow? That's your amygdala damping down nicely; well done!') But you still have to persuade the patient into the scanner in the first place. Furthermore, as moving can ruin the results, cooperation is required from the participants. Even for those who manage to keep still, it is possible for a participant trained in cognitive countermeasures to fool a scanner.[5]

Indirect measurement

Already discussed with respect to specific neuromethods, this is the crucial question of what exactly counts as brain activity. PET measures glucose levels in brain cells; fMRI measures blood supply changes in response to neural activity. Both assess the brain's demand for fuel, which is like judging a crowd by how many burgers it munches. EEG and MEG measure electromagnetic emissions, but not individual action potentials from neurons—and as we have seen, action potentials are only part of the story of neurotransmission. Then there are the chemical dimensions to be considered: neurotransmitters, synaptic proteins, and so on.

Here's an analogy for the case of fMRI: what if each individual neuron were represented by one human being? A single fMRI voxel would typically cover the responses of a population of about 100,000, the size of Cheltenham in England, Ithaca in New York, or the Pacific island nation of Kiribati.[6] At any moment, there is a lot going on in any group of 100,000 people, and the same is true of neurons, yet only the overall 'activity' in each voxel is measured by the scanner. A scan of the entire brain, meanwhile, would cover around 86 billion people.[7] In 2010, that's over 60 times the size of the world's biggest country, China, and more than 12 times the size of Earth's population.[8]

Imagine an alien spacecraft visiting Earth to look for signs of life, having picked up the TV signals we are constantly sending into space. They're worried about the propensity to violence evident in those signals, so they've brought their own scanner to find out which areas of Earth are responsible. It's an FMRI machine too, but this one scans for Fighting, Murder, Rape and intentional Injury. It treats the Earth as a single, brainlike system, as if each of the seven billion human beings (as of 2011) were a neuron. It has a spatial resolution—its 'voxel' size—of 50 square kilometres—about the size of Cheltenham.[9] It has a temporal resolution of one week—much slower than the timescale of human activity, just as fMRI scanners are slow compared to neurons. A total planetary scan takes ten weeks. The aliens want to find out which areas of Earth are particularly violent, so they set their scan running, collect their data, and analyse the clusters of statistically significant voxels.

The aliens' machine is smart, but all the clever gadgetry in the universe won't save them from failure, because their methods are based on a false assumption. It's the same assumption made by some imaging studies: that areas reflect functions in a simple and singular way. For instance, a quick literature search for articles on the human medial prefrontal cortex (mPFC) reveals a fascinating suggestion that this region may mediate aspects of social identity and the deep human preference for 'people like us'.[10] The same search links the mPFC to autism, phobia, addiction, depression, emotion regulation, strategic reasoning, risk processing, pain processing, trauma, and stress responses.[11] Likewise, the aliens' violence detector tells them which areas of Earth are violent, but nothing about what else is going on in these afflicted places. Even during a genocide, people still eat, sleep, make love, make music, do scientific research.[12]

Timing can also be crucial. If the aliens come calling in the early 1970s, when the Khmer Rouge are slaughtering the people of Cambodia, they'll get significant 'activation' in South Asia. If they arrive in 1994, and scan between April and June, they'll undoubtedly detect the Rwandan genocide, and label Africa, as others have before them, a heart of darkness. In 1916, they might decide that Europe is a good place to avoid. Few neuroimaging experiments sample across cultures, control for time of day, or take note of their participants' current workload, stress levels, or whether they were out partying the night before the experiment.

The Rwandan example also highlights the issue of scale. The aliens' detector is only picking up mass human activity, just as fMRI scanners pick up mass brain activity—or more precisely, changes in blood supply demanded by that activity. In Rwanda, however, although around 800,000 people died, their extinction was not down to tribal conflict or spontaneous popular uprising; it was deliberately organized by a small and determined core of powerful extremists. The aliens' detector cannot resolve such fine details, so their understanding of violence on Earth will remain superficial. Similarly for our current neuroimaging techniques. If we are to realize the DNE visions of the brain supremacy, like dream recording and artificial experience, we need to do much better.

The problems of indirect measurement need a lot more work. It remains to be seen whether modifying one dimension of brain function—for example changing brain chemistry by taking a drug—is sufficient to produce the desired degree of control over neural experience. Simultaneous modification of both chemical and electromagnetic dimensions is made challenging by their very different timescales. Yet as optogenetic methods are already demonstrating, the ability to manipulate genes and proteins more precisely will close that gap. Many problems will be solved, moreover, as DNE programming technologies are developed. We have accomplished only a little of what is possible.

The risks of interpretation

The brain supremacy is only in part about neuroscience, its restraints and capabilities. It is also about the perception of neuroscience: its interpretation by commentators and opinion-formers, its reception by politicians, corporations, and citizens, the support of taxpayers and the influence of many vested interests. To prosper, scientists are encouraged to raise their discipline's public profile, taking research from the lab into the public sphere. Science communication can reap an excellent harvest of publicity. But it also has risks.

Neuroimaging techniques, particularly fMRI, have proved exceptional at gaining media attention. They offer fantastic views of an extremely complicated system at work and play, and promise insights into something we humans find fascinating: us. Like any way of seeing, however, they simplify the thing perceived in the process of representing it. (If your only tool is a big shiny hammer, problems may tend to look like nails.)

An example already mentioned is the possibility of fMRI being used for mind-reading. Here is a typical description from the BBC:[13]

> **Brain scans could be useful as lie detectors to show if a witness lies when identifying a suspect in a crime investigation, US researchers believe.**
>
> Scientists at Stanford University were able to tell when a person recognised a mug shot by reading their brain waves.
>
> Functional magnetic resonance imaging (fMRI) revealed tell-tale brain activity during the memory recall task, Proceedings journal reports.
>
> But experts warn the technology is not foolproof and can give false results.

And such false positives could have serious legal consequences, say Dr Jesse Rissman and his team, who conducted the research.

Setting aside the reference to the non-existent journal *Proceedings*, the absence of a link to the source article and the mention of 'reading brain waves' (this is fMRI, not EEG), the BBC piece is a concise and balanced summary of the findings and associated ethical issues.[14] Yet it is science-lite which tells us little of the methods. It does not mention, for instance, how many people took part. We need to know, not least because an experiment involving, say, 100 participants is probably worth more attention than one with only five.

The article itself, 'Detecting individual memories through the neural decoding of memory states and past experience', can be found in the American journal *PNAS*.[15] Its abstract, which gives some details of the methods, is excellent: lucid, well written, easy to read and there for all to see. To get the numbers, however, you need to read the 'supplementary information', which like the main article is not open access, so most people will need to pay $10 to read it.[16] (Only $10? You'd pay $32 over at *Nature*!) There we learn that 23 volunteers participated in total, roughly as many men as women, 'recruited from the Stanford University community and surrounding areas'. (Friends, family, students, strangers?) As the researchers note, that's quite a small, specialized group from which to draw any general conclusion, let alone one with the profound implications of 'Brain scans could be useful as lie detectors'.

Why does all this matter? Because understanding what a brain scanner is actually doing, and how fMRI experiments are done, takes the sensational edge off a great deal of science-lite interpretation. And that edge, exciting though it may be, introduces inaccuracies which should be anathema to scientists and funding bodies alike (at present, 'impact' is a factor in funding decisions, but what about the quality of the impact?) Working out whether the ability to 'read brain waves' makes our privacy even more of an endangered species—and brings us closer to the brain supremacy's goal of DNE recording—will be much easier if we start with an accurate view of the methods involved and the long chains of inferences on which they depend.

The scientists' concern was with memory, and the fact that brains respond differently to new and familiar stimuli. Could this 'familiarity signal' be used to detect whether someone has or lacks particular memories—whether stimuli are new to the person perceiving them? The researchers used fMRI to obtain brain activity patterns and computer classification techniques to find patterns in them (such as the familiarity signal). They looked at how closely people's brain responses to a stimulus matched the familiarity signal. If the match was good, the person could have a memory of the stimulus.

So does fMRI allow us to do mind-reading? Not yet. Detecting whether a memory is present is not the same as reading the contents of that memory. Nor does detecting a memory mean that it is true.

Recognizing that their research has implications for the legal system, the researchers call for more work to be done before companies rush to market fMRI lie detection techniques. Alas, the call comes too late; both these and other (EEG-based) methods are already being touted, and in some cases accepted, as forensic evidence.[17] At the time of the BBC report, a legal case was under way in the United States, centred on whether someone had lied, in which brain scans were being put forward as evidence. A few weeks later US judge Tu Pham set an important legal precedent by ruling that the brain scans were not acceptable evidence, but this will not stop attempts to use fMRI in similar future cases.[18] Since companies are already rushing to market, more research is urgently required to figure out whether the methods work before some unfortunate innocent finds themselves on death row (*PNAS* is a US publication) because someone thinks their brain waves say they lied.

Rissman et al.'s own research built and trained a computer model, using some of their fMRI data as inputs and the participants' responses as the training signal.[19] The model was then tested on further data. Without knowing what the participants themselves had said, it was able to discriminate new from familiar stimuli, even when it was trained on all but one of a group of people and then tested on the final group member. (A lie detector which only works on the person it was trained on is not much use.) This kind of computational approach, using brute-force statistics to number-crunch enormous quantities of brain data, will be increasingly important in the brain supremacy.

Note, however, that what the classifier learned to distinguish was subjective experience: whether the person thought the image they were seeing was one they had seen before. Its ability to say whether the person had actually seen the image was much more limited. That is, the study was able to uncover brain signals which correlate with people's beliefs about what they saw, but not signals reflecting the reality of their past experience. A second experiment confirmed that the classifier could do its task for explicit memories, which participants are aware of having, but was hopeless on implicit ones.[20] Ideally, mind-reading machines would be able to pick up on the brain's record of experiences without them having to be consciously recalled.[21]

Oh dear. Bang goes the dream of a lie detector? As the authors say: 'an ideal memory detection technology would also be able to reveal whether a person had actually experienced a particular entity, without regard to his or her subjective report. Our data indicate that neural signatures of objective memory, at least for the simple events assessed here, are extremely challenging to detect reliably with current fMRI methods.' They comment: 'This may limit the ultimate utility of fMRI-based memory detection approaches for real-world application.'

Indeed it may. Especially as moving beyond a simple lab test to a real-world application involving such high stakes as a court case is likely to bring in all sorts of additional complications which will affect a person's brain responses (high anxiety, for example). At the moment, therefore, claims of mind-reading need to be treated with care. fMRI can provide information about what kind of memory is being recalled, or which of several memories set up by the experimenters is being mulled over by a participant. What it cannot yet do is tell true memories from false ones, which can feel so true to their possessors.[22]

Research, however, is progressing at an extraordinary rate, and 'never' is an unwise word to use about science. Few would have predicted the present capabilities of fMRI, and who knows what subtle distinctions in your neurochatter Son-of-fMRI may be able to detect. I remember a conversation in our lab, years ago, about the limits of early neuroimaging studies. We'd read a review which noted that the supposed position of an area of the brain called the anterior cingulate could vary by about a centimetre between different experiments. How we jeered. (If you had a map of the world which put London in France you wouldn't be impressed.) That, however, was two decades ago. Neuroimaging has come a very long way, and the speed of advance is if anything accelerating.

Confounding variables

Neuroimaging research is often vulnerable to the problem of confounding factors: overlooked features which may affect the brain's activity but which haven't been controlled for. Mostly these are not relevant to understanding the results of an experiment, but in some cases they might be the path to a new hypothesis. Sometimes we just don't understand what we're looking at in sufficient depth to say one way or the other.

Because of the time and number of data points required, many studies cannot afford to control for many potentially confounding variables. Take two well-known psychological phenomena: social desirability (the urge to please the researcher) and self-confirmation (the desire to look good). As we have understood at least since Stanley Milgram's work on obedience to authority, these are powerfully—but variably, depending on participant personality—in play in a laboratory situation.[23] Outside the lab things may well be different. Could these social factors affect how easily brain activity patterns can be decoded, or confound interpretation of social neuroscientific studies?

We don't know, yet. We're only just starting to look.[24] Tempting though it can be to confuse absence of evidence with evidence of absence, there are some questions on which science cannot legitimately pronounce—among them many in psychology and neuroscience—

because adequate research hasn't yet been done. There is much we don't know about how social factors affect human brain function, in and out of laboratories and scanners. The obstacle here is not only the expense required to answer all these questions, but also the stubbornness with which some scientists continue to disparage the relevant social psychological research, as if 'all that wishy-washy nonsense', as I have heard it called, does not apply to their work and need not be considered. It does, and it must, because social factors can have big effects.

For instance, the well-known phenomenon of stereotype threat has been shown to affect performance on tasks from basic visual learning and mental rotation to mathematics and intelligence tests.[25] If participants are primed with the belief that they are the sort of person who does badly on the test, they tend to live down to the expectations imposed on them. A study in which students were given 15 hard maths problems to solve found that while the control group averaged 6.52 problems correct, the group under stereotype threat averaged only 4.04, a drop of 38%.[26] Many experiments in brain research would be more than happy with that size of difference. Social factors cannot be ignored, however difficult they are to take into account.

Types of participants

Computational analysis may be able to associate different patterns of brain activity with different kinds of subjective experience. This may allow researchers to generalize to similar patterns not previously presented in the experiment, and perhaps to use information about the signals given off by brains like yours to work out what your brain responses mean. This would be a step closer to true mind-reading.

Yet whether information mostly gleaned from Western students would apply equally well to a !Kung bushman or a Thai woman we just don't know. Cross-cultural neuroscience is woefully limited at present, and most human beings are neither Westerners nor students. In the near future, brain activity patterns may be matched against growing databases of known associations from across the world, allowing researchers to infer that someone is looking at a bird or sucking a peppermint whatever the race, age, gender, or educational background of the participant. To get to that point will require an immense amount of data to be gathered and stored.

It is not beyond the bounds of possibility, furthermore, that before too long you may find yourself thinking instructions to your car, house, mobile phone, or cash machine, or their equivalents, wherever and whoever you are. Indeed, this form of brain–machine interfacing is already starting to happen with EEG, which can distinguish, for example, the brain patterns associated with thinking 'go left' or 'go right', allowing the severely disabled to navigate, video gamers to play by 'thought control', and so on.[27] That is tremendously exciting progress, and ongoing research into older technologies like EEG, and newer methods like terahertz wave scanning, suggests no technical reason why further advances will not be possible.[28] We cannot yet read a partner's mind, or write a book by thought alone, but perhaps in my lifetime we will. If those powers are to be made available worldwide, cross-cultural studies have a lot of catching up to do.

The problem of normal

At present we don't have an adequate idea of what is 'normal' in terms of the human brain. Psychological tests like the WAIS measures of cognition and the Big Five measures of personality have been run on thousands of people, providing a large database of human variation, but they have their limitations.[29] A decade ago, in a letter to *The Lancet*, I suggested a similar database for neuroscience, making the point that the field needed far more information about far more brains.[30] That is still true. Although attempts to address the issue are in progress, we need data from thousands of individuals, of different ages and from different cultures, to be able to derive comprehensive norms for brain structure and function.[31] Since fMRI researchers use magnets of varying strengths, several kinds of software, different methods of mapping the functional signals onto the anatomical brains, and so on, and since information about participants varies considerably in quality, amalgamating data from different studies is a seriously non-trivial task.[32]

The challenge of context

Recall the example of Edmund, the violently fantasizing office worker. Chapter 3 considered the possibility that intention-reading technology might be used to prevent him attacking his co-worker. Detecting intention by itself, however, is not enough. If Edmund buys a melon on the way home from work and acts out his urges, his intention to swing the axe does not signal a murder. He may take out his anger on the melon as a substitute for his colleague, or stop and think when he sees how the axe has mangled the fruit. He may pull a muscle. Whatever happens, there is no inevitable connection between the violence he commits at home and future violence against his annoying colleague—otherwise every gamer who scythes his way through virtual opponents for hours on end would be a real-life killer. To minimize false positive alarms, an intention-monitoring system should be able to distinguish the context of the action, allowing the destruction of melons and computer men, but not the reach-and-swing that threatens irksome workmates. That, however, is far more easily said than done.

The problem of meaning

This is not least because of the problem, already mentioned, of definition. Just as fuzzy categories in mental illness give you poorly delineated 'genes for' psychiatric problems, so matching neuroscience to violence is a complicated business because deciding what counts as violence is harder than it looks—witness the perennial debate over physically disciplining children. Explosive, impulsive violence of the kind that fuels pub brawls may be easier to detect and prevent than premeditated violence of the kind associated with predators and psychopaths, but there will always be difficult cases and differing opinions.

The methodological difficulties are soluble, in principle, with suffi-ciently elaborate technology. Some problems, however, may be beyond a purely technical fix. The use of lie detection offers an example: as noted earlier, it currently cannot distinguish what really took place from what the scanned person believes happened. In other words, a liar who comes to believe the lie will pass the test.

The problem is that beliefs are only rarely solid and inflexible. The philosopher Ludwig Wittgenstein, whose late masterpiece the *Philo-sophical Investigations* should be required reading for every neuroscien-tist—it would save so many the labour of reinventing his ideas—observed that even very familiar mental furniture can be made to waver, to strike us as strange and doubtful:

> I want to remember a tune and it escapes me; suddenly I say 'Now
> I know it' and I sing it. What was it like to suddenly know it? Surely it
> can't have occurred to me *in its entirety* in that moment!—Perhaps you
> will say: 'It's a particular feeling, as if it were *there*'—but is it there?
> Suppose I now begin to sing it and get stuck?—But may I not have
> been *certain* at that moment that I knew it? So in some sense or other it
> was *there* after all!—But in what sense?[33]

Beliefs can be much more malleable than we think. Even apparently rigid convictions can change astonishingly fast. When political change sucks popular support away from a terrorist movement, the ex-sup-porters were not necessarily faking the strength of their earlier com-mitment. They may or may not be equally passionate about the new dawn, but if dogmatic adherence to the advocates of violence no longer offers sufficient benefits, it's amazing how the certainty can seep away. A current fashion among psychologists is to remark on the ease with which human emotion can override rational capacities. It is however just as fascinating to see how quickly passion can be subsumed by rational self-interest.

Given this flexibility, it is unsurprising that people's attitudes to their beliefs are far more subtle than a mere committed/uncommitted dichot-omy. If I, as an intellectual exercise, argue strongly for a case that I do not actually believe, I will quickly find myself thinking, 'Perhaps there's some sense in that after all'.[34] Social psychological research shows that I am not alone; asked to defend a position, people tend to shift towards it.[35] If it is so easy to make oneself believe something, at least temporarily, then those who want to use scanners for lie detection have a hugely difficult task ahead of them.

Likewise with issues of criminal responsibility and mental illness. The trouble lies outside the scanner, with the woolly definitions of the psychological symptoms with which the neuroimaging signals are being associated. Garbage in, garbage out, no matter how precise the machine which processes the garbage. Until we have a clearer perspective on what is and is not to be called 'responsible', 'psychopathic', 'normal', 'schizophrenic', and so on, we cannot be sure which claims— even about groups, let alone individuals—are accurate. That makes testing those claims extremely difficult.

The challenge of complexity

Brain manipulation at the level required for DNE programming is far beyond what neuroscience can currently promise.[36] Ethical constraints mean that most research is done in rats, mice, and simpler organisms (notably those tiny unsung neuroheroes C. elegans and D. melanogaster, the nematode and the fruit fly).[37] These cannot report the experience of manipulation any more than they can consent to receive it, and translating to the human scale, where genetic manipulation is not currently allowed, is not straightforward. Electrical, magnetic, and deep brain stimulation do not affect individual circuits; nor does neurosurgery. The same is true of chemical enhancements, such as taking modafinil to ward off fatigue. Whether illegally traded, prescribed by a GP, or bought in a supermarket, ingested chemicals exert widespread effects in multiple areas of the brain and body. Coffee, for example, has been linked to changes in insulin and glucose metabolism, cholesterol, liver function, cell growth, immune inflammatory responses, and Alzheimer's, among others.[38]

The sunny confidence with which proponents of cognitive enhancement greet the prospect of changing bad habits, removing unwanted memories, and sharpening our powers of retention and concentration must therefore be tempered with awareness of just how difficult it will be to translate brain manipulation into human brains. Not just because of the ethical issues, but because of the exponentially greater complexity of the systems involved. *C. elegans* has 302 neurons; you have around 86 billion.[39] The most advanced current brain-change techniques still more closely resemble changing the Earth's entire weather system than making it rain on Number 4, Acacia Avenue, Cheltenham, UK because Number 4's begonias need watering. Did I say begonias? Far too large-scale. The precision needed to microengineer the mind is more akin to the power to prevent one raindrop from drowning the minuscule spiderling on Number 4's windowsill.

Once again language misleads us. It is easy to say, for example, that neurons communicate by releasing neurotransmitter molecules which cross the synapse and activate receptors on postsynaptic neurons. It is less easy to grasp what that actually implies: where the receptors cluster thickly, in an area of the neuron's cell membrane called the postsynaptic density, an article in *Nature Neuroscience* has identified 1,461 proteins, mutations of which 'cause 133 neurological and psychiatric diseases', according to current knowledge.[40] Each of these, in principle, could be a separate target for manipulation, and each has the protein's equivalent of a social life. The thought of how much research is required to sort through that lot, even in fast-breeding animals and with ever-quicker gene processing, is enough to give the most liberal funding agency a headache. And the postsynaptic density is by no means the whole story, even for synapses, let alone for neurons, brain regions, or whole human beings.

In practice, of course, we will not attempt to unravel the entire system before we try to control it. The clinical motivation demands solutions for all the people suffering from those 133 diseases—and from everything else that can go wrong with a human brain. If we waited till we fully understood what we were doing, neurology would not exist as a branch of medicine, and both neuroscience and human health would be much the poorer. Instead, researchers will refine existing technologies according to perceived clinical priorities, attempting to ease the heavy burdens of mental distress, chronic pain, addiction, and the neurodegenerative disorders. They will also pursue the analysis agenda, using neuromethods, statistics, and computational brute force to better understand how healthy brains work. And some of them will follow the dream of enhancement, hoping to endow us with superhuman capacities to read and reprogram our minds, and the minds of others.

Some form of the brain supremacy is now probably unstoppable. Its development is likely to be rapid—so rapid that within the next few decades we may look back in wonder at the primitive notions of today's research. If we do not already have the technology, we soon will. What will we do with it? How can we best shape the future of neuroscience, and hence our own futures? That is the topic of the next and final chapter.

15

Creating the Brain Supremacy

My own view is that it is far better to understand the Universe as it
really is than to pretend to a Universe as we might wish it to be

(Carl Sagan, physicist)

Futures are not solidly predestined. If we want the benefits of the
brain supremacy without its nastier possibilities, now is the time to
act. Small changes made sooner will have more impact, for much less
effort, than later ones. We cannot rely on the current systems proving
adequate to this brave new world, whether they involve the governments who regulate scientific research, the media who translate it for
public consumption, the ethical and cultural opinion-formers (from
professors to *Daily Mail* columnists), or the universities and companies
who produce the data. Their investment, too often, is in the status quo
or the near future, not the longer term, and their agendas are not
always yours or mine.

The brain and the web

The acceleration of modern neuroscience has coincided with the globalization of communication technologies, which is currently standardizing
human experience according to a largely Western template.[1] In their
early days personal computers were transformative and the internet
a glorious revolution. Today both can seem increasingly oppressive:

gateways to spam, porn, and marketing; tools watching you while you think you're using them; means for corporations and governments to outsource labour to consumers; and channels providing a deluge of social expectations for your already anxious and overloaded mind. Just as we reach for unprecedented powers of self-fashioning, we face enormous pressure to conform to our cultures' expectations. The agony aunts of yesteryear were few and avoidable. Now everyone seems to know better than his or her neighbour, and to feel the need to say so. Worse, we have the whole world's most accomplished people against whom to measure ourselves, and fail.[2]

The social power exerted via the web is startling for anyone who needs to use the internet—which increasingly means almost all of us. Freedom to speak and act exists, provided nothing you say or do causes offence to someone with cyberpower. The result: fragmented online communities of very like-minded individuals. From Twitter and Facebook to ad-laden blogs and websites, the proliferation of online opinion, amplified and focused by anonymity and the ease of transmission, makes public censure impossible to ignore, so it is easier for birds of a feather to flock together in forums where they can reinforce each other's outlooks. Provided your thoughts are in tune with those of your online community, the web can provide a valuable social boost, especially if real life is not all you have been led to expect. In the longer term, and when combined with the new ability to rework ourselves as well as our Facebook pages, it may be less conducive to originality, as we succumb to the massive pressure to be normal.[3]

We are still working through the new technology's impact on creativity—and there is still time to absorb its consequences. But we will have to do so quickly and with care if we are to handle the bigger challenge of the brain supremacy.

Science grew up in the age of mastery, in which humans used the natural sciences to achieve unprecedented control of their surroundings. Now it must master the world of the brain supremacy, in which the target of control is human nature. This new environment, to which it is not so well adapted, will force scientists, and the rest of us, to evolve new ways of thinking. Unlike previous revolutions, it will also provide new, direct ways of doing so. Earlier attempts to build human utopias, like communism, were brought down by the stubborn resilience of human nature. The utopias envisaged by proponents of brain enhancement are not so limited.

The wisdom of Athene and the gift of Prometheus

> When the facts change I change my opinions. What do you do?
>
> (attributed to the economist John Maynard Keynes)

At its heart, the scientific method tests beliefs—hypotheses—against the way the world is. It sounds so simple, and therein lies its fabulous power; but as always with pearls of great price, the setting matters. The choice of hypotheses and experiments, which literature is read and cited, which grants are funded, which professors appointed, what else is currently fashionable in the field: all this and more feeds into the exercise of the method.

When the test is done, the experimenter hopes to find his hypothesis confirmed. If the world gives a thumbs-down, however, he has a choice. The scientific route, and also the wise one, is to change the hypothesis so that its predictions better match what actually happens, adapting beliefs to the dictates of nature. For humans struggling to control the world around them this submission of mind to reality was an effective strategy for aligning beliefs with the phenomena they modelled, maximizing their accuracy and predictive power. Earthquakes, volcanoes, and many other features of nature are not susceptible to wishful thinking by humans, so learning to predict their dangers allows us to accommodate them better (or live with the risk).

I call this option the Athenian path. The ancient Greeks' goddess of wisdom—powerfully armed and skilled in the arts of life, adept at persuasion, yet yielding to the commands of Zeus, king of the gods—seems a fitting symbol for the mind which adapts to a world it cannot control. It is this flexibility which holds the key to science's achievements, allowing it to develop ever more accurate models, more powerful predictions, and hence more efficient technologies. It is the strength of a web of provisionally trusted beliefs, not the brittle strength of rigidly held convictions; once again, dogmatism should have no place in science. An Athenian thinker can relinquish even the longest-held scientific belief, should the evidence demand it. My Greek dictionary is silent on the etymology of 'Athene', but it is tempting to speculate that the word comes from 'thein' ($\theta\acute{\eta}\nu$), 'expressing strong conviction', since the prefix a- negates the meaning of what follows.[4] 'No strong convictions' leaves room for open-mindedness, an essential ingredient of research advances. Athenian science is science as wisdom.

Discarding a cherished belief, however, can be intensely painful, especially when a person feels under threat; most people find it easier to defend their favourite ideas than to abandon them. If an experiment fails to produce the desired result, researchers will at the very least run extensive equipment checks and come up with a slew of modifications to their original ideas in order to explain the apparent contradiction. A few will go further and falsify their data rather than abandon their hypotheses. (How many cases of scientific fraud exist we do not know. It rarely comes to public attention, either because science attracts only superlative human beings or because scientists and their regulatory bodies haven't to date paid all that much attention to wrongdoing in the ranks.)

There is also a third way of reconciling beliefs to painful facts: the process I have elsewhere called world-shaping.[5] This occurs when, instead of changing the belief to match observed reality, a person changes reality to fit his or her ideas of what it should be.

This is the engineer's choice, technology. Its benefits, as we know, have been immense. The Greeks' embodiment of this very human tendency to change what is, because of ideas about what might be, was Prometheus, who brought fire—and hence freedom—to mankind. The etymology is again revealing: 'promeitheis' ($\pi\rho o\mu\eta\theta\acute{\eta}s$) meant being provident, having forethought. Such forethought implies a mental model, and that in turn implies that sometimes such models may be preferred to the world they do not accurately represent. If you can see ahead to what may be coming, you can use the intervening time to change the future.[6] Promethean science is science as mastery.

Fire tamed made survival easier, leaving time to think, observe, and predict the natural world. Athene the observational scientist adapted our ancestors to a world they could not control; Prometheus the engineer allowed them to begin to control it. Both capacities left early humans with spare time and energy, and this leisure allowed them to set out on the path of technology, dreaming of how their surroundings might be different. Now the brain supremacy will turn the Promethean fire on the dreamers themselves. We can already buy cosmetic surgery to alter our appearance and pills to help with minds and moods—but these are only crude attempts at interference. Soon, if we can afford it, we may be able to change ourselves and our children in ways which have never before been possible.

The key question for the brain supremacy is whether we should do so, and how.

Changing human nature

Human nature has often resisted imposed change. Seeing the brain supremacy as providing tools to overcome that obstacle, improving oneself—and others—on demand, assumes that such alteration is not only possible (with negligible ill effects), but beneficial and morally desirable. Who is best placed to judge these benefits? The individual modified? What if that person wants to enhance traits we find morally repugnant? Yet if not the individual, who? We are affected by the choices of others, so perhaps we should be allowed to influence them, especially if they are likely to do us harm.

This is the central dilemma coiled at the heart of Western liberalism: how to treat people who hate and despise your ideals. Should we tolerate the intolerant, accept all comers to the marketplace of ideas, and offer freedom of belief to those whose beliefs revolt us? We may have become better at managing the language of diversity, but we haven't removed the underlying instincts of hostility to people who choose to be different. As globalization shrinks the world we lose our power to pretend they don't exist. Then we are at risk of succumbing to otherization, the suite of ancient, visceral responses to threatening strangers which evolved to protect ingroup members and exploit outsiders.[7] That way lies trouble: stereotyping, harassment, social exclusion, collective punishment, and all manner of injustice, in extreme cases up to and including murder.[8]

The brain supremacy promises an alternative solution. If someone intends to do you harm, change their intention. If they wish to destroy your degenerate way of life, adjust their desire. If they believe you are evil, change their belief. You will need to do so without their consent, of course, but only until they have been brought to understand your point of view. Then they will see that you acted in their best interests as well as your own. (If this promise is even partially fulfilled, it will make the methods described in my first book, *Brainwashing*, look feeble by comparison.)

Whether science can deliver that solution, no one can currently predict. We are just beginning to learn how to alter memories, with and without drugs; we do not yet know how to break down strong beliefs by brain manipulation.[9] But once the possibility has been imagined it cannot be un-thought, and its potential advantages make it very desirable. The goal of precision brain change—and all the failed attempts along the way—has inspired much work already, and that will continue.

Much depends, once again, on what we try to change. Human traits and brain states vary in terms of how malleable they are, from fleeting thoughts and easily abandoned false beliefs through to habits, learned responses, instinctive reactions, and the structural features of temperament and personality. We can think of these as having been formed at different times, from evolutionarily moulded instincts like the vomiting reflex, through traits like trustfulness which are shaped in childhood, to the learned routines of adult work. The earlier these characteristics are set—the more they correspond to what we think of as human nature—the more drastic and/or earlier manipulations may have to be to change them.

The most grandiose claims of the brain supremacy are that one day it may alter our deepest traits. Not just to modify traumatic memories, but to make human memory more efficient and controllable. Not just to ease the symptoms of depression, but to cure personality disorders. Not just to challenge traditional views of the self, but to give us the tools to change that self's foundations, should we choose.

Another important question is how—and on whom—these techniques would be initially tested and used? History gives a grim answer: on volunteers, yes, but also on enemies, or patients unable to give informed consent, or social outcasts.[10] That must change. Brain research, more than most sciences, needs a good memory for past mistakes, given the power to which it offers access.

This is why the brain supremacy will be different from previous scientific revolutions. They have changed us mightily, but indirectly. Our attempts to solve the hardest problems facing our species have become ever more dependent on science and technology, and many people blame science and technology for creating yet more alarmingly serious problems.[11] Without the internal combustion engine, the plastics industries, our other demands for oil, and above all our increasing population—so the argument goes—the planet would be fine, instead of under visible and growing strain.[12]

Yet we rely on Prometheus, expecting technological solutions to all our problems. Indeed, the roots of our difficulties spring less from technofixes than from the Promethean psychology of millions of individuals seeking ways to reduce their anxieties and boost their feelings of control.[13] We the people insist on free choice, yet yearn to be like others. We expect an unending flow of novelties, yet want everything to be both cheap and harmless. We tend to think in short-term, self-centred fashion, and we are fiercely averse to any losses or restrictions imposed by others. If we were once, at base, apes with extra capacities (most obviously language), now we are apes with iPods, our extra capacities even more enhanced—and expensive.

Unfortunately, our resources are more limited than our desires. As the physicist Stephen Hawking has remarked, if we carry on as we are, 'It will be difficult enough to avoid disaster on planet Earth in the next hundred years'.[14] His preferred solution is travel to other planets, but that simply replicates the problem across space. To solve it once and for all, we need to return to the more scientific, Athenian approach, and instead of world-shaping shape ourselves to fit the world's constraints (see Figure 19). But that goes against very powerful instincts.

Since most writers on brain enhancement are scientists or philosophers, it is hardly surprising that the capacities most frequently mentioned as possible targets are precisely those Promethean skills which underlie science and technology, like intelligence and memory. The irony of the brain supremacy, however, is that it could give us the tools to make us more Athenian—better scientists, less emotional about our convictions, and readier to accept our limitations—by undermining the Promethean instincts which have brought us our past achievements and current predicament.

Within my lifetime we may develop the ability to alter facets of human nature such as empathy, aggression, conformity, the desire for control, and the tendency to compare oneself with others. Surgery could reduce the desire for control, for example, or a pill could artificially satisfy it. Using such methods, we may be able to modulate emotional responses before they drown out the smaller, saner voices on the brain's decision-making committees. We may find ways of moderating hubris and dogmatism (though whether the people who most need them would take the treatments is another matter). And we may be able to make our brains more manageable, able to review their ideas and abandon any which are out of date, inflexibly grounded in unhelpful emotions, or otherwise causing problems. In other words, the brain supremacy could make us all more scientific.

Perhaps even more crucially, we may be able to rebalance our reward systems, so that certain kinds of pleasure lose their appeal (like drugs and tobacco) and others (like getting a hug) produce a warmer glow. Much depends on whether the techniques for making

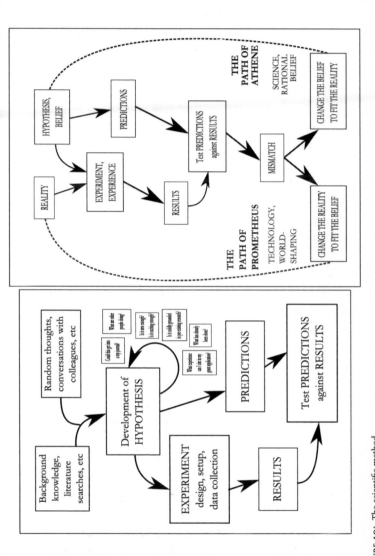

FIGURE 19: The scientific method.

In the left image, arrows indicate typical sequences of events, although in practice constraints at any stage can influence others (for example, restrictions on available equipment may require the researcher to rethink which predictions are tested). The right image shows a simplified outline of the method, together with the two options available when experimental results conflict with a prediction. On the left is the path of Prometheus, or world-shaping: the technological choice to adjust some aspect of reality in order to make it better fit a mental model. On the right is the path of Athene, or wisdom: the scientific choice to adjust hypotheses about the world in order to make them better fit perceived reality.

such changes, which may initially become available for clinical use on individuals, can then be applied more crudely to humans en masse. What could the power to revalue the hunger for money, status, or belonging do to Western society? Should we use such power on our enemies, our leaders, or ourselves? With less of the drive to control and change the world—including the social world of other people—would humanity be better off, or worse?

This is why neuroscience is of critical interest to anyone with a stake in the current modus vivendi of consumer capitalism. We could make ourselves even more enslaved to the forces which currently dictate our destiny, but we also have the chance to make genuine improvements to the human species. Either option is potentially dangerous, since brains are so complex that the law of unintended consequences will forcefully apply. This revolution needs to be handled with care.

Preparing for the future

Earning trust requires more than just focusing on the science.
We have to communicate it effectively too

(Paul Nurse, president of the Royal Society)

To be ready for the coming changes we need to be prepared to look carefully, sometimes critically, at neuroscience and its place in society. One obvious problem is that at present neuroscientists, like scientists in general, are very unrepresentative of the public they serve—and which provides their research material. Science is about accurately reflecting reality, and for the science of the brain supremacy that must include the nuances of social reality.

A minor but illuminating example comes from a TV documentary on negative perceptions of science, 'Science under Attack', presented by the President of the Royal Society, Sir Paul Nurse.[15] In a programme asking why the public doesn't trust science, his expert interviewees were exclusively white males, though he did exchange a few words with two women—one black, one white, both waitresses—and a male

Asian taxi driver. The unstated implication is clear: scientific authority has not yet been transferred from high-status men to females and ethnic minorities, and science has not yet escaped its history as a gentleman's club.[16] Could this exclusivity have something to do with the lack of public trust? (Some negative perceptions of science can be accurate, even when the perceivers are not themselves trained scientists.)

Visibly bringing more varied personnel into science's upper strata, where they can be seen to exert authority instead of waiting on it, is likely to broaden the profession's appeal. It would surely also be good for science, with new voices and different backgrounds bringing new ways of thinking. A white heterosexual male researcher may be just as technically adept at investigating social problems as his minority counterparts. However, such a researcher, especially one operating under the common but mistaken belief that his powers of reasoning make him less prone to psychological biases (a delusion so widespread that psychologists call it the fundamental attribution error), may not even perceive the existence of the problems. A woman, a transgender or disabled person, or a working-class lad adversely affected by social phenomena may be more likely to identify the problems, and more motivated to spend the time researching them.

Yet *pace* Stephen Hawking disabled scientists are rare, as are non-heterosexual and working-class scientists, and high-profile women researchers (Figure 20 shows sample data for women).[17] The precise quotient of minorities needed to make science more representative is not the point at issue; any improvement would be welcome. My argument is rather that worrying about perceptions of science can imply that the problem lies with the perceivers, instead of in the ranks of science itself. It doesn't. Research into human nature—and the crucial decision-making about which studies to pursue—is currently done by a marginal subset of humans. That needs to change.

As many scientific commentators have remarked, more political engagement, more awareness of media strategies, and especially more awareness, debate, and understanding of science are also urgently

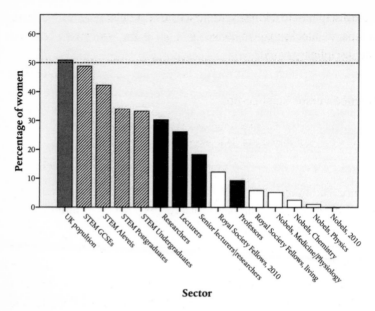

Sector

FIGURE 20: Women in science.

The graph shows the proportion of female participants in science at various levels, with the dashed horizontal line indicating equality (50%). For ease of comparison most measures are for the UK. The leftmost bar (solid grey) shows the proportion of women in the UK population. The next four bars (striped) show UK female participation in science, technology, engineering, and medical (STEM) subjects at four levels of education: the GCSE (age 16), the A-level (age 18), and undergraduate and postgraduate university degrees. The four solid black bars give proportions for UK academic scientists: researchers, lecturers, senior staff, and professors. Finally, the white bars indicate female participation in two of science's top accolades: election to a Royal Society Fellowship (UK) and winning a Nobel Prize (worldwide). As seniority rises, the percentage of women decreases.

required. Better science teaching, in schools and beyond, is a priority. For example, the UK national curriculum talks of 'Life processes and living things', 'Materials and their properties', and 'Physical processes' rather than the biology, chemistry, and physics of my teenage exams; but the artificial boundaries remain.[18] Yet as this book has shown, researchers need to bring together methods and principles from all three disciplines to address specific scientific problems. Teaching them in separate blocks may be convenient, but is it appropriate in today's interdisciplinary world?

Science versus science-lite

Scientific truth is too beautiful to be sacrificed
for the sake of light entertainment or money

(Richard Dawkins, biologist)

Science communication could also make itself more effective by abandoning its apparent belief that people are only interested in science if enough gimmicks are laid on and enough complexities airbrushed out. People like answers to 'why' and 'how' questions that stretch their minds; we are a curious species. Science communication for adults—teaching beyond school—could also benefit from less of a youth focus. Radio Four's *In Our Time*, which regularly tackles scientific topics in some depth, achieves weekly audiences of over two million, so it can be done.[19]

If you want to understand how brains work and you don't have a relevant background, science-lite reports are not much help. Nor are the research papers they draw upon. The concepts involved are not necessarily hard in themselves; brain research is not quantum mechanics, though it sometimes uses it. But they require deep context: large amounts of background information which few people have the time to go through. Science-lite is flourishing for the same reason prostitution does: both offer fun without commitment. Science, on the other hand, is hard work.

Unfortunately, science-lite, with its brevity and its emphasis on findings, tends to promote the idea that research is easier and more fun than we might think. This science con—the myth we feed our young that science is all about exciting ideas and startling discoveries—implies that the necessary boring toil can be downplayed or bypassed altogether. It can't. Flicking data round cyberspace is fine, but the notion that it can substitute for lengthy, sometimes mind-numbing labour is as misplaced in science as in, say, nursing or mining. Research has its glorious moments, but it is often unavoidably dull, frustrating, and beset by bureaucracy. It can also be infuriatingly political and viciously competitive. The chances of fame and riches are low compared with many other professions, and the work, despite its annoyances, has an addictive quality which makes it voraciously demanding of time, effort, and life-energies.

The science con leads youngsters to think they could be the next Einstein. In practice they've more chance of winning the lottery.[20] Even getting a job at postdoctoral level can prove impossible, given the competition; and this results in a lot of highly trained people being made to feel like failures through no fault of their own.[21] The science con also hides, and therefore devalues, the expertise, time, and energy which goes into research. No wonder people complain that science is expensive, when they are never shown the effort it takes.

The science con may be useful in the short term for raising the public profile of science, but its long-term effects may not be so positive. Furthermore, whether it succeeds in bridging the gap between science and the public is debatable.[22] And that gap must be bridged if we are to handle the brain supremacy, which will involve the most complicated science that humanity has yet encountered. To achieve this, we need to move away from the science con. Instead of presenting research as easy and fun, scientists, the media, teachers, and government will need to emphasize its challenging and even elitist nature as a difficult and expensive exercise—which happens to teach some very useful life skills and to be hugely rewarding in itself.

Accessibility, in the age of the internet, need not mean dumbing down. There are plenty of specialist sites offering science tutorials for any level, from absolute beginner to postdoc and beyond. Science is something anyone can learn about, though not without effort. What makes it appear to recede into the Olympian realm of genius is its immense specialization, in discourse and practices. Yet once the dragon of jargon has been domesticated by familiarity (and good communication), we find that many of the core ideas are surprisingly simple, though they combine to produce complexities unfathomable by even the greatest scientists.[23] To get those ideas across requires contributions from governments and the media, researchers and science communicators, and of course an interested, well-informed public.

Being more realistic about science will only work if the cultural norms surrounding science change. In the eighteenth century, cultural norms saw scientific talks as fashionable events, and great thinkers of the day, even in the arts, were expected to be abreast of the latest research.[24] Today science is still marketed as entertainment, but scientists often complain that ignorance of science is acceptable in a way that ignorance of literature or politics would not be. Ignorance, of course, is not in itself a problem, *if* the person is willing to learn. When society's public figures show some basic acquaintance with science— and regard their knowledge as unremarkable—then science will garner the status that its defenders feel it deserves.

More importantly, the brain supremacy will gain the scrutiny it needs, with far greater public understanding of just what it is that neuroscientists do and the fabulous neuromethods with which they do it. Many scientists hope that a more scientifically literate public will mean more support for generous science budgets, but may not be so keen on the increase in criticism which may accompany it. Yet why should the public not have more of a say in funding decisions? Why should they not have more knowledge and control of how science is regulated, used, and sometimes distorted by governments and corporations? In a society where the membership criteria for elite scientific bodies, the candidates for top prizes, the biggest grants, and even misconduct cases were as readily discussed as their equivalents in business, the arts or politics, the brain supremacy would be more likely to offer benefits to many, rather than to the usual powerful few.

We are living on the edge of a transformative era. The brain supremacy will enhance or supplant old understandings of selves, human relationships, moral codes, and even what is and is not real. Oh brave new world, that has such science in it!—and the promise of so much more to come. The choice of *how* it will change us, of whether it follows Prometheus or Athene, belongs to every citizen, not just to scientists, business leaders, and governments. Yet so few members of the public take part in public events and debates on science that citizens' opinions can be drowned out by more powerful vested interests. On the plus side, anyone wanting to alter the course of the brain supremacy will be able to make a considerable difference.

The brain supremacy belongs to all of us. We can accept its gifts, or leave them for others to exploit. The choice is ours. Now is the time to make it.

More about the Figures

Figures 1a-c: Data are from the publicly available Google N-grams corpus of books published in English. The dataset includes about 360 billion English words and comprises about 4% of all published books (Michel et al., 2011). The time-span of 1900–2008 was chosen because nineteenth-century usage of 'neuroscience' is minimal, and because the dataset was produced in mid-2009. Graphs were retrieved, with smoothing set to zero, from http://ngrams.googlelabs.com/. They were manually digitized using the open-source programme Engauge (http://sourceforge.net/projects/digitizer/) and reconstructed using SPSS (http://www.spss.com/uk/). For further details see Google's website or the article by Michel and colleagues.

Figure 1d: Data are from the LexisNexis database, http://www.lexisnexis.co.uk/ (search criteria were: US news, duplicates off, 'neuroscience' in headline).

Figure 4: The images originate in Brodmann (1909), known as 'Localisation in the Cerebral Cortex'; see also the English translation (Brodmann, 1994). Courtesy of Wikimedia/Creative Commons licence.

Figure 6: Neuroimaging coordinates are given as points in a 3-D space (x, y, z). The x dimension (medial/lateral) is positive towards the right and negative towards the left of the brain. The y dimension (anterior/posterior) is positive towards the front and negative towards the back of the brain. The z dimension (superior/inferior) is positive towards the top and negative towards the bottom of the brain. Images were generated using MRIcron (http://www.cabiatl.com/mricro/mricron/index.html).

Figure 20: Data are taken from the UK government's office for National Statistics, the Royal Society and Nobel Prize websites (http://royalsociety.org/, http://nobelprize.org/) and Kirkup et al. (2010). Note that the graph is for illustrative purposes only, since the periods spanned by the measures vary:

the population data is from 2007, the GCSE and A-level data from 2009, the Royal Society and Nobel data are as of 2010, the overall Nobel laureate counts include the period 1901–2010, and all other data are from the academic year 2007–8.

Plate 4B: The word reading task involved showing 20 volunteers a succession of single words ('targets' such as 'COMET'). Each trial (presentation of the target) was preceded by a blank screen and followed by a 'resting' interval during which the participant kept their gaze on a single, central point, marked by a cross. The task was to read the word silently, pressing a button whenever it was the name of an animal. (Peter Hansen, personal communication.)

In fact the experimenters were not interested in how well participants knew their natural history, but in the earliest stages of brain processing during word recognition. To study this rapid response a technique called priming was used, which works as follows. Shortly before the target word is presented, an identically-pronounced non-word ('komet'), is very briefly shown to the participant. This 'prime' is not itself consciously perceived, yet it changes the person's reaction to the target word. For instance, an English reader can interpret the word 'bank' differently when primed with the words 'money' or 'river', even though the reader doesn't consciously 'see' the prime itself.

To make sure that the prime is not perceived, a masking stimulus of the same size as the target and prime (#####) is presented immediately before and after the prime. Because the prime is shown so very briefly, what the participant sees is a blank screen, followed by the mask, followed by the target. Masking works due to a curious feature of human brains: unlike computers, they do not process each input independently and accurately. Rather, each stimulus affects how the one immediately before it is presented. For very brief stimuli, like a prime (presented for only 60 ms in this study), showing a mask immediately afterwards can interfere with processing to such an extent that it prevents the prime from being consciously seen at all.

In the experimental condition shown in the image above, the targets were five letter words (e.g. 'COMET') and the primes were non-words pronounced in the same way as the target but spelled differently (e.g. 'komet'). On each individual trial, the mask (#####) was shown for half a second (500 milliseconds), followed by the prime (60 ms), the mask again (for 16 ms), and the target (for 300 ms). The image shows intense activity in visual (occipital) cortex, as well as in frontal areas associated with speech production. Data are compared with a resting condition.

Plate 4C: The image was 95% desaturated using www.picnik.com.

Plate 5: Note that the MEG analysis was done separately for a range of frequencies. The image shown in the plate is for the beta frequency band (15–25 Hz). For further details see Wheat et al. (2010); also note 18, Chapter 8.

Glossary

5-HT—serotonin, a **neurotransmitter** involved in, among other things, mood and anxiety.

5-HT$_{1A}$ receptor—one of a number of subtypes of serotonin **receptor**. It can function either as an **autoreceptor** or as a **heteroreceptor**.

acetylation—a chemical reaction, involving an acetyltransferase enzyme, which adds an acetyl group ($COCH_3$) to a molecule. In epigenetics, histone acetylation is associated with increasing **gene expression**.

action potential—an explosive change in the electrical potential across a **neuron**'s surface membrane, which is transmitted along the cell to a **synapse**, where it triggers the release of **neurotransmitter**.

ASL—arterial spin labelling, an **MRI**-derived method of measuring cerebral blood flow. It makes use of the fact that blood flowing into brain tissue changes the magnetic status of that tissue.

autoreceptor—a **receptor** for a **neurotransmitter** which is located on the 'sender' cell (the one emitting the neurotransmitter), thereby providing a feedback signal which influences the cell's activity and release of neurotransmitter. See also **heteroreceptor**.

BOLD—blood-oxygen-level dependent, a term used to describe the signal detected by an **fMRI** scanner, which reflects the change from oxygenated to deoxygenated blood as active **neurons** consume oxygen.

cerebrospinal fluid (CSF)—sometimes referred to as the extracellular volume, this liquid permeates the brain and allows for the movements of electrical charges in and out of cells which constitute neuronal signalling.

CERN—the European Organization for Nuclear Research (*Conseil Européen pour la Recherche Nucléaire*), which runs the **Large Hadron Collider**.

cortex (pl. cortices)—the outer layer of a brain, also known as grey matter, made up of **neurons** and their cross-connections. Long-distance connections between different brain areas form the inner 'white matter'. In human brains the cortex is typically made up of six layers.

CT—computer tomography, one of the older neuroimaging methods, related to the X-ray.

desensitization (of **receptors**)—a process in which a **neuron**'s receptors become less responsive to their stimulating molecules following high levels of stimulation.

DNA—deoxyribonucleic acid, a complex molecule made up of sugar molecules linked together by phosphate groups (PO_4^{3-}) and cross-linked to a second sugar-phosphate chain by the four bases adenosine (A), thymine (T), guanine (G), and cytosine (C) to form the double helix which encodes genetic information.

DNE—digitised neural experience, information about neural function and subjective experience capable of being stored, transmitted, and manipulated by potential future technologies.

dopamine—a **neurotransmitter**, involved among other things in movement and cognition. Dysfunction of dopamine-producing **neurons** is thought to be the primary problem in Parkinson's disease.

doxycycline—an antibiotic, chemically similar to tetracycline, used in genetic manipulation.

DTI—diffusion tensor imaging, a technique derived from **MRI** which measures diffusion of water along neuronal fibres in the brain.

ecological validity—a measure of how realistic a laboratory experiment is.

EEG—electroencephalography, a technique for recording the electrical emissions, or 'brain waves', given off by active brain regions.

electrophysiology—the investigation of (in this context) brain function using electrical recording and stimulation.

epigenetics—a science developed to explain why genetics has cost so much and (so far) delivered so little in the way of useful medical treatment. Epigenetics studies the physiological mechanisms which regulate **gene expression**.

false positive—an apparently significant result where in fact there is none. For example, pregnancy tests sometimes indicate that a woman is pregnant when she is not.

fluorodeoxyglucose (FDG)—a radioactive molecule used in **PET** scanning to monitor neuronal glucose consumption, a proxy measure for brain activity.

fMRI—functional magnetic resonance imaging, a neuroimaging method for 'looking inside' living human brains. See **MRI**.

gamma-ray emission—the production of high-energy radiation from a collision between a positron and an electron. Gamma rays are produced and monitored in **PET** scanning when radioactive tracer molecules decay and emit positrons.

gene expression—the set of processes whereby a cell 'reads off' a gene to build a product (usually a protein). See also **transcription**.

glia (also called glial cells, microglia)—often thought of as a 'support system' for **neurons**, providing nutrients and maintaining the brain's chemical balance. However, recent studies suggest that glia play a more active role in brain signalling than was previously thought.

glycolysis—a chemical reaction in which glucose is decomposed, releasing energy to fuel cell metabolism.

Golgi stain—a technique for staining brain tissue which has been preserved ('fixed'), e.g. using formaldehyde, by applying potassium dichromate and silver nitrate. The result highlights only a few cells, allowing their structure to be seen in detail.

heteroreceptor—a **receptor** protein embedded in the membrane of a 'recipient' cell, i.e. one stimulated by the release of **neurotransmitter** from a nearby **neuron**. See also **autoreceptor**.

histology—the study of small-scale brain anatomy (e.g. cell types, cortical layers); also, the preparation of brain samples post mortem, for example to confirm where a microelectrode was placed during an experiment.

horseradish peroxidase (HRP)—an enzyme which can be used to stain **neurons**, which readily absorb it and transport it along their axons.

hydroxyl group—a negatively charged ion made up of oxygen and hygdrogen (formula OH^-). Water (H_2O) in brain tissue tends to disassociate into hydroxyl groups and protons (H^+).

IMCOTT—'It's more complicated than that'.

ion channel—a protein built around a hole, or pore, through which ions like sodium, calcium, or chloride can pass under certain conditions. Ion channels are found in neuronal cell membranes, and allow **neurons** to control and modify the electrical potential across the membrane.

Large Hadron Collider (LHC)—one of the world's most impressive scientific machines, a particle accelerator designed to test predictions of theoretical physics.

MEG—magnetoencephalography, a neuroimaging technique which measures magnetic fields emitted by living brains.

methylation—a chemical reaction which adds a methyl group (CH_3) to a molecule. In epigenetics, DNA methylation is associated with reduced levels of **gene expression**.

MRI—a neuroimaging technique which uses strong magnetic fields and radio pulses to map changes in the magnetisation of protons in brain tissues. The same principles are also used in **fMRI**, and in variants such as **DTI** and **ASL**.

neurogenetics—the scientific study of the roles of genes in the brain, often using transgenic animals to test hypotheses about how genes affect neuronal function.

neuron—a brain cell. Neurons maintain an electrical potential across the cell membrane, which can be altered by the activation of **receptors** and **ion channels** in the membrane, and which forms the electrical basis of signals transmitted between cells via **synapses**.

neurotransmitter—a substance released by a **neuron** into its **synapses** which is able to bind to **receptors** on nearby cells, thereby transferring a signal from one neuron to another.

NIH—the National Institutes of Health, the US government organisation responsible for funding biomedical research.

Nissl stain—a cell staining technique which highlights **RNA**, and hence shows details of the cell body. It was developed by Franz Nissl (1860–1919).

optical imaging—a set of imaging techniques which work by shining light (e.g. from a laser) through brain tissue and measuring the extent of interference. Different chemicals absorb photons to different extents, and active **neurons** and **glia** scatter photons differently from inactive cells, and these observations are used to compute an image of the brain tissue.

optogenetics—the manipulation of cell function using light, and specially engineered genes which code for light-sensitive **ion channel** proteins.

PET—positron emission tomography, one of the older neuroimaging methods. It uses radioactive tracer molecules, injected into the body, to monitor brain biochemistry.

PFC—prefrontal cortex, the area of brain traditionally associated with our highest cognitive functions.

phase-locking—the process of synchronisation whereby **neurons** which are active simultaneously adjust their production of **action potentials** so that they come to fire 'in sync' and at the same frequency.

phosphorylation—a chemical reaction which adds a phosphate group (formula $PO_4{}^{3-}$) to a molecule, such as glucose.

promoter—a segment of **DNA** located near a gene which regulates **gene expression**.

receptor—a specialised protein embedded in a **neuron**'s surface membrane which changes shape when activated by a **neurotransmitter** molecule. Receptors can be either inhibitory (activation makes the cell less likely to fire) or excitatory (activation increases the chances of the cell firing). Both types can be activated by the same neurotransmitter. Receptors can also be presynaptic (located on the cell emitting the neurotransmitter) or postsynaptic (located on the recipient cell).

RNA—ribonucleic acid, an important intermediate step in **gene expression**. Gene **transcription** 'reads off' a cell's **DNA** to produce RNA, which is then 'translated' into protein (or in some cases other) products. RNA is similar to **DNA** in structure, although the base thymine (T) is replaced by uracil (U).

spatial resolution—when viewing an object, the amount of detail available to a method; how far it can 'zoom in'. For example, histological techniques have higher spatial resolution than neuroimaging methods like **fMRI**, because modern microscopes can see deep inside a single cell whereas **fMRI** cannot distinguish individual **neurons**.

SQUID—superconducting quantum interference device, the key component of a magnetoencephalography (**MEG**) scanner.

superconducting metal—a metal in which resistance to the flow of electrical current has dropped to zero.

synapse—a tiny gap between two neighbouring **neurons**, across which **neurotransmitter** is released to send signals between them. The synaptic cleft contains numerous molecules, including **receptors** on the recipient cell which detect the neurotransmitter release, transporter molecules which help to recycle neurotransmitter, and so on.

temporal resolution—when observing a phenomenon which changes over time, the smallest unit of time over which a difference can be detected. For example, temperature records measured once every day have a temporal resolution of 24 hours, in that they cannot detect any fluctuations during a single day. In neuroimaging, **MEG** and **EEG** have higher temporal resolution than **fMRI** and **PET**.

TES—transcranial electrical stimulation, a set of techniques for stimulating the brain electrically through the skull (see also note 2, Chapter 11).

*tet*O—the tetracycline operator, a segment of **DNA** useful in **neurogenetics** because it is regulated by antibiotics such as tetracycline and **doxycycline**, allowing **gene expression** to be controlled in experimental animals merely by changing the levels of antibiotic in an animal's diet.

TMS—transcranial magnetic stimulation, a method of brain stimulation which applies a focused magnetic field through the skull.

transcription (of genes)—a biochemical process which converts **DNA** into **RNA**. It is one of the steps in **gene expression**.

tTS—tetracycline-dependent Transcriptional Suppressor, a protein which can be used to suppress **transcription**, conditionally on the presence of antibiotics such as tetracycline and **doxycycline**.

two-photon imaging—a method of precisely controlling where and when a substance is released in brain tissue. The substance in question, e.g. the **neurotransmitter** glutamate, is chemically bound to 'caging compounds'. These bonds are dissolved when ultraviolet light is applied, thus releasing the glutamate.

volume currents—also called secondary currents, these are electrical flows generated in the **cerebrospinal fluid** in response to 'primary' currents flowing within **neurons**.

voxel—a unit of volume used in neuroimaging, a cubical 3D equivalent of the pixel. Brain scans are divided into voxels to facilitate analysis, standardization, and comparison. One voxel contains around 100,000 **neurons**.

List of websites

Websites mentioned in the notes and figure legends are given here in alphabetical order of topic. The number of the source note or figure is given in brackets.

Alcmaeon and Anaxagoras
Alcmaeon of Croton—http://plato.stanford.edu/entries/alcmaeon/ (note 5, Chapter 5)
Anaxagoras of Clazomenae—http://history.hanover.edu/texts/presoc/anaxagor.html (note 5, Chapter 5)

Animal research
Understanding Animal Research
—http://www.understandinganimalresearch.org.uk/ (note 26, Chapter 5)
Nature open-access resources on animal research—www.nature.com/news/specials/animalresearch/index.html (note 2, Chapter 10)

The Atlantic Salmon fMRI report
http://prefrontal.org/blog/2009/09/the-story-behind-the-atlantic-salmon/ (note 23, Chapter 7)

The BBC
Brain–computer interfacing—www.bbc.co.uk/news/technology-10647555 (note 27, Chapter 14)
Brain scans and marketing—http://news.bbc.co.uk/1/hi/sci/tech/8569087.stm (note 4, Chapter 1)
Michelle Roberts article on fMRI—http://news.bbc.co.uk/1/hi/health/8672400.stm (notes 10, Chapter 7; 13, Chapter 14).

Caenorhabditis elegans
http://www.wormbook.org/index.html (note 37, Chapter 14)
http://ims.dse.ibaraki.ac.jp/research/C_elegans_en.html (note 39, Chapter 14)

CERN
Standard Model—http://public.web.cern.ch/public/en/Science/StandardModel -en.html. (note 1, Chapter 6)
Large Hadron Collider—http://public.web.cern.ch/public/en/LHC/Milestones-en.html (note 3, Chapter 6)

David Chalmers on consciousness
http://consc.net/papers/facing.html (note 28, Chapter 8)

Chow (mouse food)
Prolab Isopro RMH 3000, available from PMI Nutrition International—http:// www.labdiet.com/pdf/5p75-5p76.pdf (note 22, Chapter 12)

Benjamin Crowell electron wavefunction image
http://www.lightandmatter.com/html_books/6mr/ch05/ch05.html (Figure 14)

Charles Darwin
Origin of Species—http://darwin-online.org.uk/pdf/1859_Origin_F373.pdf (note 25, Chapter 3)

Ronan Deazley, who studies legal issues surrounding photography
http://www.gla.ac.uk/schools/law/staff/ronandeazley/ (note 23, Chapter 3)

Mark Dow, artist
http://markdow.deviantart.com/art/Brain-Brodmann-43568326 (Plate 3)

Drosophila melanogaster
www.ceolas.org/fly/intro.html (note 37, Chapter 14)

EEG and MEG
http://www.mrc-cbu.cam.ac.uk/research/eeg/eeg_intro.html (note 2, Chapter 9)

Elements in the human body
http://chemistry.about.com/cs/howthingswork/f/blbodyelements.htm (note 4, Chapter 7)

Engauge digitizer
http://sourceforge.net/projects/digitizer/ (Figure 1)

Epigenetics journals
Epigenetics—www.landesbioscience.com/journals/epigenetics (note 19, Chapter 13)
Epigenetics and Chromatin—www.epigeneticsandchromatin.com (note 19, Chapter 13)

The Eurobarometer survey of public views of science

http://ec.europa.eu/public_opinion/archives/ebs/ebs_340_en.pdf (note 16, Chapter 4)

Eye surgery data

http://uk.opticalexpress.com/laser-eye-surgery/how-optical-express-compares-with-other-providers.html (note 24, Chapter 11)

Genetics—DNA transcription

RIKEN-OSC video (available via *Nature*)—www.youtube.com/user/Nature VideoChannel#p/a/u/1/J3HVVi2k2No (note 5, Chapter 12)

University of Utah interactive website—http://learn.genetics.utah.edu/content/begin/dna/transcribe/ (note 8, Chapter 12)

Glycolysis

http://glycolysis.co.uk/ (note 8, Chapter 6)

Google N-grams word frequency dataset

http://ngrams.googlelabs.com (Figure 1; note 10, Chapter 1)

The *Guardian*

Brain–computer interfacing—www.guardian.co.uk/science/2011/apr/17/brain-implant-paralysis-movement (note 27, Chapter 14)

EDGE report—www.guardian.co.uk/science/2011/jan/15/uncertainty-failure-edge-question (note 3, Chapter 12)

Genetics—www.guardian.co.uk/commentisfree/2011/apr/17/human-genome-genetics-twin-studies (note 31, Chapter 7)

Mortarboard blog—http://www.guardian.co.uk/education/mortarboard/2011/may/27/black-professor-shortage-failure-to-nurture-talent (note 17, Chapter 15)

Nanotechnology—www.guardian.co.uk/science/2003/apr/29/nanotechnology.science (note 31, Chapter 11)

Nature Video on connectomics—www.guardian.co.uk/science/video/2011/mar/09/brain-nerve-cells-connectomics (notes 18, Chapter 1; 30, Chapter 7)

Rockstrom sustainability report—www.guardian.co.uk/sustainable-business/living-above-our-limits (note 27, Chapter 4)

Science careers—www.guardian.co.uk/science/blog/2011/mar/18/career-science-studentship-phd-application (note 21, Chapter 15)

Stephen Hawking interview with *BigThink*

http://bigthink.com/ideas/21570 (note 14, Chapter 15)

Higher Education Statistics Agency (HESA)
www.hesa.ac.uk/index.php?option=com_content&task=view&id=1978&Ite-mid=278 (note 17, Chapter 15)

Ray Kurzweil
www.singularity.com/ (note 28, Chapter 4)

LexisNexis media database
www.lexisnexis.co.uk/ (Figure 1; note 10, Chapter 1)

Magnetism
Magnetic field strengths—www.spaceweather.com/glossary/imf.html (note 8, Chapter 9)
World Health Organisation information on electromagnetic emissions—www.who.int/peh-emf/about/WhatisEMF/en/index3.html (note 7, Chapter 9)

Magistretti chapter on brain metabolism
www.acnp.org/g4/gn401000064/ch064.html (note 7, Chapter 6)

'Marilyn Monroe' neurons
Nature News—www.nature.com/news/2010/101027/full/news.2010.568.html (note 1, Chapter 7)
TIME—http://newsfeed.time.com/2010/10/29/what-dreams-may-come-dream-recording-device-possible/#ixzz13rzjxYOQ (note 1, Chapter 7)
WIRED Science—www.wired.com/wiredscience/2010/10/brain-focus-recording/ (note 1, Chapter 7)

Albert Michelson, 'Light waves and their uses'
http://www.archive.org/details/lightwavesandthoomichgoog (note 21, Chapter 13)

MRIcron fMRI imaging software
http://www.cabiatl.com/mricro/mricron/index.html (Figure 6)

Thomas Nagel, 'What is it like to be a bat?'
http://evans-experientialism.freewebspace.com/nagel.htm (note 5, Chapter 4)

Nanotechnology
Guardian report—www.guardian.co.uk/science/2003/apr/29/nanotechnology.science (note 31, Chapter 11)
Center for Responsible Nanotechnology—www.crnano.org/dangers.htm (note 31, Chapter 11)
ETC Group—www.etcgroup.org/en/archives (note 31, Chapter 11)

National Health Service (NHS) neurosurgery data
www.nhs.uk/conditions/head-injury-severe-/pages/treatment.aspx (note 1, Chapter 10)
www.cks.nhs.uk/patient_information_leaflet/head_injury_minor (note 1, Chapter 10)

Nature
Animal research open-access resources—www.nature.com/news/specials/animalresearch/index.html (note 2, Chapter 10)

Connectomics video—www.guardian.co.uk/science/video/2011/mar/09/brain-nerve-cells-connectomics (notes 18, Chapter 1; 30, Chapter 7)

Genetics' Central Dogma video from RIKEN-OSC—www.youtube.com/user/NatureVideoChannel#p/a/u/1/J3HVVi2k2No (note 5, Chapter 12)

'Marilyn Monroe' neurons—www.nature.com/news/2010/101027/full/news.2010.568.html (note 1, Chapter 7)

Optogenetics video (from *Nature Methods*)—www.nature.com/nmeth/video/moy2010/index.html (note 2, Chapter 13)

Jennifer Rohn on science careers—www.nature.com/news/2011/110302/full/471007a.html (note 21, Chapter 15)

The Neurocritic blog
http://neurocritic.blogspot.com/2010/10/media-hsdd-hyperactive-sexual-disorder.html (note 27, Chapter 11)

Matthew Nisbet on science literacy
http://scienceblogs.com/framing-science/2007/07/the_misunderstood_meanings_of.php (note 22, Chapter 15)

Nobel Prizes
General—http://nobelprize.org/ (Figure 20; note 4, Chapter 6)

Golgi and Cajal—http://nobelprize.org/nobel_prizes/lists/year/?year=1906 (note 22, Chapter 5)

Brian Josephson—http://www.nobelprize.org/nobel_prizes/physics/laureates/1973/index.html (note 20, Chapter 9)

Numbers of prizes—http://nobelprize.org/nobel_prizes/lists/all/ (note 20, Chapter 15)

The Organisation for Economic Co-operation and Development (OECD)
http://stats.oecd.org/Index.aspx?DataSetCode=HEALTH (note 20, Chapter 7)

Parkinson's disease videos from Neuroslicer on YouTube
Before deep brain stimulation—http://youtu.be/xejclvwbwsk
After deep brain stimulation—http://youtu.be/IOHtUzWo2cg (note 19, Chapter 11)

PET scanning
PET imaging—http://sitemaker.umich.edu/pet.chemistry/positron_emission_tomography (note 8, Chapter 6)
PET radiation dose—http://rpop.iaea.org/RPOP/RPoP/Content/Information-For/HealthProfessionals/6_OtherClinicalSpecialities/PETCTscan.htm#PETCT_FAQo1 (note 6, Chapter 6)
PET scan prices—http://interactive.snm.org/index.cfm?PageID=972 (note 6, Chapter 6)

Picnik image software
www.picnik.com (Plate 4C)

Plato's *Phaedrus* from Project Gutenberg
www.gutenberg.org/ebooks/1636 (note 32, Chapter 7)

Population Data
Population Reference Bureau's 2010 World Population Data Sheet—www.prb.org/pdf10/10wpds_eng.pdf (note 26, Chapter 4)
Regional population data—www.citypopulation.de/index.html (notes 6, 8, Chapter 14)
US Census Bureau world population data—www.census.gov/ipc/www/idb/worldpop.php (notes 4, Chapter 2; 20, Chapter 15)
US Census Bureau world population clock—www.census.gov/main/www/popclock.html (note 8, Chapter 14)
Wikipedia on Cheltenham—http://en.wikipedia.org/wiki/List_of_English_districts_by_area#10_-_100_km.C2.B2 (note 9, Chapter 14)

The PubMed research database
www.ncbi.nlm.nih.gov/pubmed/ (note 1, Chapter 13)

Jennifer Rohn on science careers
www.nature.com/news/2011/110302/full/471007a.html (note 21, Chapter 15)

The Royal Society
General—http://royalsociety.org/ (Figure 20; notes 25, Chapter 6; 16, Chapter 15)
Brain Waves—http://royalsociety.org/brainwaves-security/ (note 22, Chapter 2)

Knowledge, Networks and Nations—http://royalsociety.org/policy/reports/knowledge-networks-nations/ (note 7, Chapter 2)

R.J. Rummel's democide website
https://www.hawaii.edu/powerkills/20TH.HTM (note 3, Chapter 2)

Julian Savulescu
www.practicalethics.ox.ac.uk/Pubs/Savulescu/enhancement.pdf (note 3, Chapter 4)

Science careers
The *Guardian*—www.guardian.co.uk/science/blog/2011/mar/18/career-science-studentship-phd-application (note 21, Chapter 15)
Jennifer Rohn in *Nature*—www.nature.com/news/2011/110302/full/471007a.html (note 21, Chapter 15)

The SCOPUS research database
www.scopus.com/ (needs a subscription) (notes 32, Chapter 12; 10, Chapter 14)

SIPRI (the Stockholm International Peace Research Institute)
www.sipriyearbook.org/view/9780199581122-gill/sipri-9780199581122-div1-16.xml (note 14, Chapter 4)

The Society for Neuroscience
www.sfn.org/skins/main/pdf/annual_report/fy2009/economy.pdf (note 10, Chapter 2)

SPSS
http://www.spss.com/uk/ (Figure 1)

Superconductivity
General—www.superconductors.org/ (note 17, Chapter 9)
Georgia State University's Hyperphysics site—http://hyperphysics.phy-astr.gsu.edu/hbase/hph.html (note 17, Chapter 9)
Room temperature superconductivity—www.physorg.com/news134828104.html (note 19, Chapter 9)

Talairach and MNI coordinates
http://imaging.mrc-cbu.cam.ac.uk/imaging/MniTalairach (note 18, Chapter 5)

TED Talks
Home page—www.ted.com/talks (note 22, Chapter 8)
Christopher deCharms—www.ted.com/talks/christopher_decharms_scans_the_brain_in_real_time.html (note 4, Chapter 14)

Tan Le—www.ted.com/talks/lang/eng/tan_le_a_headset_that_reads_your_
brainwaves.html (note 27, Chapter 14)

The *Daily Telegraph*
'Mind-reading' computers—www.telegraph.co.uk/science/science-news/
7421180/Telepathic-computer-can-read-your-mind.html (note 3, Chapter 1)
On science communication—http://www.telegraph.co.uk/culture/tvandradio/
8371699/Who-says-Britainis-dumbing-down.html (note 19, Chapter 15)
The suicide of Shaun Dykes—www.telegraph.co.uk/news/uknews/3108987/
Suicide-teenager-urged-to-jump-by-baying-crowd.html (note 8, Chapter 15)

Thalamus anatomy
University of Memphis—http://neuro.psyc.memphis.edu/neuropsyc/np-ugp-
thalamus.htm (note 13, Chapter 5)
The Brain from Top to Bottom—http://thebrain.mcgill.ca/flash/a/a_06/
a_06_cr/a_06_cr_mou/a_06_cr_mou.html (note 13, Chapter 5)

Tuskegee syphilis trial
The Tuskegee Syphilis Study Legacy Committee's report—http://www.hsl.vir-
ginia.edu/historical/medical_history/bad_blood/ (note 10, Chapter 15)

The UK Government
Department for Business, Innovation and Skills—www.dius.gov.uk/~/media/
publications/I/Internet-version-SET-Statistics-Nov-2009-v2 (note 11, Chapter 2)
The Office for National Statistics report on internet access—http://www.statis-
tics.gov.uk/pdfdir/iahinro810.pdf (note 21, Chapter 3)
The UK Science Curriculum—http://curriculum.qcda.gov.uk/key-stages-1-and-
2/subjects/science/keystage2/index.aspx (note 18, Chapter 15)

UK lottery odds
www.murderousmaths.co.uk/books/bkmm6xlo.htm (note 20, Chapter 15)

Vernor Vinge
www-rohan.sdsu.edu/faculty/vinge/misc/singularity.html (note 28, Chapter 4)

Wechsler Adult Intelligence Scales (WAIS)
www.pearsonassessments.com/haiweb/cultures/en-us/productdetail.htm?pid=
015-8980-808&Community=CA_Psych_Settings_Forensics (note 29, Chapter 14)

Wim Wenders, 'Unto the end of the world'
www.wim-wenders.com/movies/movies_spec/untiltheendoftheworld/un-
tiltheendoftheworld.htm (note 9, Chapter 3)

WIRED *Science*

Lobotomy—www.wired.com/wiredscience/2011/03/lobotomy-history (note 24, Chapter 2)

'Marilyn Monroe' neurons—www.wired.com/wiredscience/2010/10/brain-focus-recording/ (note 1, Chapter 7)

Optogenetics video—http://www.wired.com/wiredscience/2011/05/optogenetic-brain-video/ (note 3, Chapter 13)

Tu Pham ruling—www.wired.com/wiredscience/tag/tu-pham/ (note 18, Chapter 14)

The World Medical Association Declaration of Tokyo

www.wma.net/en/30publications/10policies/c18/index.html (note 18, Chapter 2)

X-ray information

X-ray radiation dose—www.radiologyinfo.org/en/pdf/sfty_xray.pdf (note 6, Chapter 6)

X-ray prices—http://blog.remakehealth.com/blog_Healthcare_Consumers-0/bid/8507/How-much-does-an-X-ray-cost (note 6, Chapter 6)

YouCut

www.majorityleader.gov/YouCut/ (note 28, Chapter 12)

Notes

Chapter 1

1. For more on the power of persuasion see Cialdini (2002) or my book *Brainwashing* (Taylor, 2006), which discusses the neuroscience and social psychology of persuasion and belief change.
2. See for example Batts (2009); Gozzi et al. (2010); Kanai et al. (2011); Stoeckel et al. (2008).
3. See http://www.telegraph.co.uk/science/science-news/7421180/Telepathic-computer-can-read-your-mind.html.
4. See http://news.bbc.co.uk/1/hi/sci/tech/8569087.stm, and Kato et al. (2009).
5. Pyysiäinen and Hauser (2010); Urgesi et al. (2010).
6. Wolf (2008).
7. Quirk and Milad (2010); Yoshida and Hirano (2010).
8. Boly et al. (2011); Deary et al. (2010); Schurger et al. (2010); Schwarzkopf and Rees (2010).
9. See for example Singer and Lamm (2009) and Fisher et al. (2005).
10. Data on book and newspaper content were taken from Google (http://ngrams.googlelabs.com/) and LexisNexis (http://www.lexisnexis.co.uk/).
11. Information about journal article numbers is taken from the bibliometric database of *Journal Citation Reports* (2004–2009).
12. For a recent review of work on modifying fear memories, see Maren (2011).
13. I discuss world-shaping at greater length in *Cruelty* (Taylor, 2009).
14. See for example Morgan III et al. (2009).
15. As a further illustration of how complicated neuroscience is turning out to be, there is evidence that the standard view of 'sender' neurons sending electrical signals down their axons and releasing neurotransmitters into synapses, where they bind to receptors on 'receiver' neurons, is too simplistic, because neurons seem also to emit neurotransmitter molecules from their axons; see Thyssen et al. (2010).

16. The saying 'neurons that fire together wire together' is often quoted in this context, so it is worth noting that 'together' need not mean 'simultaneously'. A recent study suggests, for instance, that in prefrontal cortex two types of receptors for the neurotransmitter dopamine may combine to stretch the time window during which 'wiring together'—learning-related changes in synapses—can occur. Activated in concert, these receptors extend the allowable gap between the first neuron and the second firing from around ten to about 30 milliseconds, giving neuronal connections more opportunity to form than was previously thought (Xu and Yao, 2010).

17. See for example Auger et al. (2011); Choi et al. (2011); Ford and Collins (2010); Goehler et al. (2007); Guyon et al. (2008); Heijtz et al. (2011); Kristensson (2011); Mélik-Parsadaniantz and Rostène (2008); Tracey (2011); Young and Korszun (2010).

18. For a visual insight into the complexities of the brain, see *Nature Video*'s commentary on two articles—Bock et al. (2011) and Briggman et al. (2011)—which is available at http://www.guardian.co.uk/science/video/2011/mar/09/brain-nerve-cells-connectomics; see also Pastrana (2011), a commentary on the same articles from *Nature Methods*.

19. Buchan (1935), p. 50.

20. Misinterpretation does not always start with the journalist; see for example Baron-Cohen (2009); Goldacre (2011a); Gonon et al. (2011).

21. For a similar approach with quantitative support, see Deslauriers et al. (2011).

22. The term 'brain scam' has been used; see for example Cordelia Fine's book on sex differences (Fine, 2010).

23. Maslow (1966), pp. 15–16.

24. See McCabe and Castel (2008), also Yarkoni et al. (2010): 'Most neuroimaging studies produce maps of brain regions that are activated by some process of interest. When researchers draw inferences about brain–behavior relationships from such maps, they often tacitly assume that these maps provide a relatively comprehensive and accurate picture of the true effects. Unfortunately, this assumption will probably fail in most cases.' Ouch! Moreover, the authority lent to explanations by neuroscience extends beyond its images to words; see Weisberg et al. (2008).

25. Taylor (2006); Taylor (2009).

26. The distinction between seeing the brain, in order to understand it, and changing the brain, while useful, is not absolute, but a fine line readily crossed. One often needs to change the brain to make its structures and behaviours more apparent, as both PET and fMRI do. Moreover, the

artificiality of a research lab will affect any brain being studied long before the machines begin their work.

Chapter 2

1. See for example any of a number of recent books commenting on human unreasonableness, flawed decision-making, statistical incompetence and so on, such as Sutherland (2007) or Ariely (2009).
2. Caramazza et al. (1981).
3. The number of dead is, of course, an estimate, covering the years 1900–1999. For a discussion of its limitations see Rummel (1997); for the revised data see R.J. Rummel's democide website at https://www.hawaii.edu/powerkills/20TH.HTM. Note that the figure excludes dead soldiers, peacetime homicides, and the damage caused by murder and by non-lethal violence. For an explanation as to why this is actually an improvement on previous centuries, in proportional if not in absolute terms, see Pinker (2011).
4. Population data are taken from the US Census Bureau (http://www.census.gov/ipc/www/idb/worldpop.php).
5. Whooping cough, caused by the bacterium *Bordetella pertussis*, is now preventable by vaccine and treatable by antibiotics.
6. See for example Niall Ferguson on Western values, Roy Porter on the Enlightenment, Elizabeth L. Eisenstein on the importance of printing, Jürgen Habermas on public debate, and Toby Huff on the spread of scientific knowledge (Ferguson, 2011; Porter, 2001; Eisenstein, 1980; Habermas, 1992; Huff, 2010). I am indebted to Gillian Wright for the Eisenstein and Porter references.
7. See for example a 2011 report on global science by the Royal Society, *Knowledge, Networks and Nations*, available from http://royalsociety.org/policy/reports/knowledge-networks-nations/.
8. More detail is available from the online paper Björk et al. (2008).
9. Kaku (1999). Terminology differs: the neurologist V.S. Ramachandran, for instance, talks of five revolutions. The first four involved Copernicus, Darwin, Freud and the science of genetics; the fifth, currently developing, will lead to what I call the brain supremacy. Ramachandran thereby puts our growing ability to transform human self-understanding on a par with the mightiest intellectual gear-changes in history.
10. This and the subsequent quotation are taken from the Society for Neuroscience's annual report, http://www.sfn.org/skins/main/pdf/annual_report/fy2009/economy.pdf.

11. Data was extracted from http://www.dius.gov.uk/~/media/publications/I/Internet-version-SET-Statistics-Nov-2009-v2.

12. I should add a caution: numerical evidence that science boosts the economy isn't as easy to get hold of as the statements imply. As a recent *Nature* editorial tartly put it, 'in the public arena, scientists should talk like scientists and desist from using dodgy numbers to bolster the already powerful case for research spending to be maintained, or even increased, during difficult economic times' (Nature Editorial, 2010b). See also MacIlwain (2010).

13. In February 2011 the UK government announced plans to cut neuroscience funding. See for example McNaughton and Robbins (2011).

14. See for example Dierolf et al. (2010), an example of the astonishing level to which X-ray tomography can now be taken.

15. Cartier et al. (2009).

16. Bardin et al. (2011); Monti et al. (2010).

17. For a sparkling introduction to the clinical terrain, see Ramachandran (2011).

18. The quotation is from the WMA Declaration of Tokyo—'Guidelines for physicians concerning torture and other cruel, inhuman or degrading treatment or punishment in relation to detention and imprisonment'. It was adopted by the 29th World Medical Assembly in October 1975, and can be accessed at http://www.wma.net/en/30publications/10policies/c18/index.html.

19. The *Oxford English Dictionary* defines 'kludge' by quoting the term's inventor, Jackson W. Granholm: 'An ill-assorted collection of poorly matching parts, forming a distressing whole'.

20. Apologies to any philosophers reading, for whom the term 'neural experience' will undoubtedly beg many questions. This book assumes a form of token–token physicalism, such that human brain activity—or perhaps in future an artificial equivalent provided by DNE recording—is essential for human minds to exist. (If you know of any aspect of a person's mental function that is unaffected by removing their nervous system, then please make your evidence public immediately.) On this view, individual patterns of neural activity are the physical substrate for individual mental events, though not all of these are experienced subjectively (Dehaene and Changeux, 2011; Wilson, 2002). Each pattern is unique and highly dynamic, but groups of patterns show features in common, allowing categories to form. In classic philosophical treatments of the mind–body problem identity tends to be absolute. In neuroscience it is statistical: two patterns of neural activity are judged to be identical if they match at the desired level of precision, even if a higher-resolution view shows differences. Neuroscience is pragmatic, and physicalism has worked well so far.

21. Bass et al. (2010); Claridge-Chang et al. (2009); Leifer et al. (2011); Stirman et al. (2011).
22. See for example http://royalsociety.org/brainwaves-security/.
23. Garnett et al. (2011); Illes et al. (2010).
24. Depatterning used repeated electric shocks to change beliefs, the idea being that the shocks would disrupt learned neural patterns, wiping the dysfunctional mental slate to allow for a fresh start. The operation of prefrontal lobotomy/leucotomy cut connections between the prefrontal lobe and other areas. For more information see Taylor (2006); also Pressman (1998), or, for a summary, see the online magazine WIRED at http://www.wired.com/wiredscience/2011/03/lobotomy-history.

Chapter 3

1. Dickens (1857/2003), *Little Dorrit*, Book I, Chapter XIII, p. 164.
2. See for example Bennett and Miller (2010); Logothetis (2008); Nemani et al. (2009); Thirion (2007).
3. See Beer and Hughes (2010); Brem et al. (2010); Filippi et al. (2010); Freeman et al. (2010); Jagiellowicz et al. (2010); Nili et al. (2010); Peters and Büchel (2010); Wittmann et al. (2010).
4. Hassabis et al. (2009).
5. Chadwick et al. (2010). 'BOLD' stands for blood-oxygen-level dependent; fMRI scanners can detect changes in the amount of oxygen in blood, as discussed in Chapter 7.
6. Just et al. (2010).
7. Kay et al. (2008). See also Naselaris et al. (2009).
8. Superconductivity is already being used to do neuroimaging, both in MEG (see Chapter 9) and in low-field MRI, which uses much weaker applied magnetic fields than those of standard fMRI.
9. The Wim Wenders film *Unto the End of the World* (1991) explores the possibility of DNE recording and playback (see http://www.wim-wenders.com/movies/movies_spec/untiltheendoftheworld/untiltheendoftheworld.htm). My thanks to Gillian Wright for this information.
10. Andersen and Cui (2009); Ciaramidaro et al. (2007).
11. Lin et al. (2011); see also Saper (2011).
12. Taylor (2009). One of the best-known researchers on bio-markers for violent criminality is Adrian Raine (Raine, 2008; Yang et al., 2008).
13. See e.g. Guastella et al. (2010a). However, an unfortunate obstacle has emerged for devotees of the so-called 'cuddle hormone': the friendliness it

appears to promote may not extend to members of disliked outgroups and may even enhance otherization (De Dreu et al., 2010).

14. Gilbert et al. (2009).
15. Akitsuki and Decety (2009); Gu and Han (2007).
16. Han et al. (2008); Singer (2006); Singer et al. (2006).
17. Singer et al. (2006).
18. See my description of callousness and sadism in Taylor (2009); also Decety et al. (2009a); Decety et al. (2009b); Newman-Norlund et al. (2009).
19. See Taylor (2006), also Taylor (2001).
20. Wyndham (1960); Wyndham (1973).
21. The UK Office of National Statistics, for example, reports that in 2010, 'More than nine million UK adults have never used the Internet', and of these, 'People who were more likely to have never used the Internet were the over 65s, the widowed, those on low incomes and those with no formal qualifications.' See http://www.ons.gov.uk/ons/rel/rdit2/internet-access—households-and-individuals/2010/news-release—9-2-million-uk-adults-have-never-used-the-internet.pdf for more details.
22. Sherry Turkle (Turkle, 2011) argues that the trend away from face-to-face communication is already apparent.
23. For an informative discussion of the legal issues surrounding photography, see Deazley (2008), or Professor Deazley's website, http://www.gla.ac.uk/schools/law/staff/ronandeazley/. I am indebted to Dr Gillian Wright for this reference.
24. Neuroimaging is already being used to study paedophilic brain responses (see for example Ponseti et al., 2012).
25. See Darwin (1859), p. 467 in the first edition, which is available from http://darwin-online.org.uk/content/frameset?itemID=F373&viewtype=text&pageseq=1.
26. 'Cui bono' —who benefits?—is a phrase associated with the Roman writer and statesman Cicero, who used it to highlight the gaps that can arise between apparent and actual interests in politics.

Chapter 4

1. Ritalin (methyl phenyl(piperidin-2-yl)acetate, commonly known as methylphenidate), a common treatment for attention deficit hyperactivity disorder (ADHD), is thought to improve some aspects of cognitive function (Agay et al., 2010; Nandam et al., 2010) and to be used by some university students and academics as a cognitive enhancer (Forlini and Racine, 2009;

Teter et al., 2003; but see also Outram, 2010). Modafinil (2-(benzhydrylsul-finyl)acetamide), used to treat the sleep disorder, narcolepsy, is likewise taken non-clinically to enhance cognition and wakefulness (Turner et al., 2004; Walsh et al., 2004).

2. See for example Farah et al. (2004); Sahakian and Morein-Zamir (2011); Steinbock (2006).

3. See Savulescu (2006). The document can be downloaded from http://www.practicalethics.ox.ac.uk/Pubs/Savulescu/enhancement.pdf.

4. See for example Benali et al. (2011); Chi and Snyder (2011); Coenen et al. (2011); Engineer et al. (2011); Esser et al. (2006); Fierro et al. (2010); Janicak et al. (2010).

5. Whether technology will be able to extend our senses beyond the normal range, or even add new senses, remains unresolved at present. Perhaps one day we will be able to answer the philosophical question famously posed by Thomas Nagel in 1974: 'What is it like to be a bat?' (Nagel (1974), text available at http://evans-experientialism.freewebspace.com/nagel.htm).

6. David Buss discusses violent fantasy in his book on the evolutionary psychology of murder (Buss, 2005). For an old but useful review of research on sexual fantasy, see Leitenberg and Henning (1995).

7. Savulescu (2006).

8. Savulescu (2006) gives the example of parents who could enhance their child's intelligence by providing a dietary supplement.

9. Åberg et al. (2009); Arden et al. (2009); Calvin et al. (2010); Deary et al. (2008); Schumacher and Martin (2009); Silvia (2008); Weiss et al. (2009). Association is not necessarily causation; studies of intelligence correlates paint a complicated picture. See for example Jokela et al. (2009); Kilgour et al. (2010); Link et al. (2008); Sabia et al. (2010).

10. The important role of motivation in intelligence also needs more consider-ation than it has received to date; see for example Duckworth et al. (2011).

11. Lynch et al. (2011).

12. Cakic (2009), p. 613.

13. The phrase is from the *Gospel of Matthew* (King James Bible), 13:12.

14. For a mighty exposition of the decline thesis, see Pinker (2011). SIPRI is the Stockholm International Peace Research Institute. See http://www.si-priyearbook.org/view/9780199581122-gill/sipri-9780199581122-div1-16.xml.

15. Persson and Savulescu (2008).

16. The Eurobarometer survey sampled over 26,000 interviews during January and February 2010. See http://ec.europa.eu/public_opinion/archives/ebs/ebs_340_en.pdf, p. 7.

17. The list is not exhaustive, because which areas are active depends on what exactly the task is (see for example Takahashi et al., 2008). The areas of cortex mentioned are the posterior cingulate and, in the parietal lobe, the angular gyrus. See also Forbes and Grafman (2010); Moll et al. (2008); Raine and Yang (2006); Shirtcliff et al. (2009).

18. Schnall et al. (2008); Wheatley and Haidt (2005). For more on the role of disgust in extremely amoral behaviour, see Taylor (2009).

19. Greene (2009); Greene et al. (2004).

20. Graham et al. (2009).

21. Hauser (2006); see also Dupoux and Jacob (2007); Mikhail (2007).

22. See for example Hurlemann et al. (2010); also Rodrigues et al. (2009).

23. De Dreu et al. (2010); De Dreu et al. (2011).

24. Avenanti et al. (2009); Cheetham et al. (2009).

25. For a discussion of the related topic of evolutionary trade-offs in brain function, see Hills and Hertwig (2011).

26. Birth and death data are taken from the Population Reference Bureau's 2010 World Population Data Sheet, available at http://www.prb.org/pdf10/10wpds_eng.pdf.

27. Rockstrom et al. (2009); see also http://www.guardian.co.uk/sustainable-business/living-above-our-limits.

28. Vinge's best-known article, written for a NASA symposium (Vinge, 1993), is available at http://www-rohan.sdsu.edu/faculty/vinge/misc/singularity.html. For more on Ray Kurzweil's ideas see http://www.singularity.com/ or Kurzweil (2005).

Chapter 5

1. See also Schoonover (2010). One of the most visually compelling techniques of recent years has been *Brainbow*, which uses genetic modification to label mouse neurons in different colours; the altered genes express fluorescent proteins. See Livet et al. (2007); also Hampel et al. (2011) and Hadjieconomou et al. (2011) for adaptations of the technique to another widely used model organism, the fruit fly.

2. The cerebrospinal fluid has other roles as well as life support. It is a reservoir of electrical charges, enabling neurotransmission, and it also appears to be involved in nerve cell development (Lehtinen et al., 2011).

3. 'Till the end of the fifteenth century and beyond, views on the conformation of the human brain were highly fanciful' (Singer, 1956).

4. Aristotle discusses physiology in *Parts of Animals*, Book II, Section vii (Aristotle, trans. 1937).

5. The idea that the brain, rather than the heart, might be the physical basis for interesting phenomena like consciousness was available to the Greek world, thanks to thinkers such as Anaxagoras of Clazomenae (http://history.hanover.edu/texts/presoc/anaxagor.html) and Alcmaeon of Croton (http://plato.stanford.edu/entries/alcmaeon/). It was, however, a minority view compared with, for example, those of Plato and Aristotle. Physicalist ideas about brain and mind can be found in many historical periods, if one looks hard enough, but their authors usually risked condemnation from religious authorities.

6. For an interesting view of the transition, seen through the lens of art, see Steiner (2010). Martinelli (1993) provides a useful summary of religious attitudes to body violation, in the context of organ donation. Many of the earliest dissections were done on criminals; see for example Singer (1956) on brain dissection.

7. Palade and Palay (1954); Robertson (1953), cited in DeFelipe (2010).

8. See for example Neher (2009). Thomas Willis's *De cerebri anatome* (1664), with illustrations by Christopher Wren, became one of the great reference texts of neuroanatomy (O'Connor, 2003).

9. Variation in structure is accompanied by variation in function. See for example Kanai and Rees (2011).

10. Pronunciation guide: for sulci, the 'c' is hard, as in 'cross', or indeed 'sulky'. For gyri, the 'g' is soft, as in 'giant'. Of the lobes, the most problematic are the parietal (pa-rye-eh-tal) and occipital (ock-sip-ital).

11. See Zilles and Amunts (2010).

12. Granular, agranular, and dysgranular cortex are differentiated by whether they have a clear Layer IV (e.g. visual cortex, with all that sensory input to process, has a thick Layer IV and hence is granular). The prefix 'a-' generally refers to a deficit (here, the lack of Layer IV; motor cortex is agranular), while the prefix 'dys-', as in everyday usage, suggests a mess. Different areas of cortex are thought to have evolved over different spans of our species' history, hence archaeo-, paleo-, and neocortex are old, middle-aged and young (most recently evolved).

13. A note on terminology: the basal ganglia and thalamus are both collective entities. For a description of thalamic parts see http://neuro.psyc.memphis.edu/neuropsyc/np-ugp-thalamus.htm. The basal ganglia include the caudate nucleus and putamen, which take input from cortex and pass it to the globus pallidus (the pale glob, as we weren't allowed to call it at college), which in turn transmits information to the thalamus. The caudate and

putamen interact with the substance nigra (so called because it looks darker than other areas, even without staining). The globus pallidus interacts with the subthalamic nucleus. For diagrams and further information, see http://thebrain.mcgill.ca/flash/a/a_06/a_06_cr/a_06_cr_mou/a_06_cr_mou. html. The nucleus accumbens, often mentioned in addiction research, is not shown there. It is located between the caudate and putamen. The term 'ventral striatum' is often used to refer to this area.

14. For human brains, Swanson (1995) gives a figure of 77% by volume; DeFelipe (2010) suggests 85%.

15. For an even better, tongue-rolling sense of the folds and crevasses in this super-crumpled evolutionary masterpiece, try the German equivalent: *Grosshirnrinde*, literally 'the big brain bark' (as in tree, not dog). It is no doubt just coincidence that German-speaking researchers have contributed so much to neuroscience, from Brodmann to Wernicke and many more.

16. The island of Reil, in Latin, becomes *insula Reili*, nowadays shortened to 'insula', the more usual name for this deep-buried fold of cortex. 'Reil' is the German anatomist Johann Christian Reil (1759–1813). Broca's area, named after Paul Broca (1824–1880), is involved in speech production. Friedreich's ataxia (Nikolaus Friedreich, 1825–1882) is a neurodegenerative disorder which affects spinal neurons, leading to motor problems such as difficulty walking and slurred speech. Some patients also develop diabetes and heart disease. Alzheimer's disease, a form of dementia, was formally described by Alois Alzheimer (1864–1915).

17. GPS is the global positioning system, a network of satellites providing time and location information.

18. See Gitelman et al. (2002). There are two systems of brain coordinates commonly used in neuroimaging. One is based on a brain atlas published by Jean Talairach and Pierre Tournoux, which analysed a single brain (Talairach and Tournoux, 1988). The other, from the Montreal Neurological Institute, is based on fMRI scans of multiple brains, the aim being to create a framework more representative of the population as a whole. A useful discussion of differences between Talairach and MNI can be found at http://imaging.mrc-cbu.cam.ac.uk/imaging/MniTalairach. The paper cited here, by Gitelman et al. (2002), uses Talairach coordinates.

19. Relating Brodmann areas to other, e.g. functional measurements can be less than straightforward, but here too advances are being made. See for example Geyer et al. (2011).

20. With reference to prefrontal cortex variation, see for example Rajkowska and Goldman-Rakic (1995).

21. The brain's duplex structure means that there are two of most structures, or else a right and a left one. 'Most' excludes, for example, the corpus callosum, which, as a two-way channel of communication between left and right hemispheres, does not need a duplicate.

22. Cajal and Golgi shared the Nobel Prize for medicine/physiology in 1906, in recognition, the citation says, 'of their work on the structure of the nervous system'. See http://nobelprize.org/nobel_prizes/lists/year/?year=1906.

23. Dendrites are short extensions of the cell, with which other neurons make synaptic connections. See notes 11 and 19, Chapter 8.

24. See for example Fu and Zuo (2011).

25. IMCOTT: the fixation process involves more distinct stages than I have implied. For the detail see Morecraft et al. (1992).

26. The website http://www.understandinganimalresearch.org.uk/ states that 3,656,080 scientific procedures using animals were carried out in Britain in 2008. Of these, 77% were on laboratory-bred rodents, 21% on non-mammals, 1.1% on large mammals like sheep and pigs, 0.7% on small mammals like rabbits and ferrets, 0.18% on specially bred dogs and cats, and 0.13% (about 4,750 procedures) on primates.

Chapter 6

1. A useful explanation of the Standard Model can be found on the website of CERN, the organisation which, among much else, built and manages the Large Hadron Collider (LHC). See http://public.web.cern.ch/public/en/Science/StandardModel-en.html.

2. Kuhn discusses normal and abnormal (paradigm-changing) science in his influential book *The Structure of Scientific Revolutions* (Kuhn, 1962).

3. *A Brief History of Time* was first published in 1988 and Brian Greene's *The Elegant Universe* in 1999 (Hawking, 1988; Greene, 1999). Brian Cox's BBC series *The Wonders of the Solar System* was aired in 2010. CERN (see note 1 above) approved the LHC's construction in late 1994, after about a decade of planning, according to their website (http://public.web.cern.ch/public/en/LHC/Milestones-en.html).

4. Data on Nobel Prize winners is available from http://nobelprize.org/.

5. Less intuitively, as we shall see, fMRI can also be thought of in this way if you count energy as 'stuff'.

6. The approximate effective dose for a typical PET scan has been estimated as eight millisieverts (http://rpop.iaea.org/RPOP/RPoP/Content/InformationFor/HealthProfessionals/6_OtherClinicalSpecialities/PETCTscan.

htm#PETCT_FAQ01). The estimate for an X-ray of the gastrointestinal tract, of 6–8 mSv, comes from http://www.radiologyinfo.org/en/pdf/sfty_xray.pdf. For comparison, the radiation dose considered to be lethal (within hours) is 20–50 grays, equivalent to 200–500 mSv, according to the Health Physics Society (http://hps.org/publicinformation/ate/q1005.html). With respect to prices, as of March 2011 a US medical site states that 'PET scan charges range from $850–$4,000' (http://interactive.snm.org/index.cfm?PageID=972), while another gives X-ray prices as 'ranging from $50 to over $200' (http://blog.remakehealth.com/blog_Healthcare_Consumers-0/bid/8507/How-much-does-an-X-ray-cost).

7. See for example Clark and Sokoloff (1999), cited in Raichle and Gusnard (2002), and Magistretti et al. (2000), available online at http://www.acnp.org/g4/gn401000064/ch064.html.

8. IMCOTT. For more detail about glycolysis, see http://glycolysis.co.uk/. For more about PET imaging, see for example http://sitemaker.umich.edu/pet.chemistry/positron_emission_tomography.

9. Fluorine-18 has nine protons and nine neutrons in its atomic nucleus. Oxygen-18 has ten neutrons and eight protons, and is created when one proton becomes a neutron as the fluorine-18 emits a positron. The commonest form of oxygen has eight protons and eight neutrons. See Shapiro (2002), pp. 38–9.

10. Boecker et al. (2008). The half-life of a radioactive material X which decays to form some other material is the time taken for the amount of X to halve. So if you have 100 molecules of radioactive F^{18}-fluorodeoxyglucose to begin with, after nearly two hours you will have 50 molecules left.

11. Raichle (2009).

12. For example, Salimpoor et al. (2011) used PET to reveal that listening to favourite pieces of music can cause dopamine release from areas of the basal ganglia, just as taking recreational drugs like cocaine and alcohol can. Also of interest is work on a portable PET scanner for rats (Schulz et al., 2011).

13. See for example Babiloni et al. (2004); Baillet et al. (1999); Herzog et al. (2010); McDonald et al. (2010).

14. Ceccarini et al. (2009); Huang et al. (2010); Nahrendorf et al. (2010).

15. Urban et al. (2010). The ventral striatum is part of the basal ganglia; see note 13, Chapter 5. The study selected social drinkers who were not dependent on or abusing alcohol and gave them either alcohol or a placebo. 'The placebo consisted of cranberry juice and soda alone, while the alcohol drink in addition contained the equivalent of three standard drinks of 100 proof vodka designed to deliver an average of .75g alcohol per kilogram

body water. The individual amount of alcohol was calculated based on the subject's amount of body water according to the equation: total body water (g/liter) = −2.097 + .1069 (height in cm) + .2466 (weight in kg). For men, the volume of the drink amounted to 500 mL, while women received 350 mL.'

16. Urban et al. (2010): 'we estimate that the alcohol challenge increased extra-cellular DA [dopamine] levels by 138% in men and 69% in women' (p. 690). The estimate relies on 'simplifying' but not unreasonable assumptions about how the radioligand used in the study behaves in synapses. See the authors' discussion, p. 693.

17. 'PET scans can be designed to capture an image twice a minute, and hence allow experiments which compare multiple conditions—but limits on radioactive exposure mean few images can be collected compared with fMRI' (Royal Society (2011), p. 14). See also Frøkjær et al. (2011) for a comparison of PET's temporal resolution ('tens of seconds', p. 98) with those of fMRI and electrophysiology.

18. Rissman et al. (2010), Supplementary Information.

19. The other four excluded participants were either unable to keep still or to do the task.

20. The last time I enquired about fMRI scan fees for a potential experiment (in 2007; see Chapter 7 for details), I was quoted £365 per hour. The Royal Society's recent review of neuroscience (Royal Society, 2011) gives a figure of £500.

21. For an example of why gender differences need to be considered, see Jacobs and D'Esposito (2011).

22. For more on the power of scientific authority, a usual starting point is Stanley Milgram's work on obedience. See Milgram (1963) for the original article or Milgram (1997) for the book-length exposition.

23. The change of term from 'subject' to 'participant' may seem a minor one, but it can rouse very strong feelings. The complaint of 'political correctness gone mad' is by no means restricted to politics. Like many well-meaning changes, this one seeks to empower one group of people (volunteers) at the expense of another (experimenters). Given how hard it is for someone who has committed vast swathes of their life to what others see as a fairly arcane pursuit not to despise those others, I'd say the likely outcome is a redirec-tion of the sense of superiority into other forms of self-expression, such as the arrogant (and unscientific) ideology of scientism. Those scientists who treat their experimental fodder with respect don't need Orwellian brow-beating. As for the others, there's no law that says researchers have to be nice.

24. See for example Hayden (2010); Kim et al. (2010); Nature Editorial (2010a); Wald and Wu (2010).

25. If current growth rates in female membership were maintained, and *ceteris paribus*, gender parity in the Royal Society would be reached some time in 2075, at the earliest. Data for the calculation were taken from the Royal Society's website: http://royalsociety.org/.

Chapter 7

1. The articles whose titles I cite were downloaded on 30 October 2010 from http://www.wired.com/wiredscience/2010/10/brain-focus-recording/ (*WIRED Science*), http://newsfeed.time.com/2010/10/29/what-dreams-may-come-dream-recording-device-possible/#ixzz13rzjxYOQ (*TIME*) and http://www.nature.com/news/2010/101027/full/news.2010.568.html (*Nature News*).

2. At the time of these headlines, late in 2010, the well-received movie *Inception* had recently highlighted the concept of dream manipulation. Marilyn Monroe (born 1926) and Josh Brolin (born 1968) are actors from such different eras that one presumes *Nature's* readership taps a rather different demographic from that of *WIRED's*.

3. The *Nature* article on which the reports are based is somewhat more soberly titled: 'On-line, voluntary control of human temporal lobe neurons' (Cerf et al., 2010).

4. The commonest six elements in the human body by mass are oxygen (65%), carbon (18%), hydrogen (10%), nitrogen (3%), calcium (1.5%), and phosphorus (1.0%). Estimates are taken from Harper et al. (1977), cited at http://chemistry.about.com/cs/howthingswork/f/blbodyelements.htm.

5. Protons are not the only material suitable for magnetic resonance analyses. Magnetic resonance spectroscopy (MRS) exploits this potential by tuning the scanner to different resonance frequencies, enabling scientists to 'scan' for the presence of different chemicals in brain areas. It has been used, for instance, to study the brain biochemistry of multiple sclerosis (Caramanos et al., 2005).

6. IMCOTT: if the magnetic field were the same all the way across the brain you wouldn't be able to tell individual areas apart, so scanners incorporate mechanisms for creating a magnetic gradient between one side and the other.

7. Researchers are already starting to design proteins to order, a necessary step on the road to nanomachines (Fleishman et al., 2011).

8. IMCOTT. Echo-planar imaging is one form of MRI, albeit a widely used one. As for microwave ovens, they too use a principle of resonance, in that

they rely on electrically charged molecules tending to align themselves with applied electromagnetic fields. However, they alternate these fields—the microwaves—extremely rapidly, causing the molecules in the food to rotate. As the molecules move they disrupt others nearby, transferring energy through the food—as when a disturbance in a crowd spreads out from its source to make the whole ensemble more agitated. The energy provided to the molecules by a fast-flipping electromagnetic field thus makes them move more, raising the food's average kinetic energy—its temperature. Far less energy is provided by fMRI pulses. Rogue researchers may sometimes cook their data, but never their participants.

9. The scanner listens to this 'echo' pulse, then sends out another pulse, and so on. Because the pulses are very short and swift, the scanner can detect the change in radio frequency brought on by a change in the magnetic field as blood deoxygenates. By applying pulses at different angles, all around the head—which is why the scanner has its square-doughnut shape—information about successive 'slices' through the brain can be collected and assembled into a 3D image of the brain.

10. The article, by journalist Michelle Roberts, is sourced from http://news.bbc.co.uk/1/hi/health/8672400.stm (published online 10 May 2010). My thanks to Michelle and to the BBC for permission to reproduce part of this article.

11. See for example Ben Goldacre on neuro-(un)realism (Goldacre, 2010).

12. IMCOTT again. For example, the blood oxygen response appears to differ across the six layers of cortex, beginning in the deeper layers and with the surface Layer I being slowest to respond (Tian et al., 2010). Most fMRI studies to date have focused on finding out which areas are active in a task, but to understand how brains work in detail we'll need to think about how cortical layers interact in an active area as well as where those areas are.

13. Tuning can be done by adjusting various scanner parameters, such as the strength of the external magnetic field and the timing of the radio pulses.

14. See for example Calamante et al. (1999), Bandettini (2009).

15. This has been a notorious quibble for fMRI researchers. Because the technology measures changes in blood oxygen levels, not neuron activity, it was argued that the two might not go together. The central assumption of fMRI, that increasing brain activity demands more oxygen, might be false. Recently, however, studies in animals have shown that fMRI signals are indeed correlated with more direct measures of neural activity. See Halpern-Manners et al. (2010); Lee et al. (2010); Schölvinck et al. (2010); cf. Lin et al. (2010). A further complication is that there are various measures of neural activity available. Researchers have also inferred, using studies in

rats, that most of the change in blood oxygen is driven by the activity of neurons processing the signals they receive, rather than by either those input signals or the outputs (spikes) which the processing produces. See for example Harris et al. (2010).

16. See for example Bennett and Miller (2010).

17. See Taylor (2006).

18. The fMRI experiment is based on a real study, designed by myself and a colleague at Birmingham University, Dr Peter Hansen, with additional advice from Professor John Stein at Oxford. We got everything ready to go, only to be prevented, by an unfortunate combination of circumstances, from carrying out the study. So it goes.

19. Any scientific experiment studies the differences between one or more experimental and control conditions, so careful selection of both is essential for good experiments. Some fMRI studies, for example, compare their experimental condition (e.g. looking at images) with 'rest'. Unfortunately, it has become clear that whatever human brains do when they are supposed to be resting, quietly doing very little is not on the agenda. As an influential review remarked in 2006, 'It seems plausible, therefore, that a baseline of unconstrained rest is likely to elicit some of the same cognitive processes and associated neural activity as are engaged by explicit social tasks. It is also likely that the cognitive activity that occurs during rest might depend on the context in which this condition occurs' (Amodio and Frith, 2006). As contexts go, scanners are not among the more restful: participants may daydream, but they may also worry about their performance, try to suppress stray thoughts, fantasize about the experimenter, etc. This is a particular problem in social neuroscience, when the experimental condition may also involve similar processes.

20. The Organisation for Economic Co-operation and Development (OECD) reports that in 2007 MRI scans were carried out on 91 in every 1,000 people in the USA, up from 56 per 1,000 in 2000. As the US population in 2007 was about 302 million, the sample size from this country and year alone is a hefty 27 million. For full data see http://stats.oecd.org/Index.aspx?Data-SetCode = HEALTH.

21. For the estimate of average neurons-per-voxel, see de-Wit et al. (2010).

22. The large numbers of voxels in an fMRI scan result in many tests of statistical significance being required to compare them across experimental conditions. The 'problem of multiple comparisons' is that purely by chance some of those results will indicate significance where none exists (i.e. they will be false positives). If for example the level of significance, or

p-value, is set at less than 0.05 (the default for many research studies), then there is a 5% probability (1 in 20 chance) that a positive result is random rather than genuinely significant. The number of comparisons used in fMRI accumulates an unacceptably large number of false positives, so to reduce these errors statistical corrections must be applied.

23. For a description of the Atlantic salmon case, which was presented at a major neuroimaging conference, *Human Brain Mapping*, in 2009, see http://prefrontal.org/blog/2009/09/the-story-behind-the-atlantic-salmon/.

24. Nemani et al. (2009).

25. Strictly speaking, since the wavefunction's equation involves complex numbers, the wavefunction itself is considered an abstract entity, not a 'real' feature of the world (what 'real' means in the context of quantum mechanics is a long-running debate). To obtain the probability map, the absolute (i.e. unsigned) square of the wavefunction's amplitude is taken. For more on how to measure wavefunctions, see Hosten (2011), which comments on Lundeen et al. (2011).

26. For example, Ringler et al. (2003) reports percentage BOLD signal changes of around 2% in a task involving painful stimulation of volunteers' fingers (by squeezing or tapping).

27. Feinberg et al. (2010).

28. Terminology: *in vivo* studies involve living organisms and are usually contrasted with *in vitro* ('in glass') studies, which may for instance use tissue slices or cultured (artificially grown and maintained) cells.

29. See for example Stevens (2009); Tomasi and Volkow (2010); van den Heuvel and Hulshoff Pol (2010).

30. See note 18, Chapter 1; also Pastrana (2011). The analogy with the genome is linguistically clumsy, but since the completion of the human genome project such analogies have become increasingly popular. Proteomes map proteins, inflammasomes map immune function, metabolomes map the products of metabolism, and so on. Maybe sounding more like genetics makes the science seem 'harder' and encourages funding success? On this trend, the term for the complete map of human knowledge, using the Greek root *gnosis*, could be 'gnome'. Perhaps not.

31. See for example http://www.guardian.co.uk/commentisfree/2011/apr/17/human-genome-genetics-twin-studies.

32. The phrase 'carving nature at her joints' is thought to originate in Plato's *Phaedrus* (265d–266a), in which Socrates describes a principle of thought as 'that of division into species according to the natural formation, where the

joint is, not breaking any part as a bad carver might'. *Phaedrus* is available online from Project Gutenberg at http://www.gutenberg.org/ebooks/1636.

33. For a discussion of discovery science with reference to functional connectivity, see Biswal et al. (2010).

Chapter 8

1. Penfield and Erickson (1941).

2. Early experiments on electricity are associated with the Italian scientist, Luigi Galvani; see for example Ball (2011b). Shelley may have learned about them through the work of Erasmus Darwin, grandfather of Charles, who conducted similar experiments.

3. Electrocution is a significant cause of both accidental death and suicide (Chan and Duflou, 2008; Shetty et al., 2010).

4. The novelist in question is Jane Austen, the book *Pride and Prejudice*.

5. IMCOTT. It is not entirely clear what a chemical bond actually is (Ball, 2011a).

6. To be pedantic, the difference is there by a combination of many chances, and the advantages they brought to innumerable organisms, over the aeons-long course of evolution since cells acquired membranes.

7. Traditionally the action potential was thought to travel along a neuron's long axon unchanged, spreading with equal effect through the axon's branches to activate synapses. That view has now been challenged (Sasaki et al., 2011), as has the concept that each neuron releases one kind of neurotransmitter (El Mestikawy et al., 2011).

8. The NMDA receptor, named for its responsiveness to the glutamate-like chemical n-methyl-d-aspartate, was a stalwart teaching example when I first encountered neuroscience. This prominence was partly because it is so important for synaptic plasticity—the change in how easily neural signals can pass from one cell to the next, which is thought to underlie learning. (When synapses change to let signals flow more readily the process is called long-term potentiation; when they adjust to flow less readily, it is known as long-term depression.)

9. IMCOTT. NMDA receptors are also interesting, however, because two distinct events must happen simultaneously before the ion channel opens. One is conventional neurotransmission: the receiving cell will 'feel' a signal from a sender when the latter's spat-out glutamate has bound to the NMDA receptor. By itself this is not enough to open the ion channel, because it is blocked by an intruder particle: a magnesium ion (Mg^{2+}), squatting over the hole and preventing access. To push the magnesium out of the way it is first necessary

to make the electrical potential across the membrane more positive—for example, by activating other kinds of receptors which allow positive ions into the cell. This repels the positively charged magnesium ion. Once the channel is clear, and the glutamate bound, the NMDA receptor will then allow entry. This voltage-dependent activation lets the receptor function like a logical device, outputting a signal only if sender neuron A (which releases glutamate to bind to NMDA receptors) and sender neuron(s) B (which stimulates non-NMDA receptors to boost the membrane potential) are both active *at the same time*. Neurons that fire together wire together, as the saying goes. In another IMCOTT, this is not always the case, as some patterns of firing can reduce the flow of signals through a synapse (long-term depression).

10. See for example Sheffield et al. (2011).

11. Dendrites also seem to play an important role in the internal computations that neurons use for deciding whether to fire off a spike or not. The simple version is that they collate and sum up the cell's electrochemical inputs, but inevitably IMCOTT. See for example Branco and Häusser (2011), which suggests that how a dendrite processes its inputs depends on its location.

12. The structure and behaviour of receptors, and the cell's consequent behaviour, can vary for cells in different brain regions and species. Neurons are not identikit structures, either in anatomy, pharmacology or electrical properties (Marder and Taylor, 2011).

13. On the oversimplification inherent in the term 'overall balance', see note 11, above. A further IMCOTT is that the electromagnetic fields generated by neurons appear capable of 'feeding back' into, and thereby altering, the voltage maintained across the cell membrane, a process known as ephaptic coupling. The Greek etymology of 'ephaptic' is close to that of 'synapse', replacing 'syn' with 'epi' to change touching *with* into touching *on*. See for more detail Anastassiou et al. (2011); Binczak et al. (2001).

14. An etymological note: the Greek from which we get electroencephalography offers a delightful put-down for neuroscientific hubris, referring to the brain as merely '(the thing) in the head': en-kephalos.

15. Pravdich-Neminsky (1913), cited in Niedermeyer and Lopes Da Silva (2004), p. 3.

16. For example, a 2011 study from Leslie Ungerleider's group at the NIH (Wu et al., 2011) aims to link the traditional anatomical process of tracing brain fibre pathways—research in which Ungerleider has been a world leader for decades—with the modern technology of MRI.

17. The electrons whose flows generate the currents detected by EEG take their name from the Greek word for amber (ἤλεκτρον).

18. An estimate from computer modelling suggests that only between ten and fifty thousand synchronously firing neurons may be required for detection by EEG or MEG (Murakami and Okada, 2006; see also Hadjipapas et al., 2009). The resulting signals vary in time (i.e. they have a measurable frequency), and some show regular patterns. For example, the alpha rhythm pulses, waxing and waning in its size, at a rate of between about eight and twelve times a second (8–12 Hertz) when the eyes are closed or the brain's owner is nicely relaxed. Meditate or daydream, and the theta rhythm predominates, as the brain ticks over at 4–7 Hz. Fall asleep in your yoga class, and if you reach slow wave sleep you'll embark on the delta rhythm, a gentle sub-4 Hz swell. Alertness and concentration, on the other hand, bring on the beta rhythm—faster pulses of 12–30 Hz—and for hard work the gamma rhythm, ranging from 30 to 100 Hz. Gamma waves seem to arise when the brain requires communion between different areas to solve a problem like matching perceptions in one sense with those in another, or with memories. As neurons across (in their terms) vast distances bring their firing into step, the gamma pulse emerges, a marker of focus.

19. Action potentials also travel along axons, whereas EPSPs and IPSPs travel along dendrites. Because of the way the cortex has developed, dendrites tend to be aligned similarly, whereas axons vary in the direction they take; dendritic signals are thus likely to reinforce each other, and axonal action potentials to cancel each other out.

20. IMCOTT. The superficial layers of cortex also contain wiring, enabling adjacent regions of cortex to synchronize their activity, as well as inhibitory interneurons which, among other things, filter out physically incompatible signals (e.g. by making sure that neurons stimulated when a person closes their fist are not firing simultaneously with neurons stimulated when the same hand is opened). Deep in the brain are also numerous clusters of brain cells—the nuclei of the thalamus, brainstem, amygdala, and so on.

21. A recent study further complicates the story by suggesting that the density of neurons may vary across cortex; work in some species of monkey found that early sensory processing areas had more densely packed neurons than 'higher-level', later-processing areas (Collins et al., 2010). EEG models' default assumption is that neuron density is similar everywhere in cortex.

22. See for example Green and Kalaska (2011); Miranda et al. (2011). Another resource for learning about potential applications is TED, which makes short talks available online (http://www.ted.com/talks).

23. Susan Greenfield's book *Tomorrow's People* and Kevin Kelly's *What Technology Wants* (Greenfield, 2004; Kelly, 2010) offer interesting views about our increasing reliance on technology.

24. See for example Niedermeyer and Lopes Da Silva (2004), pp. 674–7.

25. The number of 170 billion includes neurons and non-neuronal cells (Azevedo et al., 2009; see also note 7, Chapter 14).

26. Electrical recording can also be done invasively on human patients for whom there is clinical justification, measuring signals from the cortical surface: this technique is also called electrocorticography. See for example its use to study the neural mechanisms of consciousness and anaesthesia by Breshears et al. (2010).

27. For an early example of the link between radiation and conspiracy theory, dating from around the time of the French Revolution, try Mike Jay's book *The Air Loom Gang* (Jay, 2003).

28. See for example Whittingstall and Logothetis (2009). Once again, language aids the deception by making things seem more solid than they are. As an example, take the implied assertion, in a paper in the journal *Intelligence* (Jausovec, 2000), that 'higher alpha power' is equivalent to 'less mental activity'. (Alpha power can be thought of as reflecting how much of the brain's resources are being channelled into producing EEG alpha waves, relative to other frequencies.) The abstract states: 'The analysis of EEG measures in Experiment 1 indicated that highly intelligent individuals showed higher alpha power (less mental activity)'. It sounds so simple; it isn't. Taken at face value this is a very controversial statement, virtually guaranteed to wind up any philosopher in the vicinity and a fair number of scientists as well, since it makes 'mental activity' seem far easier to define than it actually is. Are the neuronal spikes of a coma victim, or a very recently dead person, mental activity? How about the signals read off a brain slice or an isolated neuron? The hard problem of consciousness—how brains make mental activity—is not so easily solved (see Chalmers, 1995, available at http://consc.net/papers/facing.html).

29. Bradberry et al. (2010).

30. Current EEG control of movement—e.g. of a wheelchair or in a game—is extremely simplistic compared with the possibilities unleashed by being able to decode hand movements. Re brain implants, they can function well in the short term, but these 'neuroprosthetics' can fail, or cause scarring of brain tissue, so their use requires careful management and follow-up (Leach et al., 2010).

31. In principle the participants could have waved their hands all over the place en route to their chosen targets, but in practice they tended to move the hand directly from A to B, following only a small number of trajectories (as the article graphics show) and making only a few of the possible movements.

Chapter 9

1. Schrödinger's cat may or may not be the traditional black animal associated with witchcraft, because when the physicist set out his famous paradox (Schrödinger, 1935) he did not specify further than 'eine Katze'.
2. See http://www.mrc-cbu.cam.ac.uk/research/eeg/eeg_intro.html for more on the differences between EEG and MEG.
3. Ahlfors et al. (2010a); Hansen et al. (2010); see also http://www.mrc-cbu.cam.ac.uk/research/eeg/eeg_intro.html. Both EEG and MEG require complex analysis and modelling to interpret their data. The models for both are currently too simple, though as so often in neuroscience, advances in computing are helping to improve the situation. At present, however, many models make unrealistic assumptions about brain shape, fail to take account of interactions between the electromagnetic fields generated by multiple neuronal sources, and so on (Ahlfors et al., 2010b). The 'brainwaves' analysed are also typically averaged over many individual electromagnetic events, so they are less than fully reflective of the quicksilver neural reality they record. Thus any single piece of research using these techniques should be seen as provisional for now, as is the case for other neuroimaging methods such as fMRI.
4. Placing electrodes directly onto the brain has been used in patients to control brain–computer interfaces: see for example Leuthardt et al. (2011).
5. At a rough estimate, a good EEG setup will deprive you of around $50,000. A MEG scanner will cost approximately 20 times that sum, which is in the same expensive region as MRI facilities.
6. The learning curve for MEG will become easier as more analysis tools are developed, a process which is already underway; see for instance Dalal et al. (2011).
7. MRI magnetic fields are commonly measured in tesla (1 tesla = 10,000 gauss). Scans at 3T are common; higher strengths, like 7T, are also being used. See Niedermeyer and Lopes Da Silva (2004), p. 116; also http://www.who.int/peh-emf/about/WhatisEMF/en/index3.html. The figure for a microwave oven is the maximum cited by the World Health Organisation for a distance of 3cm.
8. Data are taken from http://www.spaceweather.com/glossary/imf.html.

9. For more technical details of MEG, see Hansen et al. (2010).

10. To clarify, Schrödinger's 'undulatory theory', which gave us the Schrödinger wavefunction of quantum entities like electrons, was set out in 1926, but no cats appear in this paper. His paradox was described in 1935 (Schrödinger, 1926; Schrödinger, 1935).

11. As Schrödinger put it: 'eine winzige Menge radioaktiver Substanz, *so* wenig, daß im Lauf einer Stunde *vielleicht* eines von den Atomen zerfällt, ebenso wahrscheinlich aber auch keines' (Schrödinger, 1935, p. 812, italics in the original).

12. This is not to say that quantum effects are irrelevant to an understanding of 'macro-world' phenomena, but that we are not naturally equipped to notice them. Investigation is revealing that they may be important for various natural processes, including such basic functions as photosynthesis (Ishizaki and Fleming, 2009).

13. Niobium, also called columbium, is a rare and valuable component in modern technologies from earrings to aerospace. Brazil and Canada are major producers, but niobium is also extracted from more highly fraught regions like the Congo. Should you ever need to torment an MEG researcher, therefore, you could always ask whether the scanner's SQUIDs are made from conflict metals. Teasing an fMRI researcher is easier, with their immense magnetic fields: just ask them which way's due north.

14. More exactly, the temperature at which niobium becomes superconducting is 9.2 degrees on the Kelvin scale, equivalent to $-263.95°C$. This is close to absolute zero (0 K), the theoretical limit at which the movement of molecules in a substance (which provides its heat) is minimal. The zero-point on the Celsius scale is the freezing point of water, 273.15 K, at which atoms still have plenty of energy to move.

15. Niobium atoms have 41 protons and 52 neutrons in the atomic nucleus, so their more distant electrons are relatively far away from, and weakly attracted to, the nucleus.

16. To understand the effect of cooling a metal, recall that electrons in an atom can exist in one of only a limited range of energy states. Changing state takes a fixed dose of energy of a particular frequency (e.g. from cosmic rays). Imagine an explorer crossing the slashed volcanic landscape of Iceland with only a collection of wooden planks to bridge the chasms. For each fissure she crosses, she must choose exactly the right length of plank (too short, no crossing; too long, and the plank's weight with her on it risks breaking through the ice). Only when the plank fits can the explorer move on. Why does resistance drop as the metal is cooled? Because at

higher temperatures atoms are more active, and that activity is expressed as emissions of energy from the atom. Imagine that the explorer is trying to make her way across the landscape while dodging a hail of planks flying in all directions. When atoms shed energy quanta, electrons which interact with those quanta are scattered. The cooler the metal, the more likely an electron is to hold its course and flow smoothly. As a metal's temperature sinks towards absolute zero there are fewer quantum planks (Plancks?) available for the electrons to use in order to change to a different energy state. Even if stray atoms should still jiggle, making energy available, it may not be the right frequency for an electron to absorb. If only children were built like this, so that when football practice was cancelled (no high-energy state available) they wouldn't absorb the quantum of cake just beforehand. If atoms get too heavy they split apart in nuclear fission, an option not available to our obese youth.

17. IMCOTT. For more detail on superconductivity and related phenomena see http://www.superconductors.org or the 'Condensed Matter' option on Georgia State University's *Hyperphysics* website: http://hyperphysics.phy-astr.gsu.edu/hbase/hph.html.

18. Superconductors have their cake and eat it, according to the dominant mathematical model of this process, 'BCS theory' (named after the physicists John Bardeen, Leon Cooper, and Robert Schrieffer). Below a certain critical temperature, electrons fall into a quantum state in which they form temporary weak bonds with other electrons ('Cooper pairs'), instead of the mutual loathing usually observed between two negative charges. A Cooper pair does not behave like two electrons, and its energy state is lower than the residual energy shed by vibrating atoms. In terms of our explorer analogy (see note 16 above), the quantum plank is always too big for the crevasse. Quanta produced by atoms, in other words, can no longer affect a Cooper pair, which means that electrons flowing in this configuration are not scattered off course. However, all electron–atom interactions involve the exchange of quanta—including collisions. Thus a Cooper pair is no longer affected by the atoms' existence *at all*, even to the extent of bumping into them. Our explorer has become a ghost, able to pass through solid matter unaffected. The electron waveform can simply flow through the metal as if there were no atoms. Hence the metal's resistance is not simply very low; when Cooper pairs form, it drops to zero, and the metal has become a superconductor.

19. See for example http://www.physorg.com/news134828104.html.

20. Josephson junctions are named after the physicist Brian Josephson, who predicted their existence in the 1960s and gained not only a Nobel prize (in 1973; see http://www.nobelprize.org/nobel_prizes/physics/laureates/1973/index.html) but the immortality of having his name attached to a number of useful, if specialist, electronic devices. Left to itself, an electron wave carrying current around a superconducting SQUID ring will split into two waves at the point where the current is applied to the SQUID, heading in opposite directions and thus interacting with each other. A typical SQUID has two Josephson junctions on opposite sides of its ring. By changing the phase of the electron wave as it passes through them, they alter the way in which the wave interacts with itself—rather as a barrier placed in a swimming pool will change how waves on its surface reinforce or interfere with each other. This allows the SQUID to pick up extremely tiny fluctuations in the surrounding magnetic field. The technique works as follows. A magnetic field is made up of quanta—called fluxons—just as light is made up of photons. When a magnetic field changes outside the SQUID, that change must be cancelled out by an equal magnetic flux—and the only way to create this is to induce an additional electrical current in the SQUID. When this brings the level of current flowing in the SQUID above a certain threshold, the critical current, the superconducting state collapses and resistance appears. The insertion of the Josephson junctions allows this to be measured. If the external magnetic field changes by some multiple of a fluxon, the electron wave will reinforce itself; if the change is some multiple of half a fluxon, there will be interference. (Don't ask, it's all in the math.) This is the level of change which the SQUID can detect, which shows its extraordinary power.

21. See for example McDonald et al. (2010); Ou et al. (2010); Wheless et al. (2004); Zanto et al. (2011).

22. Zotev et al. (2008a); Zotev et al. (2008b).

23. Ou et al. (2009); Plis et al. (2010).

24. The clash of cultures involved in the popularization of neuroimaging will be considerable, and the ethical risks need serious attention. When it comes to messing with people's heads, research and clinical ethics are greatly preferable to the profit motive, in the same way as being operated on by a doctor who wants to heal you is preferable to being sliced open by a doctor who wants to sell your kidneys on the open market. When it comes to brains, as commercialized psychiatry's love of a pill for every ill has surely shown, the pursuit of profit can be very damaging.

Chapter 10

1. Very severe epilepsy which cannot be treated in any other way can be eased by lobectomy, in which the area of brain where the abnormal activity begins its spread across the brain is removed (Bell et al., 2011; Tanriverdi et al., 2009). Neurosurgery is also used to treat severe cases of neurodegenerative disorders like Parkinson's disease and multiple sclerosis, and the worst head injuries. To give an idea of the disparity between injuries and surgery, in the UK, the National Health Service estimates that about 4,000 people have neurosurgery per year (for severe head injuries), while around 700,000 are treated for head injuries as a whole. See http://www.nhs.uk/conditions/head-injury-severe-/pages/treatment.aspx and http://www.cks.nhs.uk/patient_information_leaflet/head_injury_minor.

2. Comments on animal research from the leading journals *Science* and *Nature* are informative here; see for example Miller (2011), Stephens (2011), and the open-access resources at http://www.nature.com/news/specials/animalresearch/index.html.

3. See for example Clark et al. (2011).

4. Taylor (2009); Wheatley and Haidt (2005).

5. Stevenson and Kording (2011).

6. See for example Branco et al. (2010); Pettit et al. (1997).

7. Pettit et al. (1997), p. 465.

8. Northoff et al. (2010).

9. See for example London et al. (2010) on variability in neuronal firing rates and Bromberg-Martin et al. (2010), which suggests that neurons of the dopaminergic system use tonic (steady) firing to code for how rewarding a stimulus is and phasic (burst) firing to signal how salient—i.e. how distinctive—it is.

10. An example: Rancz et al. (2011) combines electrophysiology, the topic of this chapter, with neurogenetics (see Chapters 12 and 13).

11. Hatfield et al. (1994).

12. Hipp et al. (2011).

13. See Fell and Axmacher (2011) on the importance of phase synchronization in memory, and Romei et al. (2011) on visual perception.

Chapter 11

1. Williams et al. (2009).

2. Brunoni et al. (2011); Rothwell (1997). Limitations on space—in a book written primarily for non-specialists—prevent an in-depth discussion of

the various kinds of electrical stimulation and the distinctions between them (e.g. TES versus tDCS). For simplicity, I have used the term TES to refer to electrical stimulation in general—i.e. as contrasted with magnetic stimulation and including similar techniques like tDCS—whereas the technical literature generally differentiates TES and tDCS. For the same reason, I have not gone into the details of repetitive versus single-pulse TMS.

3. Dell'Osso et al. (2011).
4. If TMS gives you a headache you may soon be able to try ultrasound (Tufail et al., 2010).
5. TES has typically used direct current stimulation; however, alternating currents can also be used (Nitsche et al., 2009; Ozen et al., 2010).
6. Sandrini et al. (2010).
7. Esser et al. (2006).
8. TMS has also been used in conjunction with other techniques, such as EEG (Bikmullina et al., 2009), where the underlying electrophysiology is better understood.
9. Bonnard et al. (2009); Kalbe et al. (2010); Silvanto and Cattaneo (2010).
10. Depending on the design of the coil, deeper penetration can be achieved.
11. Cerebellar TMS can however be done; see for example Colnaghi et al. (2010).
12. For an example of a longer-term TMS treatment study, see Janicak et al. (2010).
13. Chen et al. (2008). See also Lipton and Pearlman (2010); Medina and Tunez (2010); O'Reardon et al. (2007).
14. See for example Borckardt et al. (2011); Borckardt et al. (2009); Nekhendzy et al. (2010). For a discussion of which technique is appropriate when, see Priori et al. (2009). Much more—and better-quality—research is needed for both electrical and magnetic stimulation. A 2010 Cochrane Review (the gold standard for medical interventions) did not find sufficient evidence that either TES or TMS was beneficial in chronic pain, for instance (O'Connell et al., 2010).
15. See for example Zhou et al. (2011), which argues for DBS of the nucleus accumbens (NAc, see note 13, Chapter 5) as a treatment for opiate addiction. 'The clinical practice of surgical ablation of the NAc in China, although controversial and currently stopped, appeared to be effective in alleviating psychological dependence on opiate drugs', the authors note, but 'DBS is a less invasive, reversible, and adjustable stereotactic neuromodulation technique.' See also Wu et al. (2010), on alcohol addiction.
16. Bewernick et al. (2010); Denys et al. (2010); Greenberg et al. (2010); Kennedy et al. (2011); Krack et al. (2010); Owen et al. (2007); Pereira et al. (2010);

Rauch et al. (2006); Ray et al. (2008); Rouaud et al. (2010); Vesper et al. (2007).

17. Ray et al. (2009).

18. Brain tissue is insensitive to trauma, perhaps because it wasn't worth evolution's while to supply pain receptors in a world where skull-penetrating injuries were so often fatal.

19. For a story showing the human costs of Parkinson's disease and the remarkable effects which can be achieved by deep brain stimulation, see the videos from Neuroslicer on YouTube showing a Parkinson's patient 'before' (http://youtu.be/xejclvwbwsk) and 'after' (http://youtu.be/IOH-tUzWo2cg) deep brain stimulation.

20. See for example Kuhn et al. (2010).

21. See for example Herzog et al. (2003); Owen et al. (2006).

22. See for example Quinkert et al. (2010).

23. As a recent review notes, 'Both research and clinical practice have focused initially on motor outcome only, but have neglected quality of life independent of motor function and, in particular, normative and psychosocial factors that are easily missed with quantitative outcome parameters (e.g. with movement scores or quality of life scores).' See Synofzik and Schlaepfer (2011), p. 9.

24. Finding numbers for how many people have had this form of eye surgery is not easy; I scanned ophthalmic professional bodies' websites in vain. However, one 'leading UK provider' alone claims to have carried out more than 700,000 operations, so 'millions' across the board is a justifiable estimate (http://uk. opticalexpress.com/laser-eye-surgery/how-optical-express-compares-with-other-providers.html). Incidentally, that provider refers to 'procedures', not operations.

25. See for example LeDoux (2002).

26. DBS also induces wariness because of its historical associations, as a form of psychosurgery, with much cruder and more dubious methods such as prefrontal lobotomy (Skuban et al., 2011; see also note 24, Chapter 2).

27. HSDD dates from DSM-IV; in earlier days it was called frigidity. It is a controversial topic even among psychiatrists. I have already cited, in note 11, Chapter 7, an incisive article by Ben Goldacre (Goldacre, 2010). The study to which he refers was presented at the Society for Neuroscience conference in 2010—yes, its wide media coverage came despite it not having been published—and its abstract can be found at the SfN website, Nowak et al. (2010). Also worth a read is The Neurocritic's blog (http://

neurocritic.blogspot.com/2010/10/media-hsdd-hyperactive-sexual-disorder.html).

28. See for example Palacios (2010).

29. A Google search for 'female Viagra' in January 2011 offers over three million results, suggesting the potential market is a large one. Modern hormone therapies join an older, herbal-based pharmacopoeia, including damiana (from a small American shrub) and gingko (from the maidenhair tree, *Gingko biloba*). Both have been hailed for their powers of sexual healing. There is little evidence for either claim.

30. A 2010 survey of 400 women diagnosed with HSDD found that 60% cited 'stress or fatigue' as a contributory factor, and 40.8% cited 'dissatisfaction with my physical appearance' (Maserejian et al., 2010).

31. In 2003 it was widely reported in the British press that the heir to the throne Prince Charles had expressed concerns to the Royal Society about nanotechnology's potentially destructive effects, raising the possibility that self-replicating nanomachines (grey goo, or, when combined with biotech, green goo) might escape human control and devastate the planet. See for example http://www.guardian.co.uk/science/2003/apr/29/nanotechnology. science; the website http://www.crnano.org/dangers.htm may also be of interest. The report which may have prompted the Prince's concern is available from http://www.etcgroup.org/en/archives.

32. Intracellular recording has already been implemented with a nanoscale device, for example, to reduce cell damage (Duan et al., 2011).

33. The journal offering a special issue on neurogenetics is *Neuron*, Volume 68, Issue 2, 21 October 2010.

Chapter 12

1. See for example Jones and Loon (2005); Robinson (2010).

2. The quotation is from Bernard (1957). I should note that describing Bernard as a physiologist is like calling Newton a physicist: accurate, but an incomplete account of his importance.

3. See http://www.guardian.co.uk/science/2011/jan/15/uncertainty-failure-edge-question.

4. See for example Graveley et al. (2011) and Kharchenko et al. (2011), which report genetics analyses, going beyond traditional DNA, of the fruit fly *Drosophila melanogaster*.

5. For a mesmerizing video of this process, see the RIKEN-OSC video (available via *Nature*) 'The Central Dogma' (http://www.youtube.com/user/

NatureVideoChannel#p/a/u/1/J3HVVi2k2No). Incidentally, even as well-established a theory as the central dogma can still be subject to challenge; see for example Li et al. (2011).

6. Poliseno et al. (2010).

7. Baker (2011).

8. RNA, ribonucleic acid, is similar to DNA in structure, although the base thymine (T) is replaced by uracil (U). If you would like to learn more about gene transcription there is an entertaining interactive website at http://learn.genetics.utah.edu/content/begin/dna/transcribe/.

9. The RNA abbreviations stand for messenger, small interfering, large intergenic noncoding, and micro RNAs, respectively. See for example Guo et al. (2010) and Huarte et al. (2010).

10. The textbook mentioned is Bear et al. (1996), in which I counted 666 pages. Glance over the index, and you will find mention of neurotransmitters such as ACh (acetylcholine), adrenaline and noradrenaline, dopamine, enkephalin, GABA (gamma-aminobutyric acid), glutamate, glycine, and serotonin. You will not find recent arrivals on the neurotransmitter list, like neuropeptide Y, cholecystokinin or adenosine; nor will you find the extraordinary range of receptor subtypes that mediate the many effects of these chemicals on neurons, glia, and blood vessels. You will find oxytocin and vasopressin, but in 1996 these neurohormones were thought of primarily as chemicals released by the brain into the blood to control body functions such as lactation and childbirth. We now know that they act via brain receptors to change neuronal activity and influence behaviours like social recognition, affiliation, and aggression (Guastella et al., 2010b; Insel, 2010). Many other body chemicals have likewise escaped relegation to the sub-neck zone: oestrogen (a sex hormone), cortisol (a stress hormone), leptin (involved in eating), and even interleukins (components of the immune system) are all now known to affect the brain (Benedict et al., 2009; Dedovic et al., 2009; Dumitriu et al., 2010; Pinteaux et al., 2009; Spulber and Schultzberg, 2010; Sugama and Conti, 2008). More will undoubtedly be discovered. The links between brain and body grow ever more many and various, as the extent of our embedded, embodied natures grows ever more apparent.

11. The third edition of Bear et al. (1996), published in 2006, has 928 pages. To illustrate the change since then, I consulted a bibliometric database (Thomson Reuters, 2004–2009). In 2006, it records 207 journals in neurosciences and neuroimaging, publishing 28,904 articles. By 2009, the last year available, those figures are 238 journals and 32,545 articles, jumping about 15% and 13% respectively.

12. Richardson-Jones et al. (2010), p. 40.

13. Richardson-Jones et al. (2010).

14. See Richardson-Jones et al. (2010), p. 40; also Barbui et al. (2011); Cipriani et al. (2009).

15. Magalhaes et al. (2010).

16. Millan et al. (2000).

17. Colgan et al. (2009).

18. Blier et al. (1998).

19. Richardson-Jones and colleagues estimate the half-life (see note 10, Chapter 6) of 5-HT$_{1A}$ receptors in their genetically modified mice at around eight days. 'Four weeks after doxycycline removal, maximal suppression is achieved and 5-HT$_{1A}$ receptor levels are undetectable' (Richardson-Jones et al., 2010, p. 41).

20. Millan et al. (2000).

21. Richardson-Jones et al. (2010), p. 42.

22. The chow used in the *Neuron* study was a standard laboratory rodent food. Its precise composition can be found at http://www.labdiet.com/pdf/5p75-5p76.pdf.

23. Creating 'knock-out' mice with no 5-HT$_{1A}$ receptors has been done. Richardson-Jones et al. cite three references in their paper: Ramboz et al. (1998), on which René Hen was a co-author, and two studies from other US research groups (Heisler et al., 1998; Parks et al., 1998).

24. The exact numbers of animals are not given as they vary with the experimental task (e.g. not all mice did every test described in the paper), but they range up to around 25 animals per group (HIGH and LOW groups).

25. Some of the system checks involved slicing up mouse brains to see whether there were any receptors, and if so how many and where. To do this a technique called autoradiography was used. It is similar to PET, in that a radioactive molecule which binds to the receptors is used. This is sloshed over the brain slice, which is then photographed with a film which darkens where there is more radioactivity (i.e. more receptors). The researchers also checked that the receptors in the LOW mice (those supposed to have fewer autoreceptors) were really fewer, again using brain slices, by applying a chemical which selectively binds to this kind of 5-HT receptor. Normal cells responded vigorously; cells with fewer 5-HT$_{1A}$ receptors didn't. To make sure that these were 5-HT neurons, the researchers stained the brain slices with a marker selective for serotonergic cells. In addition, to check that changes in receptor levels translated into effects in the whole brain, the mice were given another receptor-stimulating chemical, one which in

normal animals induces hypothermia. The HIGH mice got cold, as normal mice do; the LOW mice's response was significantly weaker. Finally, the researchers had another group of mice that lacked the tTS gene but were kept on doxycycline. That allowed them to control for any effects of the antibiotic itself on mouse behaviour.

26. Microdialysis involves inserting a tiny probe into the brain area of interest. The probe is designed to resemble a blood vessel, and like a blood vessel it can absorb chemicals from the cerebrospinal fluid surrounding neurons, thereby allowing researchers to assess the levels of these chemicals in the area.

27. The project which produced Richardson-Jones et al. (2010) was worked on by 'the authors of the paper plus a couple technicians' (i.e. 14 people) over a period of five years (René Hen, personal communication). Projects generate multiple publications, of course (see e.g. Richardson-Jones et al., 2011), so generally the amount of effort required to achieve the first publication on a project is considerably greater than that needed to generate subsequent papers.

28. See www.majorityleader.gov/YouCut/.

29. Blier et al. (1998).

30. Richardson-Jones et al. (2010), p. 49.

31. An alternative proposed by the authors is that, since 5-HT_{1A} autoreceptors are inhibitory, reducing their levels may reduce their capacity to limit serotonin release (Richardson-Jones et al., 2010, p. 49).

32. Needless to say, Blier himself is not so sure about what the results of the *Neuron* study show. His commentary on the paper is well worth reading (Blier, 2010). He argues, among other caveats, that 'a different degree of 5-HT_{1A} autoreceptor desensitization may well be present in SSRI-treated 1A-High and 1A-Low mice. The spontaneous firing rate of 5-HT neurons may thus be differentially affected by the long-term SSRI regimen in 1A-Low and 1A-High mice.' IMCOTT, in short. Richardson-Jones et al. (2010) is a piece of the puzzle of depression, not a final narrative, and work on that puzzle is ongoing; see for example Hahn et al. (2010), one of the 26 publications to have cited Richardson-Jones et al. when I checked on SCOPUS (subscription required) http://www.scopus.com/ in early June 2011.

33. The analogy to the human case is limited by the very factor which gives the mouse model such analytical power: the adult onset of the receptor deficiency induced by withdrawing doxycycline from the diet. Natural human genetic variation, by contrast, is encoded from conception.

Chapter 13

1. In the PubMed database of research articles (http://www.ncbi.nlm.nih.gov/pubmed/; searched 16 May 2011), the original report by Boyden et al. (2005) had been cited by other studies only 11 times up to the end of 2007. In 2008 things change: 29 citations, and 36 more in 2009. Figures for 2010 are not given because, due to processing delays, they are likely to be incomplete.

2. See http://www.nature.com/nmeth/video/moy2010/index.html.

3. The execution of optogenetic methods is complex, and one fine-grained description of neurogenetics in this book is plenty, so I will not go into further detail. Interested readers may wish to watch a video on the topic, such as the one provided by *WIRED Science* at http://www.wired.com/wiredscience/2011/05/optogenetic-brain-video/, or consult the research literature, for example Boyden et al. (2005); Nagel et al. (2003) (which described the channelrhodopsin protein), and for more recent developments Liu and Tonegawa (2010), Han et al. (2011), or Berndt et al. (2011).

4. Archaerhodopsin-3 is a proton pump: a molecule which actively transfers hydrogen ions out of the cell. This makes the interior more negative, which tends to suppress cell signalling. The protein triggered by blue light is also a proton pump. The chloride channel, which is a passive opening rather than an active pump, is inhibitory since it allows the influx of Cl^- ions into the cell. See Chow et al. (2010); Gradinaru et al. (2010).

5. Zhang et al. (2010) gives how-to details for mammalian brains.

6. See for example Adamantidis et al. (2007); Han et al. (2009b).

7. Some species of snake have specialized ion channels for infrared detection; see Gracheva et al. (2010).

8. Ye et al. (2010).

9. Examples of optogenetics used in combination with other approaches include: for deep brain stimulation Gradinaru et al. (2009), for electrophysiology Cardin et al. (2010), for fMRI Lee et al. (2010), and for neurogenetics Zhu et al. (2009).

10. Adamantidis et al. (2007); Franks et al. (2009); Higley and Sabatini (2010); Tecuapetla et al. (2010).

11. Synchronized neuronal networks are associated with attention (Cardin et al., 2009).

12. See Gourine et al. (2010) for an example of ontogenetic research on glia.

13. Zhang et al. (2007).

14. The etymology sheds light here: epigenetics (from the Greek: *epi* = on, upon) builds upon and goes beyond genetics.

15. See Handel and Ramagopalan (2010). Jean-Baptiste Lamarck (1744–1829) is best known for his suggestion that organisms might be able to pass characteristics acquired during their lifetime (as opposed to features encoded in their genes) to their offspring, an idea long scorned by the Darwinian consensus. It is not thought, however, that epigenetic changes can last for enough generations to be significant in long-term evolution.

16. Zaranek et al. (2010).

17. Coufal et al. (2009); see also Day and Sweatt (2011).

18. Schmeck Jr (1987).

19. The first, eponymous journal was *Epigenetics* (http://www.landesbioscience. com/journals/epigenetics/). In 2008 an open-access rival started publication: *Epigenetics and Chromatin* (http://www.epigeneticsandchromatin.com/).

20. Bollati and Baccarelli (2010); Feng et al. (2010); Lim et al. (2010); McGowan and Szyf (2010).

21. Whether Kelvin actually said, 'There is nothing new to be discovered in physics now' is disputed, as famous quotations frequently are. I cannot find any such statement in the 1900 or 1894 meeting reports of the British Association for the Advancement of Science, in Kelvin's lecture to the Royal Institution of 27 April 1900, or in his 1894 Popular Lectures vol. 2, all possible sources according to online references. The physicist Albert Michelson is often cited in a similar context as saying that 'future discoveries must be looked for in the sixth place of decimals' (Michelson (1902), p. 24, available from http://www.archive.org/details/lightwavesandthoo-michgoog), but this is advocating greater experimental precision, not supporting the claim of 'nothing new'. In the 27 April 1900 lecture, Kelvin himself acknowledged the existence of 'two clouds on the horizon' of scientists' current understanding of energy: the failure to detect the ether, and 'the Maxwell–Boltzmann doctrine regarding the partition of energy' (Kelvin, 1901, p. 2). These and other 'clouds' such as radioactivity and the photoelectric effect helped to stimulate development of what was to become known as 'the new physics'. So the pompous closed-mindedness implied by the quotation may be a little unfair to the noble Lord.

22. Nature Editorial (2011).

23. The mechanisms by which intergenerational epigenetic effects occur are beginning to be identified. See Sandovici et al. (2011); Vucetic et al. (2010) on diet, Launay et al. (2009); Youngentob and Glendinning (2009) on smoking and drinking, and McGowan et al. (2008); McGowan et al. (2009); Murgatroyd et al. (2009) on childhood experiences.

24. IMCOTT. Other mechanisms have been identified. A 2010 review notes that five 'broad and interrelated mechanisms are known to affect chromatin structure: DNA methylation, histone modification, remodelling by chromatin-remodelling complexes, insertion of histone variants, and the effects of non-coding RNAs' (Dulac, 2010).
25. Jargon note: DNA is a nucleic acid. Sugar + base combinations are called nucleosides, or nucleotides if the phosphates are included.
26. Baker (2011).
27. The methyl and acetyl groups, unlike phosphate, are not ions—their bonds are covalent—so by convention their abbreviations do not show their electrical charges.
28. Gregg et al. (2010a); Gregg et al. (2010b). See also Sato and Stryker (2010); Schalkwyk et al. (2010).
29. Ballestar (2010); Best and Carey (2010); De Smet and Loriot (2010); Ding et al. (2010); Goodfellow et al. (2010); McGowan and Szyf (2010); Movassagh et al. (2010); West et al. (2010).
30. For a recent discussion of germline transmission, see Lange and Schneider (2010).
31. For a review of epigenetics with respect to mental health, see McGowan and Szyf (2010).
32. The abbreviation NR3C1 stands for Nuclear Receptor (subfamily) 3 (group) C (member) 1.
33. Anacker et al. (2010); Dedovic et al. (2009); Hawes et al. (2009); McCrory et al. (2010); Tanriverdi et al. (2007).
34. Darnaudery and Maccari (2008).
35. McGowan et al. (2009).
36. Fish et al. (2004); Gunnar and Quevedo (2008); Veenema (2009).
37. McGowan and Szyf (2010), p. 70. However, it is not yet known when during development the important changes occur. As the authors note, 'it remains unclear whether the epigenetic aberrations documented in brain pathologies were present in the germ line, whether they were introduced during embryogenesis, or whether they were truly changes occurring during early childhood' (p. 70).
38. Batstra et al. (2003); Blood-Siegfried and Rende (2010); Flick et al. (2006).
39. A related issue concerns the extent to which epigenetic changes in response to, for example, abusive upbringing are pathologies, as opposed to adaptations to difficult circumstances (Heiming et al., 2009; Heiming and Sachser, 2010). This is a version of the 'problem of normal' discussed in Chapter 14.

40. Combes and Whitelaw (2010); McGowan and Szyf (2010); Weaver (2007).

Chapter 14

1. See note 20, Chapter 2. The prospect of DNE recording raises interesting philosophical issues. For example, if such a transcript were to be transferred, not into ordinary storage media, but into a purpose-built artificial nervous system, would the result comprise a conscious machine, a silicon clone of the person recorded, or what? Questions like this are one reason why I chose to do science rather than philosophy.

2. As mentioned in Chapter 8, how ecologically valid a task is reflects how 'real-world' it is. The artificial nature of psychology experiments is a cause for concern; see for example Rai and Fiske (2010).

3. The same objections apply to other neuroimaging methods, though to varying extents; EEG and MEG are less distorting experiences than fMRI since the person is wearing a cap or reclining under a machine rather than being engulfed by a scanner. Efforts to make neuroimaging more portable, and hence less distant from everyday experience, are ongoing; see for example Schulz et al. (2011) on a head-mounted PET system for rats, and Theis et al. (2011) on magnetic resonance without the need for large magnetic fields.

4. See for example a talk given to the TED forum by Christopher deCharms in 2008 (http://www.ted.com/talks/christopher_decharms_scans_the_brain_in_real_time.html).

5. Ganis et al. (2011).

6. For the estimate of average neurons per voxel, see de-Wit et al. (2010). Regional population data are taken from http://www.citypopulation.de/index.html. The values are: Cheltenham, UK, 98,875; Ithaca, NY, 101,564; Kiribati, 99,500 (estimates are for mid-2010, except for the population of Cheltenham which is taken from the 2001 census).

7. Based on a post mortem analysis of four reasonably *compos mentis* brains from men 'deceased from nonneurological causes and without cognitive impairment', aged from 50 to 71, from a brain bank in Brazil, 'We find that the adult male human brain contains on average 86.1 ± 8.1 billion NeuN-positive cells ('neurons') and 84.6 ± 9.8 billion NeuN-negative ('nonneuronal') cells' (Azevedo et al., 2009). The estimate of 86 billion holds, in other words, for 'neuronists' who grant non-neuronal cells like glia only second-class citizenship in the brain's republic. Yet the roles of glia in brain functions appear increasingly substantial: see for example Allaman et al. (2011); Attwell et al. (2010), and Suzuki et al. (2011). If glia are included, that roughly doubles the numbers.

8. The population of China in mid-2010 was estimated as 1,338,613,000 by http://www.citypopulation.de/index.html. The world population, as of 8 July 2010 (17:12 UTC), is estimated by the US Census Bureau to be 6,854,627,896. See http://www.census.gov/main/www/popclock.html.

9. I chose the figure of 50 km^2 simply because of the example of Cheltenham in my earlier analogy; this English borough, containing a little over 100,000 people, covers an area of around 46 km^2 (according to Wikipedia, at http://en.wikipedia.org/wiki/List_of_English_districts_by_area#10_-_100_km.C2.B2).

10. Data were obtained from a search of the SCOPUS research database, http://www.scopus.com/ (subscription required), on 13 July 2010. Results were restricted to a single year, 2009. See also Volz et al. (2009).

11. See for example Coricelli and Nagel (2009); Hermann et al. (2009); Koenigs and Grafman (2009); Koya et al. (2009); Shalom (2009); Straube et al. (2009); Urry et al. (2009); Xue et al. (2009).

12. A few researchers have even disgraced their professions by using the abnormal conditions pertaining during genocide to facilitate their studies. See for example Muller-Hill (2001) on perhaps the most notorious example in the West, from the Nazi regime.

13. The article, by journalist Michelle Roberts, is sourced from http://news.bbc.co.uk/1/hi/health/8672400.stm (published online 10 May 2010). My thanks to Michelle and to the BBC for permission to reproduce this article.

14. The media aversion to providing hyperlinks to original research is remarked upon by science commentator Ben Goldacre in *The Guardian* (Goldacre, 2011b).

15. Rissman et al. (2010). PNAS is short for *Proceedings of the National Academy of Sciences of the United States of America*.

16. Information is correct at the time of writing, early in 2011, but there is considerable pressure to make scientific information more available to wider audiences so PNAS may yet change its policy. Many journals have already, for example, made their contents available, often with a delay.

17. Miller (2010); Royal Society (2011), pp. 18, 74. See also Schauer (2010).

18. The case is summarized by *WIRED* at http://www.wired.com/wiredscience/tag/tu-pham/, which includes a link to the full legal ruling. Judge Tu Pham did not say that brain scans could never be used in similar circumstances, but that these particular scans were inadequate (the judge took account of criticisms from other neuroscientists).

19. The training honed the mathematical model used by the researchers, teaching it to rely more on features of the brain response commonly

found in new images, as distinguished from features shared by new and familiar images. Note the assumption that there are such features, i.e. that all new images have something in common which allows the brain to tell them apart from old hat visual experience. Once training was over, the model was tested by giving it brain responses that it had not been trained on, and seeing how well it classified them as 'new' or 'previously seen'. See also Mendelsohn et al. (2010).

20. To see whether their classifier could sort brain responses into 'new' or 'familiar' when the person wasn't consciously recognizing images, the authors asked a separate group of people to do a second experiment, in which the participants didn't know they were doing a memory task. First, they were shown pictures of faces and asked to rate them on attractiveness. Next, in the scanner, they were shown some of the same pictures, mixed in with some new ones, and asked to decide whether the faces were male or female. The idea was that this would distract them from consciously recognizing familiar faces. It's not quite as simple a task as it seems, because to standardize the images their background and hair have been removed. Not quite what you're facing, so to speak, when you meet an old friend in the street. The classifier was unable to distinguish new and familiar images under these conditions.

21. The distinction between implicit and explicit memories has been funda- mental to memory research in neuroscience and psychology for decades. This being science, however, the distinction has not escaped challenge. See for example Henke (2010), who argues that types of memory should be distinguished by the kinds of neuronal processing they employ, rather than by whether consciousness is involved.

22. In the abstract, incidentally, you may have noted the absence of the phrase 'lie detection'. You won't find it in the article either, except in the refer- ences, but there is sufficient mention of forensic technologies in the initial introduction, the final discussion, and the press release to make the point obvious.

23. Milgram (1963; 1997); see also note 22, Chapter 6.

24. Psychology has studied the 'demand characteristics' of the lab environ- ment; see for example Wooffitt (2007). Neuroscience, however, has to date not taken nearly enough notice of this work—as indeed is the case for its recognition of social psychological effects in general.

25. Examples of common stereotype threats studied in the research literature include the belief that black Americans are better at sport than their white counterparts, and that women are less good than men at mathematics,

physics, and other sciences. See Croizet et al. (2004); Rydell et al. (2009); Miyake et al. (2010).

26. Rydell et al. (2009); see also Rydell et al. (2010).

27. See for example the TED talk by Tan Le (http://www.ted.com/talks/lang/eng/tan_le_a_headset_that_reads_your_brainwaves.html), and reports from the BBC (http://www.bbc.co.uk/news/technology-10647555) and *The Guardian* (http://www.guardian.co.uk/science/2011/apr/17/brain-implant-paralysis-movement).

28. Bakopoulos et al. (2008); Harris et al. (2007).

29. For the Big Five, the standard citation is the manual, Costa and McCrae (1992). The Wechsler Adult Intelligence Scales test various aspects of cognitive function, such as working memory and information processing ability. The current version is WAIS-IV (released in 2008; see http://www.pearsonassessments.com/haiweb/cultures/en-us/productdetail.htm?pid=015-8980-808&Community=CA_Psych_Settings_Forensics). It includes ten core tests, which can take up to an hour and a half to do, assessing verbal comprehension (Similarities, Vocabulary, Information), perception processing (Block Design, Matrix Reasoning, Visual Puzzles), working memory (Digit Span, Arithmetic) and processing speed (Symbol Search, Coding). WAIS tests are standard methods in research—the lab where I did my postdoc on dyslexia ran them routinely on participants. They are also used clinically, for example to detect mild cognitive impairment (which may indicate incipient Alzheimer's) or to decide whether a schoolchild deserves 'special needs' assistance. To determine what is and is not normal performance on the tests, 2,200 people were sampled, their responses plotted, and the extremes defined statistically.

30. Taylor (2000).

31. See for example Giedd and Rapoport (2010).

32. With respect to lie detection, on fMRI reliability see Spence (2008).

33. Wittgenstein (1974), Part I, Section 184, p. 74^e.

34. This flexibility is so pronounced that one assumes it has advantages for social living, promoting group cohesion by allowing group members to, in effect, make themselves more alike psychologically. It is often useful to take on the ideological shades of those around you. However, believing's chameleon tendency can be a real disadvantage too. As I learned when researching my previous book, *Cruelty* (Taylor, 2009), it can speed the growth of dangerous beliefs about other people, under certain conditions, and it also allows those beliefs to harden into extreme, even lethal forms.

35. A prominent theory of why this happens is that the conflict between a person's belief and what they are saying is experienced as the

uncomfortable state of cognitive dissonance, which provokes attempts to reduce it (Cooper, 2007; Festinger, 1957). Neural signals associated with dissonance have been identified (van Veen et al., 2009; see also Goel et al., 2010). For particular relevance to science, Munro (2010) is of interest.

36. For one thing, our ability to manipulate brains will depend on our ability to read them, and as pointed out in earlier chapters that requires much more development. See also Farah et al. (2009).

37. The nematode *Caenorhabditis elegans* is around a millimetre long, lives in soil, and eats bacteria. For all you need to know, see http://www.wormbook.org/index.html. The fruit fly *Drosophila melanogaster*, also known as the vinegar fly, can reach around 3 mm and, although its name means 'dew-lover', its preferred diet includes fruit sugars and microorganisms which grow on decaying fruit. See http://www.ceolas.org/fly/intro.html.

38. Allred et al. (2009); Arendash et al. (2009); Atanasov et al. (2006); Chung et al. (2007); Fukushima et al. (2009); Hanhineva et al. (2010); Kalthoff et al. (2010); Paur et al. (2010); Shin et al. (2010); Tao et al. (2008); Uto-Kondo et al. (2010); Vitaglione et al. (2010).

39. http://ims.dse.ibaraki.ac.jp/research/C_elegans_en.html; see also Azevedo et al. (2009).

40. Bayés et al. (2011).

Chapter 15

1. Ferguson (2011).

2. Upward social comparison has been associated with depression; see for example Bazner et al. (2006).

3. I am of course not the first to note these concerns. See for example Carr (2010); Greenfield (2004); Lanier (2010).

4. The Greek lexicon referenced is the mighty Liddell and Scott, the standard reference (Liddell and Scott, 1901).

5. World-shaping is described in more detail in Taylor (2009).

6. This is the essence of human freedom, according to the philosopher Daniel Dennett (Dennett, 2003).

7. As I describe in *Cruelty* (Taylor, 2009), otherization is the set of processes acting to increase the social distance between persons or groups. It may involve no more than stereotyping, avoidance, and verbal denigration, but once triggered it can, under certain circumstances, escalate, both personally and at the group level, to become as extreme as murder or genocide.

8. See Taylor (2009). Evidence that people have such impulses is not hard to find; the charming folk who cheer on hesitant suicides in public places are only one of many instances. See for example the *Daily Telegraph*, 30 September 2008, on the death of British teenager Shaun Dykes (http://www.telegraph.co.uk/news/uknews/3108987/Suicide-teenager-urged-to-jump-by-baying-crowd.html).

9. For traditional methods of changing beliefs, see Taylor (2006). For new methods of changing memories biochemically, e.g. by altering protein synthesis, see for example Chen et al. (2011); Day and Sweatt (2010); Han et al. (2009a); Lee et al. (2008); Nader and Einarsson (2010); Rossato et al. (2010); Sacktor (2011); Shema et al. (2007); Stefanko et al. (2009). Note my assumption that memories and beliefs have much in common at the biochemical level. For a method for humans, not involving toxic drugs, see Schiller et al. (2010).

10. For example, the Tuskegee and Guatemala syphilis trials did not include what we would now consider adequate informed consent (Minogue and Marshall (2010); see also the Tuskegee Syphilis Study Legacy Committee's report, available from http://www.hsl.virginia.edu/historical/medical_history/bad_blood/. Tuskegee involved poor black people; Guatemala used prisoners. See also Cuddy et al. (2008); Harris and Fiske (2006); Harris and Fiske (2007); Harris and Fiske (2009); and my discussion in Taylor (2009).

11. See for example Snapp et al. (2010).

12. Scientists are at the forefront of such concerns (Godfray et al., 2010; McDonald et al., 2011; Rockstrom et al., 2009).

13. Research suggests that the sense of being in control is a major contributor to well-being at the national level (Fischer and Boer, 2011).

14. The online interview with Stephen Hawking is available at http://bigthink.com/ideas/21570.

15. 'Science under Attack', an edition of the BBC's science programme *Horizon* presented by Sir Paul Nurse, was first aired on BBC2 (and the BBC's high-definition channel) on 24 January 2011.

16. The Royal Society's website lists 106 Original Fellows, of whom 41 were titled. The remnant includes such names as Robert Hooke, Elias Ashmole, and the three Johns Aubrey, Evelyn, and Dryden, who were not exactly peasant labourers. Data were taken from http://royalsociety.org/.

17. The paucity of disabled participants extends beyond science to academia in general, as figures from the UK Higher Education Statistics Agency for 2009–2010 attest: of full-time and part-time academic staff whose disability status was reported, 2.8% declared a disability. Women made up 44.0% of

staff, ethnic minorities 12.0%. See http://www.hesa.ac.uk/index.php?
option=com_content&task=view&id=1978&Itemid=278; also Gewin (2011)
and, on the low numbers of senior black academics, the *Guardian*'s Mortarboard blog (http://www.guardian.co.uk/education/mortarboard/2011/may/
27/black-professor-shortage-failure-to-nurture-talent).

18. See http://curriculum.qcda.gov.uk/key-stages-1-and-2/subjects/science/key-
    stage2/index.aspx.

19. See http://www.telegraph.co.uk/culture/tvandradio/8371699/Who-says-Britain-
    is-dumbing-down.html.

20. The chances of winning the UK lottery are usually estimated as being about
    14 million to one (http://www.murderousmaths.co.uk/books/bkmm6xlo.
    htm). There has, obviously, only ever been one Albert Einstein. To estimate
    the chances of reaching a comparable status, that of a Nobel science laureate,
    we can take a cross-section from the year 2010, in which the world popula-
    tion was approximately 6.8 billion (estimated by the US Census Bureau to be
    6,854,627,896, as of 8 July 2010; see http://www.census.gov/ipc/www/idb/
    worldpop.php). In the same year there were six science Nobel laureates
    (http://nobelprize.org/nobel_prizes/lists/all/), which makes the chance of
    someone alive in 2010 being a laureate about one in a billion. Even were
    the world population to be restricted to a realistic age range (science Nobel
    prizewinners have been from 25 to 88 years old), you are still more likely to
    win the lottery.

21. See for example http://www.guardian.co.uk/science/blog/2011/mar/18/career-
    science-studentship-phd-application, and Jennifer Rohn's article and com-
    ments at http://www.nature.com/news/2011/110302/full/471007a.html.

22. See for example Matthew Nisbet on science literacy (http://scienceblogs.
    com/framing-science/2007/07/the_misunderstood_meanings_of.php).

23. No less a figure than Albert Einstein agrees that 'most of the fundamental
    ideas of science are essentially simple, and may, as a rule, be expressed in a
    language comprehensible to everyone' (Einstein and Infield, 1938, cited by
    Elias A. Zerhouni in Wallace, 2008, p. 135).

24. Holmes (2009).

Bibliography

Åberg, M.A.I., Pedersen, N.L., Torén, K., Svartengren, M., Bäckstrand, B., Johnsson, T., Cooper-Kuhn, C.M., Åberg, N.D., Nilsson, M., and Kuhn, H.G. (2009), 'Cardiovascular fitness is associated with cognition in young adulthood', *Proceedings of the National Academy of Sciences of the United States of America*, 106, pp. 20906–11.

Adamantidis, A.R., Zhang, F., Aravanis, A.M., Deisseroth, K., and de Lecea, L. (2007), 'Neural substrates of awakening probed with optogenetic control of hypocretin neurons', *Nature*, 450, pp. 420–4.

Agay, N., Yechiam, E., Carmel, Z., and Levkovitz, Y. (2010), 'Non-specific effects of methylphenidate (Ritalin) on cognitive ability and decision-making of ADHD and healthy adults', *Psychopharmacology*, 210, pp. 511–19.

Ahlfors, S., Han, J., Belliveau, J., and Hämäläinen, M. (2010a), 'Sensitivity of MEG and EEG to source orientation', *Brain Topography*, 23, pp. 227–32.

Ahlfors, S.P., Han, J., Lin, F.H., Witzel, T., Belliveau, J.W., Hamalainen, M.S., and Halgren, E. (2010b), 'Cancellation of EEG and MEG signals generated by extended and distributed sources', *Human Brain Mapping*, 31, pp. 140–9.

Akitsuki, Y. and Decety, J. (2009), 'Social context and perceived agency affects empathy for pain: an event-related fMRI investigation', *Neuroimage*, 47, pp. 722–34.

Allaman, I., Bélanger, M., and Magistretti, P.J. (2011), 'Astrocyte-neuron metabolic relationships: for better and for worse', *Trends in Neurosciences*, 34, pp. 76–87.

Allred, K.F., Yackley, K.M., Vanamala, J., and Allred, C.D. (2009), 'Trigonelline is a novel phytoestrogen in coffee beans', *Journal of Nutrition*, 139, pp. 1833–8.

Amodio, D.M. and Frith, C.D. (2006), 'Meeting of minds: the medial frontal cortex and social cognition', *Nature Reviews Neuroscience*, 7, pp. 268–77.

Anacker, C., Zunszain, P.A., Carvalho, L.A., and Pariante, C.M. (2010), 'The glucocorticoid receptor: pivot of depression and of antidepressant treatment?', *Psychoneuroendocrinology*, 36, pp. 415–25.

Anastassiou, C.A., Perin, R., Markram, H., and Koch, C. (2011), 'Ephaptic coupling of cortical neurons', *Nature Neuroscience*, 14, pp. 217–23.

Andersen, R.A. and Cui, H. (2009), 'Intention, action planning, and decision making in parietal-frontal circuits', *Neuron*, 63, pp. 568–83.

Arden, R., Gottfredson, L.S., Miller, G., and Pierce, A. (2009), 'Intelligence and semen quality are positively correlated', *Intelligence*, 37, pp. 277–82.

Arendash, G.W., Mori, T., Cao, C., Mamcarz, M., Runfeldt, M., Dickson, A., Rezai-Zadeh, K., Tane, J., Citron, B.A., Lin, X., Echeverria, V., and Potter, H. (2009), 'Caffeine reverses cognitive impairment and decreases brain amyloid-beta levels in aged Alzheimer's disease mice', *Journal of Alzheimer's Disease*, 17, pp. 661–80.

Ariely, D. (2009), *Predictably Irrational: the Hidden Forces that Shape Our Decisions.* London: HarperCollins.

Aristotle (trans. 1937), 'Parts of Animals'. In *Aristotle: Parts of Animals. Movement of Animals. Progression of Animals*, trans. A.L. Peck and E.S. Forster. Cambridge, MA: Harvard University Press, pp. 52–435.

Atanasov, A.G., Dzyakanchuk, A.A., Schweizer, R.A., Nashev, L.G., Maurer, E.M., and Odermatt, A. (2006), 'Coffee inhibits the reactivation of glucocorticoids by 11beta-hydroxysteroid dehydrogenase type 1: a glucocorticoid connection in the anti-diabetic action of coffee?', *FEBS Letters*, 580, pp. 4081–5.

Attwell, D., Buchan, A.M., Charpak, S., Lauritzen, M., MacVicar, B.A., and Newman, E.A. (2010), 'Glial and neuronal control of brain blood flow', *Nature*, 468, pp. 232–43.

Auger, C.J., Coss, D., Auger, A.P., and Forbes-Lorman, R.M. (2011), 'Epigenetic control of vasopressin expression is maintained by steroid hormones in the adult male rat brain', *Proceedings of the National Academy of Sciences of the United States of America*, 108, pp. 4242–7.

Avenanti, A., Minio-Paluello, I., Bufalari, I., and Aglioti, S.M. (2009), 'The pain of a model in the personality of an onlooker: influence of state-reactivity and personality traits on embodied empathy for pain', *Neuroimage*, 44, pp. 275–83.

Azevedo, F.A.C., Carvalho, L.R.B., Grinberg, L.T., Farfel, J.M., Ferretti, R.E.L., Leite, R.E.P., Filho, W.J., Lent, R., and Herculano-Houzel, S. (2009), 'Equal numbers of neuronal and nonneuronal cells make the human brain an isometrically scaled-up primate brain', *Journal of Comparative Neurology*, 513, pp. 532–41.

Babiloni, F., Mattia, D., Babiloni, C., Astolfi, L., Salinari, S., Basilisco, A., Rossini, P.M., Marciani, M.G., and Cincotti, F. (2004), 'Multimodal integration of EEG,

MEG and fMRI data for the solution of the neuroimage puzzle', *Magnetic Resonance Imaging*, 22, pp. 1471–6.

Baillet, S., Garnero, L., Marin, G., and Hugonin, J.P. (1999), 'Combined MEG and EEG source imaging by minimization of mutual information', *IEEE Transactions on Biomedical Engineering*, 46, pp. 522–34.

Baker, M. (2011), 'Genomics: genomes in three dimensions', *Nature*, 470, pp. 289–94.

Bakopoulos, P., Karanasiou, I., Zakynthinos, P., Pleros, N., Avramopoulos, H., and Uzunoglu, N. (2008), 'Towards brain imaging using THz technology', *IST 2008—IEEE Workshop on Imaging Systems and Techniques Proceedings*.

Ball, P. (2011a), 'Beyond the bond', *Nature*, 469, pp. 26–8.

Ball, P. (2011b), *Unnatural: the Heretical Idea of Making People*. London: Bodley Head.

Ballestar, E. (2010), 'Epigenetics lessons from twins: prospects for autoimmune disease', *Clinical Reviews in Allergy and Immunology*, 39, pp. 30–41.

Bandettini, P.A. (2009), 'What's new in neuroimaging methods', *Annals of the New York Academy of Sciences*, 1156, pp. 260–93.

Barbui, C., Cipriani, A., Patel, V., Ayuso-Mateos, J.L., and van Ommeren, M. (2011), 'Efficacy of antidepressants and benzodiazepines in minor depression: systematic review and meta-analysis', *British Journal of Psychiatry*, 198, pp. 11–16, sup 1.

Bardin, J.C., Fins, J.J., Katz, D.I., Hersh, J., Heier, L.A., Tabelow, K., Dyke, J.P., Ballon, D.J., Schiff, N.D., and Voss, H.U. (2011), 'Dissociations between behavioural and functional magnetic resonance imaging-based evaluations of cognitive function after brain injury', *Brain*, 134, pp. 769–82.

Baron-Cohen, S. (2009), 'Media distortion damages both science and journalism', *New Scientist*, 2701, pp. 26–7.

Bass, C.E., Grinevich, V.P., Vance, Z.B., Sullivan, R.P., Bonin, K.D., and Budygin, E.A. (2010), 'Optogenetic control of striatal dopamine release in rats', *Journal of Neurochemistry*, 114, pp. 1344–52.

Batstra, L., Hadders-Algra, M., and Neeleman, J. (2003), 'Effect of antenatal exposure to maternal smoking on behavioural problems and academic achievement in childhood: prospective evidence from a Dutch birth cohort', *Early Human Development*, 75, pp. 21–33.

Batts, S. (2009), 'Brain lesions and their implications in criminal responsibility', *Behavioral Sciences and the Law*, 27, pp. 261–72.

Bayés, À., van de Lagemaat, L.N., Collins, M.O., Croning, M.D.R., Whittle, I.R., Choudhary, J.S., and Grant, S.G.N. (2011), 'Characterization of the proteome, diseases and evolution of the human postsynaptic density', *Nature Neuroscience*, 14, pp. 19–21.

Bazner, E., Bromer, P., Hammelstein, P., and Meyer, T.D. (2006), 'Current and former depression and their relationship to the effects of social comparison processes. Results of an internet based study', *Journal of Affective Disorders*, 93, pp. 97–103.

Bear, M.F., Connors, B.W., and Paradiso, M.A. (1996), *Neuroscience: Exploring the Brain*. Baltimore, MD: Lippincott Williams and Wilkins.

Beer, J.S. and Hughes, B.L. (2010), 'Neural systems of social comparison and the "above-average" effect', *Neuroimage*, 49, pp. 2671–9.

Bell, B., Lin, J.J., Seidenberg, M., and Hermann, B. (2011), 'The neurobiology of cognitive disorders in temporal lobe epilepsy', *Nature Reviews Neurology*, 7, pp. 154–64.

Benali, A., Trippe, J., Weiler, E., Mix, A., Petrasch-Parwez, E., Girzalsky, W., Eysel, U.T., Erdmann, R., and Funke, K. (2011), 'Theta-burst transcranial magnetic stimulation alters cortical inhibition', *Journal of Neuroscience*, 31, pp. 1193–203.

Benedict, C., Scheller, J., Rose-John, S., Born, J., and Marshall, L. (2009), 'Enhancing influence of intranasal interleukin-6 on slow-wave activity and memory consolidation during sleep', *FASEB Journal*, 23, pp. 3629–36.

Bennett, C.M. and Miller, M.B. (2010), 'How reliable are the results from functional magnetic resonance imaging?', *Annals of the New York Academy of Sciences*, 1191, pp. 133–55.

Bernard, C. (1957), *An Introduction to the Study of Experimental Medicine*, trans. H. Greene. New York: Dover Publications.

Berndt, A., Schoenenberger, P., Mattis, J., Tye, K.M., Deisseroth, K., Hegemann, P., and Oertner, T.G. (2011), 'High-efficiency channelrhodopsins for fast neuronal stimulation at low light levels', *Proceedings of the National Academy of Sciences of the United States of America*, 108, pp. 7595–600.

Best, J.D. and Carey, N. (2010), 'Epigenetic opportunities and challenges in cancer', *Drug Discovery Today*, 15, pp. 65–70.

Bewernick, B.H., Hurlemann, R., Matusch, A., Kayser, S., Grubert, C., Hadrysiewicz, B., Axmacher, N., Lemke, M., Cooper-Mahkorn, D., Cohen, M.X., Brockmann, H., Lenartz, D., Sturm, V., and Schlaepfer, T.E. (2010), 'Nucleus accumbens deep brain stimulation decreases ratings of depression and anxiety in treatment-resistant depression', *Biological Psychiatry*, 67, pp. 110–16.

Bikmullina, R., Kicic, D., Carlson, S., and Nikulin, V.V. (2009), 'Electrophysiological correlates of short-latency afferent inhibition: a combined EEG and TMS study', *Experimental Brain Research*, 194, pp. 517–26.

Binczak, S., Eilbeck, J.C., and Scott, A.C. (2001), 'Ephaptic coupling of myelinated nerve fibers', *Physica D: Nonlinear Phenomena*, 148, pp. 159–74.

Biswal, B.B., Mennes, M., Zuo, X.-N., Gohel, S., Kelly, C., Smith, S.M., Beckmann, C.F., Adelstein, J.S., Buckner, R.L., Colcombe, S., Dogonowski, A.-M., Ernst, M., Fair, D., Hampson, M., Hoptman, M.J., Hyde, J.S., Kiviniemi, V.J., Kötter, R., Li, S.-J., Lin, C.-P., Lowe, M.J., Mackay, C., Madden, D.J., Madsen, K.H., Margulies, D.S., Mayberg, H.S., McMahon, K., Monk, C.S., Mostofsky, S.H., Nagel, B.J., Pekar, J.J., Peltier, S.J., Petersen, S.E., Riedl, V., Rombouts, S.A.R.B., Rypma, B., Schlaggar, B.L., Schmidt, S., Seidler, R.D., Siegle, G.J., Sorg, C., Teng, G.-J., Veijola, J., Villringer, A., Walter, M., Wang, L., Weng, X.-C., Whitfield-Gabrieli, S., Williamson, P., Windischberger, C., Zang, Y.-F., Zhang, H.-Y., Castellanos, F.X., and Milham, M.P. (2010), 'Toward discovery science of human brain function', *Proceedings of the National Academy of Sciences of the United States of America*, 107, pp. 4734–9.

Björk, B.-C., Roos, A., and Lauri, M. (2008), 'Global annual volume of peer reviewed scholarly articles and the share available via different Open Access options', *ELPUB 2008 Conference on Electronic Publishing*.

Blier, P. (2010), 'Altered function of the serotonin 1A autoreceptor and the antidepressant response', *Neuron*, 65, pp. 1–2.

Blier, P., Piñeyro, G., El Mansari, M., Bergeron, R., and De Montigny, C. (1998), 'Role of somatodendritic 5-HT autoreceptors in modulating 5-HT neurotransmission', *Annals of the New York Academy of Sciences*, 861, pp. 204–16.

Blood-Siegfried, J. and Rende, E.K. (2010), 'The long-term effects of prenatal nicotine exposure on neurologic development', *Journal of Midwifery and Women's Health*, 55, pp. 143–52.

Bock, D.D., Lee, W.-C.A., Kerlin, A.M., Andermann, M.L., Hood, G., Wetzel, A.W., Yurgenson, S., Soucy, E.R., Kim, H.S., and Reid, R.C. (2011), 'Network anatomy and *in vivo* physiology of visual cortical neurons', *Nature*, 471, pp. 177–82.

Boecker, H., Henriksen, G., Sprenger, T., Miederer, I., Willoch, F., Valet, M., Berthele, A., and Tölle, T.R. (2008), 'Positron emission tomography ligand activation studies in the sports sciences: measuring neurochemistry *in vivo*', *Methods*, 45, pp. 307–18.

Bollati, V. and Baccarelli, A. (2010), 'Environmental epigenetics', *Heredity*, 105, pp. 105–12.

Boly, M., Garrido, M.I., Gosseries, O., Bruno, M.-A.l., Boveroux, P., Schnakers, C., Massimini, M., Litvak, V., Laureys, S., and Friston, K. (2011), 'Preserved feedforward but impaired top-down processes in the vegetative state', *Science*, 332, pp. 858–62.

Bonnard, M., Spieser, L., Meziane, H.B., de Graaf, J.B., and Pailhous, J. (2009), 'Prior intention can locally tune inhibitory processes in the primary motor cortex: direct evidence from combined TMS-EEG', *European Journal of Neuroscience*, 30, pp. 913–23.

Borckardt, J.J., Reeves, S.T., Frohman, H., Madan, A., Jensen, M.P., Patterson, D., Barth, K., Smith, A.R., Gracely, R., and George, M.S. (2011), 'Fast left prefrontal rTMS acutely suppresses analgesic effects of perceived controllability on the emotional component of pain experience', *Pain*, 152, pp. 182–7.

Borckardt, J.J., Smith, A.R., Reeves, S.T., Madan, A., Shelley, N., Branham, R., Nahas, Z., and George, M.S. (2009), 'A pilot study investigating the effects of fast left prefrontal rTMS on chronic neuropathic pain', *Pain Medicine*, 10, pp. 840–9.

Boyden, E.S., Zhang, F., Bamberg, E., Nagel, G., and Deisseroth, K. (2005), 'Millisecond-timescale, genetically targeted optical control of neural activity', *Nature Neuroscience*, 8, pp. 1263–68.

Bradberry, T.J., Gentili, R.J., and Contreras-Vidal, J.L. (2010), 'Reconstructing three-dimensional hand movements from noninvasive electroencephalographic signals', *Journal of Neuroscience*, 30, pp. 3432–7.

Branco, T., Clark, B.A., and Häusser, M. (2010), 'Dendritic discrimination of temporal input sequences in cortical neurons', *Science*, 329, pp. 1671–5.

Branco, T. and Häusser, M. (2011), 'Synaptic integration gradients in single cortical pyramidal cell dendrites', *Neuron*, 69, pp. 885–92.

Brem, S., Bach, S., Kucian, K., Guttorm, T.K., Martin, E., Lyytinen, H., Brandeis, D., and Richardson, U. (2010), 'Brain sensitivity to print emerges when children learn letter-speech sound correspondences', *Proceedings of the National Academy of Sciences of the United States of America*, 107, pp. 7939–44.

Breshears, J.D., Roland, J.L., Sharma, M., Gaona, C.M., Freudenburg, Z.V., Tempelhoff, R., Avidan, M.S., and Leuthardt, E.C. (2010), 'Stable and dynamic cortical electrophysiology of induction and emergence with propofol anesthesia', *Proceedings of the National Academy of Sciences of the United States of America*, 107, pp. 21170–5.

Briggman, K.L., Helmstaedter, M., and Denk, W. (2011), 'Wiring specificity in the direction-selectivity circuit of the retina', *Nature*, 471, pp. 183–8.

Brodmann, K. (1909), *Vergleichende Lokalisationslehre der Grosshirnrinde in ihren Prinzipien dargestellt auf Grund des Zellenbaues*. Leipzig: Johann Ambrosius Barth Verlag.

Brodmann, K. (1994), *Brodmann's 'Localisation in the Cerebral Cortex'*, trans. L.J. Garey. London: Smith-Gordon.

Bromberg-Martin, E.S., Matsumoto, M., and Hikosaka, O. (2010), 'Distinct tonic and phasic anticipatory activity in lateral habenula and dopamine neurons', *Neuron*, 67, pp. 144–55.

Brunoni, A.R., Nitsche, M.A., Bolognini, N., Bikson, M., Wagner, T., Merabet, L., Edwards, D.J., Valero-Cabre, A., Rotenberg, A., Pascual-Leone, A., Ferrucci, R., Priori, A., Boggio, P.S., and Fregni, F. (2011), 'Clinical research with transcranial direct current stimulation (tDCS): challenges and future directions', *Brain Stimulation*, in press, corrected proof; doi:10.1016/j.brs.2011.03.002.

Buchan, J. (1935), *A Prince of the Captivity*. London: Hodder and Stoughton.

Buss, D.M. (2005), *The Murderer Next Door: Why the Mind Is Designed to Kill*. New York: Penguin.

Cakic, V. (2009), 'Smart drugs for cognitive enhancement: ethical and pragmatic considerations in the era of cosmetic neurology', *Journal of Medical Ethics*, 35, pp. 611–15.

Calamante, F., Thomas, D.L., Pell, G.S., Wiersma, J., and Turner, R. (1999), 'Measuring cerebral blood flow using magnetic resonance imaging techniques', *Journal of Cerebral Blood Flow and Metabolism*, 19, pp. 701–35.

Calvin, C.M., Deary, I.J., Fenton, C., Roberts, B.A., Der, G., Leckenby, N., and Batty, G.D. (2010), 'Intelligence in youth and all-cause-mortality: systematic review with meta-analysis', *International Journal of Epidemiology*, 40, pp. 626–44.

Caramanos, Z., Narayanan, S., and Arnold, D.L. (2005), '1H-MRS quantification of tNA and tCr in patients with multiple sclerosis: a meta-analytic review', *Brain*, 128, pp. 2483–506.

Caramazza, A., McCloskey, M., and Green, B. (1981), 'Naive beliefs in "sophisticated" subjects: misconceptions about trajectories of objects', *Cognition*, 9, pp. 117–23.

Cardin, J.A., Carlen, M., Meletis, K., Knoblich, U., Zhang, F., Deisseroth, K., Tsai, L.H., and Moore, C.I. (2009), 'Driving fast-spiking cells induces gamma rhythm and controls sensory responses', *Nature*, 459, pp. 663–7.

Cardin, J.A., Carlen, M., Meletis, K., Knoblich, U., Zhang, F., Deisseroth, K., Tsai, L.H., and Moore, C.I. (2010), 'Targeted optogenetic stimulation and recording of neurons *in vivo* using cell-type-specific expression of Channelrhodopsin-2', *Nature Protocols*, 5, pp. 247–54.

Carr, N. (2010), *The Shallows: How the Internet is Changing the Way We Think, Read and Remember*. London: Atlantic Books.

Cartier, N., Hacein-Bey-Abina, S., Bartholomae, C.C., Veres, G., Schmidt, M., Kutschera, I., Vidaud, M., Abel, U., Dal-Cortivo, L., Caccavelli, L., Mahlaoui, N., Kiermer, V., Mittelstaedt, D., Bellesme, C., Lahlou, N., Lefrere, F., Blanche, S., Audit, M., Payen, E., Leboulch, P., l'Homme, B., Bougneres, P., Von Kalle, C., Fischer, A., Cavazzana-Calvo, M., and Aubourg, P. (2009),

'Hematopoietic stem cell gene therapy with a lentiviral vector in X-linked adrenoleukodystrophy', *Science*, 326, pp. 818–23.

Ceccarini, G., Flavell, R.R., Butelman, E.R., Synan, M., Willnow, T.E., Bar-Dagan, M., Goldsmith, S.J., Kreek, M.J., Kothari, P., Vallabhajosula, S., Muir, T.W., and Friedman, J.M. (2009), 'PET imaging of leptin biodistribution and metabolism in rodents and primates', *Cell Metabolism*, 10, pp. 148–59.

Cerf, M., Thiruvengadam, N., Mormann, F., Kraskov, A., Quiroga, R.Q., Koch, C., and Fried, I. (2010), 'On-line, voluntary control of human temporal lobe neurons', *Nature*, 467, pp. 1104–8.

Chadwick, M.J., Hassabis, D., Weiskopf, N., and Maguire, E.A. (2010), 'Decoding individual episodic memory traces in the human hippocampus', *Current Biology*, 20, pp. 544–7.

Chalmers, D.J. (1995), 'Facing up to the problem of consciousness', *Journal of Consciousness Studies*, 2, pp. 200–19.

Chan, P. and Duflou, J. (2008), 'Suicidal electrocution in Sydney—a 10-year case review', *Journal of Forensic Sciences*, 53, pp. 455–9.

Cheetham, M., Pedroni, A.F., Antley, A., Slater, M., and Jäncke, L. (2009), 'Virtual milgram: empathic concern or personal distress? Evidence from functional MRI and dispositional measures', *Frontiers in Human Neuroscience*, 3, doi:10.3389/neuro.09.029.2009.

Chen, D.Y., Stern, S.A., Garcia-Osta, A., Saunier-Rebori, B., Pollonini, G., Bambah-Mukku, D., Blitzer, R.D., and Alberini, C.M. (2011), 'A critical role for IGF-II in memory consolidation and enhancement', *Nature*, 469, pp. 491–7.

Chen, R., Cros, D., Curra, A., Di Lazzaro, V., Lefaucheur, J.-P., Magistris, M.R., Mills, K., Rösler, K.M., Triggs, W.J., Ugawa, Y., and Ziemann, U. (2008), 'The clinical diagnostic utility of transcranial magnetic stimulation: report of an IFCN committee', *Clinical Neurophysiology*, 119, pp. 504–32.

Chi, R.P. and Snyder, A.W. (2011), 'Facilitate insight by non-invasive brain stimulation', *PLoS ONE*, 6, p. e16655.

Choi, M., Ku, T., Chong, K., Yoon, J., and Choi, C. (2011), 'Minimally invasive molecular delivery into the brain using optical modulation of vascular permeability', *Proceedings of the National Academy of Sciences of the United States of America*, 108, pp. 9256–61.

Chow, B.Y., Han, X., Dobry, A.S., Qian, X.F., Chuong, A.S., Li, M.J., Henninger, M.A., Belfort, G.M., Lin, Y.X., Monahan, P.E., and Boyden, E.S. (2010), 'High-performance genetically targetable optical neural silencing by light-driven proton pumps', *Nature*, 463, pp. 98–102.

Chung, J.H., Choi, S.Y., Kim, J.Y., Kim, D.H., Lee, J.W., Choi, J.S., and Chung, H.Y. (2007), '3-methyl-1,2-cyclopentanedione down-regulates age-related

NF-kappaB signaling cascade', *Journal of Agricultural and Food Chemistry*, 55, pp. 6787–92.

Cialdini, R.B. (2002), *Influence: Science and Practice*, 4th edition. Needham Heights, MA: Allyn and Bacon.

Ciaramidaro, A., Adenzato, M., Enrici, I., Erk, S., Pia, L., Bara, B.G., and Walter, H. (2007), 'The intentional network: how the brain reads varieties of intentions', *Neuropsychologia*, 45, pp. 3105–13.

Cipriani, A., Furukawa, T.A., Salanti, G., Geddes, J.R., Higgins, J.P., Churchill, R., Watanabe, N., Nakagawa, A., Omori, I.M., McGuire, H., Tansella, M., and Barbui, C. (2009), 'Comparative efficacy and acceptability of 12 new-generation antidepressants: a multiple-treatments meta-analysis', *Lancet*, 373, pp. 746–58.

Claridge-Chang, A., Roorda, R.D., Vrontou, E., Sjulson, L., Li, H., Hirsh, J., and Miesenböck, G. (2009), 'Writing memories with light-addressable reinforcement circuitry', *Cell*, 139, pp. 405–15.

Clark, D.D. and Sokoloff, L. (1999), 'Circulation and energy metabolism of the brain'. In *Basic Neurochemistry: Molecular, Cellular and Medical Aspects*, eds. G.J. Siegel, B.W. Agranoff, R.W. Albers, S.K. Fisher and M.D. Uhler, 6th edition. Philadelphia: Lippincott-Raven, pp. 637–70.

Clark, K.L., Armstrong, K.M., and Moore, T. (2011), 'Probing neural circuitry and function with electrical microstimulation', *Proceedings of the Royal Society B: Biological Sciences*, 278, pp. 1121–30.

Coenen, V.A., Schlaepfer, T.E., Maedler, B., and Panksepp, J. (2011), 'Cross-species affective functions of the medial forebrain bundle—implications for the treatment of affective pain and depression in humans', *Neuroscience and Biobehavioral Reviews*, 35, pp. 1971–81.

Colgan, L.A., Putzier, I., and Levitan, E.S. (2009), 'Activity-dependent vesicular monoamine transporter-mediated depletion of the nucleus supports somatic release by serotonin neurons', *Journal of Neuroscience*, 29, pp. 15878–87.

Collins, C.E., Airey, D.C., Young, N.A., Leitch, D.B., and Kaas, J.H. (2010), 'Neuron densities vary across and within cortical areas in primates', *Proceedings of the National Academy of Sciences of the United States of America*, 107, pp. 15927–32.

Colnaghi, S., Ramat, S., D'Angelo, E., and Versino, M. (2010), 'Transcranial magnetic stimulation over the cerebellum and eye movements: state of the art', *Functional Neurology*, 25, pp. 165–71.

Combes, A.N. and Whitelaw, E. (2010), 'Epigenetic reprogramming: enforcer or enabler of developmental fate?', *Development, Growth and Differentiation*, 52, pp. 483–91.

Cooper, J. (2007), *Cognitive Dissonance: Fifty Years of a Classic Theory*. London: Sage.

Coricelli, G. and Nagel, R. (2009), 'Neural correlates of depth of strategic reasoning in medial prefrontal cortex', *Proceedings of the National Academy of Sciences of the United States of America*, 106, pp. 9163–8.

Costa, P.T., Jr and McCrae, R.R. (1992), *Revised NEO Personality Inventory (NEO-PI-R) and NEO Five-Factor Inventory (NEO-FFI) Manual*. Odessa, FL: Psychological Assessment Resources.

Coufal, N.G., Garcia-Perez, J.L., Peng, G.E., Yeo, G.W., Mu, Y., Lovci, M.T., Morell, M., O'Shea, K.S., Moran, J.V., and Gage, F.H. (2009), 'L1 retrotransposition in human neural progenitor cells', *Nature*, 460, pp. 1127–31.

Croizet, J.-C., Despres, G., Gauzins, M.-E., Huguet, P., Leyens, J.-P., and Meot, A. (2004), 'Stereotype threat undermines intellectual performance by triggering a disruptive mental load', *Personality and Social Psychology Bulletin*, 30, pp. 721–31.

Cuddy, A.J.C., Fiske, S.T., Glick, P., and Mark, P.Z. (2008), 'Warmth and competence as universal dimensions of social perception: the Stereotype Content Model and the BIAS Map'. *Advances in Experimental Social Psychology*, 40, pp. 61–149.

Dalal, S.S., Zumer, J.M., Guggisberg, A.G., Trumpis, M., Wong, D.D., Sekihara, K., and Nagarajan, S.S. (2011), 'MEG/EEG source reconstruction, statistical evaluation, and visualization with NUTMEG', *Computational Intelligence and Neuroscience*, 2011, p. 758973.

Darnaudery, M. and Maccari, S. (2008), 'Epigenetic programming of the stress response in male and female rats by prenatal restraint stress', *Brain Research Reviews*, 57, pp. 571–85.

Darwin, C.R. (1859), *On the Origin of Species by Means of Natural Selection, or the Preservation of Favoured Races in the Struggle for Life*, 1st edition. London: John Murray.

Day, J.J. and Sweatt, J.D. (2010), 'DNA methylation and memory formation', *Nature Neuroscience*, 13, pp. 1319–23.

Day, J.J. and Sweatt, J.D. (2011), 'Epigenetic mechanisms in cognition', *Neuron*, 70, pp. 813–29.

De Dreu, C.K.W., Greer, L.L., Handgraaf, M.J.J., Shalvi, S., Van Kleef, G.A., Baas, M., Ten Velden, F.S., Van Dijk, E., and Feith, S.W.W. (2010), 'The neuropeptide oxytocin regulates parochial altruism in intergroup conflict among humans', *Science*, 328, pp. 1408–11.

De Dreu, C.K.W., Greer, L.L., Van Kleef, G.A., Shalvi, S., and Handgraaf, M.J.J. (2011), 'Oxytocin promotes human ethnocentrism', *Proceedings of the National Academy of Sciences of the United States of America*, 108, pp. 1262–6.

De Smet, C. and Loriot, A. (2010), 'DNA hypomethylation in cancer: epigenetic scars of a neoplastic journey', *Epigenetics*, 5.

de-Wit, L., Machilsen, B., and Putzeys, T. (2010), 'Predictive coding and the neural response to predictable stimuli', *Journal of Neuroscience*, 30, pp. 8702–3.

Deary, I.J., Batty, G.D., and Gale, C.R. (2008), 'Bright children become enlightened adults', *Psychological Science*, 19, pp. 1–6.

Deary, I.J., Penke, L., and Johnson, W. (2010), 'The neuroscience of human intelligence differences', *Nature Reviews Neuroscience*, 11, pp. 201–11.

Deazley, R. (2008), *Rethinking Copyright: History, Theory, Language*. Cheltenham: Edward Elgar Publishing.

Decety, J., Echols, S., and Correll, J. (2009a), 'The blame game: the effect of responsibility and social stigma on empathy for pain', *Journal of Cognitive Neuroscience*, 22, pp. 985–97.

Decety, J., Michalska, K.J., Akitsuki, Y., and Lahey, B.B. (2009b), 'Atypical empathic responses in adolescents with aggressive conduct disorder: a functional MRI investigation', *Biological Psychology*, 80, pp. 203–11.

Dedovic, K., Duchesne, A., Andrews, J., Engert, V., and Pruessner, J.C. (2009), 'The brain and the stress axis: the neural correlates of cortisol regulation in response to stress', *Neuroimage*, 47, pp. 864–71.

DeFelipe, J. (2010), 'From the connectome to the synaptome: an epic love story', *Science*, 330, pp. 1198–201.

Dehaene, S. and Changeux, J.-P. (2011), 'Experimental and theoretical approaches to conscious processing', *Neuron*, 70, pp. 200–27.

Dell'Osso, B., Priori, A., and Altamura, A.C. (2011), 'Efficacy and safety of transcranial direct current stimulation in major depression', *Biological Psychiatry*, 69, pp. e23–e24.

Dennett, D.C. (2003), *Freedom Evolves*. London: Allen Lane.

Denys, D., Mantione, M., Figee, M., van den Munckhof, P., Koerselman, F., Westenberg, H., Bosch, A., and Schuurman, R. (2010), 'Deep brain stimulation of the nucleus accumbens for treatment-refractory obsessive-compulsive disorder', *Archives of General Psychiatry*, 67, pp. 1061–8.

Deslauriers, L., Schelew, E., and Wieman, C. (2011), 'Improved learning in a large-enrollment physics class', *Science*, 332, pp. 862–4.

Dickens, C. (1857/2003), *Little Dorrit*, revised edition. London: Penguin.

Dierolf, M., Menzel, A., Thibault, P., Schneider, P., Kewish, C.M., Wepf, R., Bunk, O., and Pfeiffer, F. (2010), 'Ptychographic X-ray computed tomography at the nanoscale', *Nature*, 467, pp. 436–9.

Ding, Y., Lv, J., Mao, C., Zhang, H., Wang, A., Zhu, L., Zhu, H., and Xu, Z. (2010), 'High-salt diet during pregnancy and angiotensin-related cardiac changes', *Journal of Hypertension*, 28, pp. 1290–7.

Duan, X., Gao, R., Xie, P., Cohen-Karni, T., Qing, Q., Choe, H.S., Tian, B., Jiang, X., and Lieber, C.M. (2012), 'Intracellular recordings of action potentials by an extracellular nanoscale field-effect transistor', *Nature Nanotechnology*, 7, pp. 174–9.

Duckworth, A.L., Quinn, P.D., Lynam, D.R., Loeber, R., and Stouthamer-Loeber, M. (2011), 'Role of test motivation in intelligence testing', *Proceedings of the National Academy of Sciences of the United States of America*, 108, pp. 7716–20.

Dulac, C. (2010), 'Brain function and chromatin plasticity', *Nature*, 465, pp. 728–35.

Dumitriu, D., Rapp, P.R., McEwen, B.S., and Morrison, J.H. (2010), 'Estrogen and the aging brain: an elixir for the weary cortical network', *Annals of the New York Academy of Sciences*, 1204, pp. 104–12.

Dupoux, E. and Jacob, P. (2007), 'Universal moral grammar: a critical appraisal', *Trends in Cognitive Sciences*, 11, pp. 373–8.

Einstein, A. and Infield, L. (1938), *The Evolution of Physics: From Early Concept to Relativity and Quanta*. Cambridge: Cambridge University Press.

Eisenstein, E.L. (1980), *The Printing Press as an Agent of Change*. Cambridge: Cambridge University Press.

El Mestikawy, S., Wallén-Mackenzie, Å., Fortin, G.M., Descarries, L., and Trudeau, L.-E. (2011), 'From glutamate co-release to vesicular synergy: vesicular glutamate transporters', *Nature Reviews Neuroscience*, 12, pp. 204–16.

Engineer, N.D., Riley, J.R., Seale, J.D., Vrana, W.A., Shetake, J.A., Sudanagunta, S.P., Borland, M.S., and Kilgard, M.P. (2011), 'Reversing pathological neural activity using targeted plasticity', *Nature*, 470, pp. 101–4.

Esser, S.K., Huber, R., Massimini, M., Peterson, M.J., Ferrarelli, F., and Tononi, G. (2006), 'A direct demonstration of cortical LTP in humans: a combined TMS/EEG study', *Brain Research Bulletin*, 69, pp. 86–94.

Farah, M.J., Illes, J., Cook-Deegan, R., Gardner, H., Kandel, E., King, P., Parens, E., Sahakian, B., and Wolpe, P.R. (2004), 'Neurocognitive enhancement: what can we do and what should we do?', *Nature Reviews Neuroscience*, 5, pp. 421–5.

Farah, M.J., Smith, M., Gawuga, C., Lindsell, D., and Foster, D. (2009), 'Brain imaging and brain privacy: a realistic concern?', *Journal of Cognitive Neuroscience*, 21, pp. 119–27.

Feinberg, D.A., Moeller, S., Smith, S.M., Auerbach, E., Ramanna, S., Glasser, M.F., Miller, K.L., Ugurbil, K., and Yacoub, E. (2010), 'Multiplexed echo planar imaging for sub-second whole brain fMRI and fast diffusion imaging', *PLoS ONE*, 5, p. e15710.

Fell, J. and Axmacher, N. (2011), 'The role of phase synchronization in memory processes', *Nature Reviews Neuroscience*, 12, pp. 105–18.

Feng, J., Zhou, Y., Campbell, S.L., Le, T., Li, E., Sweatt, J.D., Silva, A.J., and Fan, G. (2010), 'Dnmt1 and Dnmt3a maintain DNA methylation and regulate synaptic function in adult forebrain neurons', *Nature Neuroscience*, 13, pp. 423–30.

Ferguson, N. (2011), *Civilization: the West and the Rest*. London: Allen Lane.

Festinger, L. (1957), *A Theory of Cognitive Dissonance*. New York: Row, Peterson and Co.

Fierro, B., De Tommaso, M., Giglia, F., Giglia, G., Palermo, A., and Brighina, F. (2010), 'Repetitive transcranial magnetic stimulation (rTMS) of the dorso-lateral prefrontal cortex (DLPFC) during capsaicin-induced pain: modulatory effects on motor cortex excitability', *Experimental Brain Research*, 203, pp. 31–8.

Filippi, M., Riccitelli, G., Falini, A., Di Salle, F., Vuilleumier, P., Comi, G., and Rocca, M.A. (2010), 'The brain functional networks associated to human and animal suffering differ among omnivores, vegetarians and vegans', *PLoS ONE*, 5, p. e10847.

Fine, C. (2010), *Delusions of Gender: the Real Science Behind Sex Differences*. Cambridge: Icon.

Fish, E.W., Shahrokh, D., Bagot, R., Caldji, C., Bredy, T., Szyf, M., and Meaney, M.J. (2004), 'Epigenetic programming of stress responses through variations in maternal care', *Annals of the New York Academy of Sciences*, 1036, pp. 167–80.

Fischer, R. and Boer, D. (2011), 'What is more important for national well-being: money or autonomy? A meta-analysis of well-being, burnout, and anxiety across 63 societies', *Journal of Personality and Social Psychology*, 101, pp. 164–84.

Fisher, H., Aron, A., and Brown, L.L. (2005), 'Romantic love: an fMRI study of a neural mechanism for mate choice', *Journal of Comparative Neurology*, 493, pp. 58–62.

Fleishman, S.J., Whitehead, T.A., Ekiert, D.C., Dreyfus, C., Corn, J.E., Strauch, E.-M., Wilson, I.A., and Baker, D. (2011), 'Computational design of proteins targeting the conserved stem region of influenza hemagglutinin', *Science*, 332, pp. 816–21.

Flick, L.H., Cook, C.A., Homan, S.M., McSweeney, M., Campbell, C., and Parnell, L. (2006), 'Persistent tobacco use during pregnancy and the likelihood of psychiatric disorders', *American Journal of Public Health*, 96, pp. 1799–807.

Forbes, C.E. and Grafman, J. (2010), 'The role of the human prefrontal cortex in social cognition and moral judgment', *Annual Review of Neuroscience*, 33, pp. 299–324.

Ford, M.B. and Collins, N.L. (2010), 'Self-esteem moderates neuroendocrine and psychological responses to interpersonal rejection', *Journal of Personality and Social Psychology*, 98, pp. 405–19.

Forlini, C. and Racine, E. (2009), 'Disagreements with implications: diverging discourses on the ethics of non-medical use of methylphenidate for performance enhancement', *BMC Medical Ethics*, 10, doi:10.1186/1472-6939-10-9.

Franks, C.J., Murray, C., Ogden, D., O'Connor, V., and Holden-Dye, L. (2009), 'A comparison of electrically evoked and channel rhodopsin-evoked postsynaptic potentials in the pharyngeal system of *Caenorhabditis elegans*', *Invertebrate Neuroscience*, 9, pp. 43–56.

Freeman, J.B., Schiller, D., Rule, N.O., and Ambady, N. (2010), 'The neural origins of superficial and individuated judgments about ingroup and outgroup members', *Human Brain Mapping*, 31, pp. 150–9.

Frøkjær, J.B., Olesen, S.S., Graversen, C., Andresen, T., Lelic, D., and Drewes, A.M. (2011), 'Neuroimaging of the human visceral pain system—a methodological review', *Scandinavian Journal of Pain*, 2, pp. 95–104.

Fu, M. and Zuo, Y. (2011), 'Experience-dependent structural plasticity in the cortex', *Trends in Neurosciences*, 34, pp. 177–87.

Fukushima, Y., Kasuga, M., Nakao, K., Shimomura, I., and Matsuzawa, Y. (2009), 'Effects of coffee on inflammatory cytokine gene expression in mice fed high-fat diets', *Journal of Agricultural and Food Chemistry*, 57, pp. 11100–5.

Ganis, G., Rosenfeld, J.P., Meixner, J., Kievit, R.A., and Schendan, H.E. (2011), 'Lying in the scanner: covert countermeasures disrupt deception detection by functional magnetic resonance imaging', *Neuroimage*, 55, pp. 312–19.

Garnett, A., Whiteley, L., Piwowar, H., Rasmussen, E., and Illes, J. (2011), 'Neuroethics and fMRI: mapping a fledgling relationship', *PLoS ONE*, 6, p. e18537.

Gewin, V. (2011), 'Equality: the fight for access', *Nature*, 469, pp. 255–7.

Geyer, S., Weiss, M., Reimann, K., Lohmann, G., and Turner, R. (2011), 'Microstructural parcellation of the human cerebral cortex—from Brodmann's post-mortem map to *in vivo* mapping with high-field magnetic resonance imaging', *Frontiers in Human Neuroscience*, 5.

Giedd, J.N. and Rapoport, J.L. (2010), 'Structural MRI of pediatric brain development: what have we learned and where are we going?', *Neuron*, 67, pp. 728–34.

Gilbert, S.J., Meuwese, J.D., Towgood, K.J., Frith, C.D., and Burgess, P.W. (2009), 'Abnormal functional specialization within medial prefrontal cortex in high-functioning autism: a multi-voxel similarity analysis', *Brain*, 132, pp. 869–78.

Gitelman, D.R., Parrish, T.B., Friston, K.J., and Mesulam, M.M. (2002), 'Functional anatomy of visual search: regional segregations within the frontal eye fields and effective connectivity of the superior colliculus', *Neuroimage*, 15, pp. 970–82.

Godfray, H.C.J., Beddington, J.R., Crute, I.R., Haddad, L., Lawrence, D., Muir, J.F., Pretty, J., Robinson, S., Thomas, S.M., and Toulmin, C. (2010), 'Food security: the challenge of feeding 9 billion people', *Science*, 327, pp. 812–18.

Goehler, L.E., Lyte, M., and Gaykema, R.P.A. (2007), 'Infection-induced viscerosensory signals from the gut enhance anxiety: implications for psychoneuroimmunology', *Brain, Behavior, and Immunity*, 21, pp. 721–6.

Goel, S., Mason, W., and Watts, D.J. (2010), 'Real and perceived attitude agreement in social networks', *Journal of Personality and Social Psychology*, 99, pp. 611–21.

Goldacre, B. (2010), 'Lost your libido? Let's try a little neuro-realism, madam', *The Guardian*, 30 October.

Goldacre, B. (2011a), 'Backwards step on looking into the future', *The Guardian*, 23 April.

Goldacre, B. (2011b), 'A case of never letting the source spoil a good story', *The Guardian*, 19 March.

Gonon, F., Bezard, E., and Boraud, T. (2011), 'Misrepresentation of neuroscience data might give rise to misleading conclusions in the media: the case of attention deficit hyperactivity disorder', *PLoS ONE*, 6, p. e14618.

Goodfellow, L.R., Earl, S., Cooper, C., and Harvey, N.C. (2010), 'Maternal diet, behaviour and offspring skeletal health', *International Journal of Environmental Research and Public Health*, 7, pp. 1760–72.

Gourine, A.V., Kasymov, V., Marina, N., Tang, F., Figueiredo, M.F., Lane, S., Teschemacher, A.G., Spyer, K.M., Deisseroth, K., and Kasparov, S. (2010), 'Astrocytes control breathing through pH-dependent release of ATP', *Science*, 329, pp. 571–5.

Gozzi, M., Zamboni, G., Krueger, F., and Grafman, J. (2010), 'Interest in politics modulates neural activity in the amygdala and ventral striatum', *Human Brain Mapping*, 31, pp. 1763–71.

Gracheva, E.O., Ingolia, N.T., Kelly, Y.M., Cordero-Morales, J.F., Hollopeter, G., Chesler, A.T., Sanchez, E.E., Perez, J.C., Weissman, J.S., and Julius, D. (2010), 'Molecular basis of infrared detection by snakes', *Nature*, 464, pp. 1006–11.

Gradinaru, V., Mogri, M., Thompson, K.R., Henderson, J.M., and Deisseroth, K. (2009), 'Optical deconstruction of parkinsonian neural circuitry', *Science*, 324, pp. 354–9.

Gradinaru, V., Zhang, F., Ramakrishnan, C., Mattis, J., Prakash, R., Diester, I., Goshen, I., Thompson, K.R., and Deisseroth, K. (2010), 'Molecular and cellular approaches for diversifying and extending optogenetics', *Cell*, 141, pp. 154–65.

Graham, J., Haidt, J., and Nosek, B.A. (2009), 'Liberals and conservatives rely on different sets of moral foundations', *Journal of Personality and Social Psychology*, 96, pp. 1029–46.

Graveley, B.R., Brooks, A.N., Carlson, J.W., Duff, M.O., Landolin, J.M., Yang, L., Artieri, C.G., van Baren, M.J., Boley, N., Booth, B.W., Brown, J.B., Cherbas, L., Davis, C.A., Dobin, A., Li, R., Lin, W., Malone, J.H., Mattiuzzo, N.R., Miller, D., Sturgill, D., Tuch, B.B., Zaleski, C., Zhang, D., Blanchette, M., Dudoit, S., Eads, B., Green, R.E., Hammonds, A., Jiang, L., Kapranov, P., Langton, L., Perrimon, N., Sandler, J.E., Wan, K.H., Willingham, A., Zhang, Y., Zou, Y., Andrews, J., Bickel, P.J., Brenner, S.E., Brent, M.R., Cherbas, P., Gingeras, T.R., Hoskins, R.A., Kaufman, T.C., Oliver, B., and Celniker, S.E. (2011), 'The developmental transcriptome of *Drosophila melanogaster*', *Nature*, 471, pp. 473–9.

Green, A.M. and Kalaska, J.F. (2011), 'Learning to move machines with the mind', *Trends in Neurosciences*, 34, pp. 61–75.

Greenberg, B.D., Rauch, S.L., and Haber, S.N. (2010), 'Invasive circuitry-based neurotherapeutics: stereotactic ablation and deep brain stimulation for OCD', *Neuropsychopharmacology*, 35, pp. 317–36.

Greene, B. (1999), *The Elegant Universe: Superstrings, Hidden Dimensions and the Quest for the Ultimate Theory*. New York: Vintage.

Greene, J.D. (2009), 'Dual-process morality and the personal/impersonal distinction: a reply to McGuire, Langdon, Coltheart, and Mackenzie', *Journal of Experimental Social Psychology*, 45, pp. 581–4.

Greene, J.D., Nystrom, L.E., Engell, A.D., Darley, J.M., and Cohen, J.D. (2004), 'The neural bases of cognitive conflict and control in moral judgment', *Neuron*, 44, pp. 389–400.

Greenfield, S. (2004), *Tomorrow's People: How 21st-Century Technology is Changing the Way We Think and Feel*. London: Penguin.

Gregg, C., Zhang, J., Butler, J.E., Haig, D., and Dulac, C. (2010a), 'Sex-specific parent-of-origin allelic expression in the mouse brain', *Science*, 329, pp. 682–5.

Gregg, C., Zhang, J., Weissbourd, B., Luo, S., Schroth, G.P., Haig, D., and Dulac, C. (2010b), 'High-resolution analysis of parent-of-origin allelic expression in the mouse brain', *Science*, 329, pp. 643–8.

Gu, X. and Han, S. (2007), 'Attention and reality constraints on the neural processes of empathy for pain', *Neuroimage*, 36, p. 256.

Guastella, A.J., Einfeld, S.L., Gray, K.M., Rinehart, N.J., Tonge, B.J., Lambert, T.J., and Hickie, I.B. (2010a), 'Intranasal oxytocin improves emotion recognition for youth with autism spectrum disorders', *Biological Psychiatry*, 67, pp. 692–4.

Guastella, A.J., Kenyon, A.R., Alvares, G.A., Carson, D.S., and Hickie, I.B. (2010b), 'Intranasal arginine vasopressin enhances the encoding of happy and angry faces in humans', *Biological Psychiatry*, 67, pp. 1220–2.

Gunnar, M.R. and Quevedo, K.M. (2008), 'Early care experiences and HPA axis regulation in children: a mechanism for later trauma vulnerability', *Progress in Brain Research*, 167, pp. 137–49.

Guo, H., Ingolia, N.T., Weissman, J.S., and Bartel, D.P. (2010), 'Mammalian microRNAs predominantly act to decrease target mRNA levels', *Nature*, 466, pp. 835–40.

Guyon, A., Massa, F., Rovère, C., and Nahon, J.-L. (2008), 'How cytokines can influence the brain: a role for chemokines?', *Journal of Neuroimmunology*, 198, pp. 46–55.

Habermas, J. (1992), *The Structural Transformation of the Public Sphere: Inquiry into a Category of Bourgeois Society*. Cambridge: Polity Press.

Hadjieconomou, D., Rotkopf, S., Alexandre, C., Bell, D.M., Dickson, B.J., and Salecker, I. (2011), 'Flybow: genetic multicolor cell labeling for neural circuit analysis in *Drosophila melanogaster*', *Nature Methods*, 8, pp. 260–6.

Hadjipapas, A., Casagrande, E., Nevado, A., Barnes, G.R., Green, G., and Holliday, I.E. (2009), 'Can we observe collective neuronal activity from macroscopic aggregate signals?', *Neuroimage*, 44, pp. 1290–303.

Hahn, A., Lanzenberger, R., Wadsak, W., Spindelegger, C., Moser, U., Mien, L.K., Mitterhauser, M., and Kasper, S. (2010), 'Escitalopram enhances the association of serotonin-1A autoreceptors to heteroreceptors in anxiety disorders', *Journal of Neuroscience*, 30, pp. 14482–9.

Halpern-Manners, N.W., Bajaj, V.S., Teisseyre, T.Z., and Pines, A. (2010), 'Magnetic resonance imaging of oscillating electrical currents', *Proceedings of the National Academy of Sciences of the United States of America*, 107, pp. 8519–24.

Hampel, S., Chung, P., McKellar, C.E., Hall, D., Looger, L.L., and Simpson, J.H. (2011), '*Drosophila* Brainbow: a recombinase-based fluorescence labeling technique to subdivide neural expression patterns', *Nature Methods*, 8, pp. 253–9.

Han, J.-H., Kushner, S.A., Yiu, A.P., Hsiang, H.-L., Buch, T., Waisman, A., Bontempi, B., Neve, R.L., Frankland, P.W., and Josselyn, S.A. (2009a), 'Selective erasure of a fear memory', *Science*, 323, pp. 1492–6.

Han, S., Fan, Y., and Mao, L. (2008), 'Gender difference in empathy for pain: an electrophysiological investigation', *Brain Research*, 1196, pp. 85–93.

Han, X., Chow, B.Y., Zhou, H., Klapoetke, N.C., Chuong, A., Rajimehr, R., Yang, A., Baratta, M.V., Winkle, J., Desimone, R., and Boyden, E.S. (2011), 'A high-light sensitivity optical neural silencer: development, and application to optogenetic control of nonhuman primate cortex', *Frontiers in Systems Neuroscience*, 5.

Han, X., Qian, X.F., Bernstein, J.G., Zhou, H.H., Franzesi, G.T., Stern, P., Bronson, R.T., Graybiel, A.M., Desimone, R., and Boyden, E.S. (2009b), 'Millisecond-timescale optical control of neural dynamics in the nonhuman primate brain', *Neuron*, 62, pp. 191–8.

Handel, A. and Ramagopalan, S. (2010), 'Is Lamarckian evolution relevant to medicine?', *BMC Medical Genetics*, 11, doi:10.1186/1471-2350-11-73, p. 73.

Hanhineva, K., Torronen, R., Bondia-Pons, I., Pekkinen, J., Kolehmainen, M., Mykkanen, H., and Poutanen, K. (2010), 'Impact of dietary polyphenols on carbohydrate metabolism', *International Journal of Molecular Sciences*, 11, pp. 1365–402.

Hansen, P., Kringelbach, M., and Salmelin, R., eds. (2010), *MEG: an Introduction to Methods*. New York: Oxford University Press.

Harper, H.A., Rodwell, V.W., and Mayes, P.A., eds. (1977), *Review of Physiological Chemistry*, 16th edition. Los Altos, CA: Lange Medical Publications.

Harris, J.S., Gu, A., and Kim, S.M. (2007), 'New THz sources for bio-medical imaging', *Proceedings of SPIE—The International Society for Optical Engineering*.

Harris, L.T. and Fiske, S.T. (2006), 'Dehumanizing the lowest of the low: neuroimaging responses to extreme out-groups', *Psychological Science*, 17, pp. 847–53.

Harris, L.T. and Fiske, S.T. (2007), 'Social groups that elicit disgust are differentially processed in mPFC', *Social Cognitive and Affective Neuroscience*, 2, pp. 45–51.

Harris, L.T. and Fiske, S.T. (2009), 'Social neuroscience evidence for dehumanised perception', *European Review of Social Psychology*, 20, pp. 192–231.

Harris, S., Jones, M., Zheng, Y., and Berwick, J. (2010), 'Does neural input or processing play a greater role in the magnitude of neuroimaging signals?', *Frontiers in Neuroenergetics*, 2, doi: 10.3389/fnene.2010.00015, p. 12.

Hassabis, D., Chu, C., Rees, G., Weiskopf, N., Molyneux, P.D., and Maguire, E.A. (2009), 'Decoding neuronal ensembles in the human hippocampus', *Current Biology*, 19, pp. 546–54.

Hatfield, E., Cacioppo, J.T., and Rapson, R.L. (1994), *Emotional Contagion*. Cambridge: Cambridge University Press.

Hauser, M. (2006), *Moral Minds: How Nature Designed Our Universal Sense of Right and Wrong*. New York: HarperCollins.

Hawes, D.J., Brennan, J., and Dadds, M.R. (2009), 'Cortisol, callous-unemotional traits, and pathways to antisocial behavior', *Current Opinion in Psychiatry*, 22, pp. 357–62.

Hawking, S. (1988), *A Brief History of Time*. London: Bantam.

Hayden, E.C. (2010), 'Sex bias blights drug studies', *Nature*, 464, pp. 332–3.

Heijtz, R.D., Wang, S., Anuar, F., Qian, Y., Björkholm, B., Samuelsson, A., Hibberd, M.L., Forssberg, H., and Pettersson, S. (2011), 'Normal gut microbiota modulates brain development and behavior', *Proceedings of the National Academy of Sciences of the United States of America*, 108, pp. 3047–52.

Heiming, R.S., Jansen, F., Lewejohann, L., Kaiser, S., Schmitt, A., Lesch, K.P., and Sachser, N. (2009), 'Living in a dangerous world: the shaping of behavioral profile by early environment and 5-HTT genotype', *Frontiers in Behavioral Neuroscience*, 3, doi:10.3389/neuro.08.026.2009.

Heiming, R.S. and Sachser, N. (2010), 'Consequences of serotonin transporter genotype and early adversity on behavioral profile—pathology or adaptation?', *Frontiers in Neuroscience*, 4, doi: 10.3389/fnins.2010.00187.

Heisler, L.K., Chu, H.-M., Brennan, T.J., Danao, J.A., Bajwa, P., Parsons, L.H., and Tecott, L.H. (1998), 'Elevated anxiety and antidepressant-like responses in serotonin 5-HT1A receptor mutant mice', *Proceedings of the National Academy of Sciences of the United States of America*, 95, pp. 15049–54.

Henke, K. (2010), 'A model for memory systems based on processing modes rather than consciousness', *Nature Reviews Neuroscience*, 11, pp. 523–32.

Hermann, A., Schäfer, A., Walter, B., Stark, R., Vaitl, D., and Schienle, A. (2009), 'Emotion regulation in spider phobia: role of the medial prefrontal cortex', *Social Cognitive and Affective Neuroscience*, 4, pp. 257–67.

Herzog, H., Pietrzyk, U., Shah, N.J., and Ziemons, K. (2010), 'The current state, challenges and perspectives of MR-PET', *Neuroimage*, 49, pp. 2072–82.

Herzog, J., Volkmann, J., Krack, P., Kopper, F., Potter, M., Lorenz, D., Steinbach, M., Klebe, S., Hamel, W., Schrader, B., Weinert, D., Muller, D., Mehdorn, H.M., and Deuschl, G. (2003), 'Two-year follow-up of subthalamic deep brain stimulation in Parkinson's disease', *Movement Disorders*, 18, pp. 1332–7.

Higley, M.J. and Sabatini, B.L. (2010), 'Competitive regulation of synaptic Ca^{2+} influx by D2 dopamine and A2A adenosine receptors', *Nature Neuroscience*, 13, pp. 958–66.

Hills, T. and Hertwig, R. (2011), 'Why aren't we smarter already', *Current Directions in Psychological Science*, 20, pp. 373–7.

Hipp, J.F., Engel, A.K., and Siegel, M. (2011), 'Oscillatory synchronization in large-scale cortical networks predicts perception', *Neuron*, 69, pp. 387–96.

Holmes, R. (2009), *The Age of Wonder: How the Romantic Generation Discovered the Beauty and Terror of Science*. London: HarperPress.

Hosten, O. (2011), 'Quantum physics: how to catch a wave', *Nature*, 474, pp. 170–1.

Huang, Y., Zheng, M.Q., and Gerdes, J.M. (2010), 'Development of effective PET and SPECT imaging agents for the serotonin transporter: has a twenty-year journey reached its destination?', *Current Topics in Medicinal Chemistry*, 10, pp. 1499–526.

Huarte, M., Guttman, M., Feldser, D., Garber, M., Koziol, M.J., Kenzelmann-Broz, D., Khalil, A.M., Zuk, O., Amit, I., Rabani, M., Attardi, L.D., Regev, A., Lander, E.S., Jacks, T., and Rinn, J.L. (2010), 'A large intergenic noncoding RNA induced by p53 mediates global gene repression in the p53 response', *Cell*, 142, pp. 409–19.

Huff, T.E. (2010), *Intellectual Curiosity and the Scientific Revolution: A Global Perspective*. Cambridge: Cambridge University Press.

Hurlemann, R., Patin, A., Onur, O.A., Cohen, M.X., Baumgartner, T., Metzler, S., Dziobek, I., Gallinat, J., Wagner, M., Maier, W., and Kendrick, K.M. (2010), 'Oxytocin enhances amygdala-dependent, socially reinforced learning and emotional empathy in humans', *Journal of Neuroscience*, 30, pp. 4999–5007.

Illes, J., Tairyan, K., Federico, C.A., Tabet, A., and Glover, G.H. (2010), 'Reducing barriers to ethics in neuroscience', *Frontiers in Human Neuroscience*, 4, doi: 10.3389/fnhum.2010.00167, p. 12.

Insel, T.R. (2010), 'The challenge of translation in social neuroscience: a review of oxytocin, vasopressin, and affiliative behavior', *Neuron*, 65, pp. 768–79.

Ishizaki, A. and Fleming, G.R. (2009), 'Theoretical examination of quantum coherence in a photosynthetic system at physiological temperature', *Proceedings of the National Academy of Sciences of the United States of America*, 106, pp. 17255–60.

Jacobs, E. and D'Esposito, M. (2011), 'Estrogen shapes dopamine-dependent cognitive processes: implications for women's health', *Journal of Neuroscience*, 31, pp. 5286–93.

Jagiellowicz, J., Xu, X., Aron, A., Aron, E., Cao, G., Feng, T., and Weng, X. (2010), 'The trait of sensory processing sensitivity and neural responses to changes in visual scenes', *Social Cognitive and Affective Neuroscience*, 6, pp. 38–47.

Janicak, P.G., Nahas, Z., Lisanby, S.H., Solvason, H.B., Sampson, S.M., McDonald, W.M., Marangell, L.B., Rosenquist, P., McCall, W.V., Kimball, J., O'Reardon, J.P., Loo, C., Husain, M.H., Krystal, A., Gilmer, W., Dowd, S.M., Demitrack, M.A., and Schatzberg, A.F. (2010), 'Durability of clinical benefit with transcranial magnetic stimulation (TMS) in the treatment of pharmacoresistant major depression: assessment of relapse during a 6-month, multi-site, open-label study', *Brain Stimulation*, 3, pp. 187–99.

Jausovec, N. (2000), 'Differences in cognitive processes between gifted, intelligent, creative, and average individuals while solving complex problems: an EEG study', *Intelligence*, 28, pp. 213–37.

Jay, M. (2003), *The Air Loom Gang: the Strange and True Story of James Tilly Matthews and His Visionary Madness*. London: Bantam Press.

Jokela, M., Elovainio, M., Singh-Manoux, A., and Kivimaki, M. (2009), 'IQ, socioeconomic status, and early death: the US National Longitudinal Survey of Youth', *Psychosomatic Medicine*, 71, pp. 322–8.

Jones, S. and Loon, B.V. (2005), *Introducing Genetics*. Cambridge: Icon.

Just, M.A., Cherkassky, V.L., Aryal, S., and Mitchell, T.M. (2010), 'A neurosemantic theory of concrete noun representation based on the underlying brain codes', *PLoS ONE*, 5, p. e8622.

Kaku, M. (1999), *Visions: How Science Will Revolutionize the 21st Century*. Oxford: Oxford Paperbacks.

Kalbe, E., Schlegel, M., Sack, A.T., Nowak, D.A., Dafotakis, M., Bangard, C., Brand, M., Shamay-Tsoory, S., Onur, O.A., and Kessler, J. (2010), 'Dissociating cognitive from affective theory of mind: a TMS study', *Cortex*, 46, pp. 769–80.

Kalthoff, S., Ehmer, U., Freiberg, N., Manns, M.P., and Strassburg, C.P. (2010), 'Coffee induces expression of glucuronosyltransferases by the aryl hydrocarbon receptor and Nrf2 in liver and stomach', *Gastroenterology*, 139, pp. 1699–710, 710 e1–2.

Kanai, R., Feilden, T., Firth, C., and Rees, G. (2011), 'Political orientations are correlated with brain structure in young adults', *Current Biology*, 21, pp. 677–80.

Kanai, R. and Rees, G. (2011), 'The structural basis of inter-individual differences in human behaviour and cognition', *Nature Reviews Neuroscience*, 12, pp. 231–42.

Kato, J., Ide, H., Kabashima, I., Kadota, H., Takano, K., and Kansaku, K. (2009), 'Neural correlates of attitude change following positive and negative advertisements', *Frontiers in Behavioral Neuroscience*, 3, doi: 10.3389/neuro.08. 006.2009, p. 6.

Kay, K.N., Naselaris, T., Prenger, R.J., and Gallant, J.L. (2008), 'Identifying natural images from human brain activity', *Nature*, 452, pp. 352–5.

Kelly, K. (2010), *What Technology Wants*. New York: Viking.

Kelvin, L. (1901). 'I. Nineteenth century clouds over the dynamical theory of heat and light', *Philosophical Magazine Series 6*, 2, pp. 1–40.

Kennedy, S.H., Giacobbe, P., Rizvi, S.J., Placenza, F.M., Nishikawa, Y., Mayberg, H.S., and Lozano, A.M. (2011), 'Deep brain stimulation for treatment-resistant depression: follow-up after 3 to 6 years', *American Journal of Psychiatry*, 168, pp. 502–10.

Kharchenko, P.V., Alekseyenko, A.A., Schwartz, Y.B., Minoda, A., Riddle, N.C., Ernst, J., Sabo, P.J., Larschan, E., Gorchakov, A.A., Gu, T., Linder-Basso, D., Plachetka, A., Shanower, G., Tolstorukov, M.Y., Luquette, L.J., Xi, R., Jung, Y. L., Park, R.W., Bishop, E.P., Canfield, T.K., Sandstrom, R., Thurman, R.E., MacAlpine, D.M., Stamatoyannopoulos, J.A., Kellis, M., Elgin, S.C.R., Kuroda, M.I., Pirrotta, V., Karpen, G.H., and Park, P.J. (2011), 'Comprehensive analysis of the chromatin landscape in *Drosophila melanogaster*', Nature, 471, pp. 480–5.

Kilgour, A.H., Starr, J.M., and Whalley, L.J. (2010), 'Associations between childhood intelligence (IQ), adult morbidity and mortality', Maturitas, 65, pp. 98–105.

Kim, A.M., Tingen, C.M., and Woodruff, T.K. (2010), 'Sex bias in trials and treatment must end', Nature, 465, pp. 688–9.

Kirkup, G., Zalevski, A., Maruyama, T., and Batool, I. (2010), *Women and Men in Science, Engineering and Technology: the UK Statistics Guide 2010*. Bradford: The UKRC.

Koenigs, M. and Grafman, J. (2009), 'Posttraumatic stress disorder: the role of medial prefrontal cortex and amygdala', Neuroscientist, 15, pp. 540–8.

Koya, E., Uejima, J.L., Wihbey, K.A., Bossert, J.M., Hope, B.T., and Shaham, Y. (2009), 'Role of ventral medial prefrontal cortex in incubation of cocaine craving', Neuropharmacology, 56 Suppl 1, pp. 177–85.

Krack, P., Hariz, M.I., Baunez, C., Guridi, J., and Obeso, J.A. (2010), 'Deep brain stimulation: from neurology to psychiatry?', Trends in Neurosciences, 33, pp. 474–84.

Kristensson, K. (2011), 'Microbes' roadmap to neurons', Nature Reviews Neuroscience, 12, pp. 345–57.

Kuhn, J., Gründler, T.O.J., Lenartz, D., Sturm, V., Klosterkötter, J., and Huff, W. (2010), 'Deep brain stimulation for psychiatric disorders', Deutsches Ärzteblatt International, 107, pp. 105–13.

Kuhn, T.S. (1962), *The Structure of Scientific Revolutions*. Chicago: University of Chicago Press.

Kurzweil, R. (2005), *The Singularity Is Near: When Humans Transcend Biology*. New York: Viking.

Lange, U.C. and Schneider, R. (2010), 'What an epigenome remembers', BioEssays, 32, pp. 659–68.

Lanier, J. (2010), *You Are Not A Gadget: A Manifesto* London: Allen Lane.

Launay, J.-M., Del Pino, M., Chironi, G., Callebert, J., Peoc'h, K., Mégnien, J.-L., Mallet, J., Simon, A., and Rendu, F. (2009), 'Smoking induces long-lasting effects through a monoamine-oxidase epigenetic regulation', *PLoS ONE*, 4, p. e7959.

Leach, J., Achyuta, A.K.H., and Murthy, S.K. (2010), 'Bridging the divide between neuroprosthetic design, tissue engineering and neurobiology', *Frontiers in Neuroengineering*, 2, doi: 10.3389/neuro.16.018.2009

LeDoux, J. (2002), *Synaptic Self: How Our Brains Become Who We Are*. London: Macmillan.

Lee, J.H., Durand, R., Gradinaru, V., Zhang, F., Goshen, I., Kim, D.S., Fenno, L.E., Ramakrishnan, C., and Deisseroth, K. (2010), 'Global and local fMRI signals driven by neurons defined optogenetically by type and wiring', *Nature*, 465, pp. 788–92.

Lee, S.-H., Choi, J.-H., Lee, N., Lee, H.-R., Kim, J.-I., Yu, N.-K., Choi, S.-L., Lee, S.-H., Kim, H., and Kaang, B.-K. (2008), 'Synaptic protein degradation underlies destabilization of retrieved fear memory', *Science*, 319, pp. 1253–6.

Lehtinen, M.K., Zappaterra, M.W., Chen, X., Yang, Y.J., Hill, A.D., Lun, M., Maynard, T., Gonzalez, D., Kim, S., Ye, P., D'Ercole, A.J., Wong, E.T., LaMantia, A.S., and Walsh, C.A. (2011), 'The cerebrospinal fluid provides a proliferative niche for neural progenitor cells', *Neuron*, 69, pp. 893–905.

Leifer, A.M., Fang-Yen, C., Gershow, M., Alkema, M.J., and Samuel, A.D. (2011), 'Optogenetic manipulation of neural activity in freely moving *Caenorhabditis elegans*', *Nature Methods*, 8, pp. 147–52.

Leitenberg, H. and Henning, K. (1995), 'Sexual fantasy', *Psychological Bulletin*, 117, pp. 469–96.

Leuthardt, E.C., Gaona, C., Sharma, M., Szrama, N., Roland, J., Freudenberg, Z., Solis, J., Breshears, J.D., and Schalk, G. (2011), 'Using the electrocorticographic speech network to control a brain–computer interface in humans', *Journal of Neural Engineering*, 8, p. 036004.

Li, M., Wang, I.X., Li, Y., Bruzel, A., Richards, A.L., Toung, J.M., and Cheung, V.G. (2011), 'Widespread RNA and DNA sequence differences in the human transcriptome', *Science*, 333, pp. 53–8.

Liddell, H.G. and Scott, R. (1901), *Greek–English Lexicon*. Clarendon Press, Oxford.

Lim, S., Metzger, E., Schule, R., Kirfel, J., and Buettner, R. (2010), 'Epigenetic regulation of cancer growth by histone demethylases', *International Journal of Cancer*, 127, pp. 1991–8.

Lin, A.-L., Fox, P.T., Hardies, J., Duong, T.Q., and Gao, J.-H. (2010), 'Nonlinear coupling between cerebral blood flow, oxygen consumption, and ATP production in human visual cortex', *Proceedings of the National Academy of Sciences of the United States of America*, 107, pp. 8446–51.

Lin, D., Boyle, M.P., Dollar, P., Lee, H., Lein, E.S., Perona, P., and Anderson, D.J. (2011), 'Functional identification of an aggression locus in the mouse hypothalamus', *Nature*, 470, pp. 221–6.

Link, B.G., Phelan, J.C., Miech, R., and Westin, E.L. (2008), 'The resources that matter: fundamental social causes of health disparities and the challenge of intelligence', *Journal of Health and Social Behavior*, 49, pp. 72–91.

Lipton, R.B. and Pearlman, S.H. (2010), 'Transcranial magnetic simulation in the treatment of migraine', *Neurotherapeutics*, 7, pp. 204–12.

Liu, X. and Tonegawa, S. (2010), 'Optogenetics 3.0', *Cell*, 141, pp. 22–4.

Livet, J., Weissman, T.A., Kang, H., Draft, R.W., Lu, J., Bennis, R.A., Sanes, J.R., and Lichtman, J.W. (2007), 'Transgenic strategies for combinatorial expression of fluorescent proteins in the nervous system', *Nature*, 450, pp. 56–62.

Logothetis, N.K. (2008), 'What we can do and what we cannot do with fMRI', *Nature*, 453, pp. 869–78.

London, M., Roth, A., Beeren, L., Hausser, M., and Latham, P.E. (2010), 'Sensitivity to perturbations *in vivo* implies high noise and suggests rate coding in cortex', *Nature*, 466, pp. 123–7.

Lundeen, J.S., Sutherland, B., Patel, A., Stewart, C., and Bamber, C. (2011), 'Direct measurement of the quantum wavefunction', *Nature*, 474, pp. 188–91.

Lynch, G., Palmer, L.C., and Gall, C.M. (2011), 'The likelihood of cognitive enhancement', *Pharmacology Biochemistry and Behavior*, 99, pp. 116–29.

MacIlwain, C. (2010), 'What science is really worth', *Nature*, 465, pp. 682–4.

Magalhaes, A.C., Holmes, K.D., Dale, L.B., Comps-Agrar, L., Lee, D., Yadav, P.N., Drysdale, L., Poulter, M.O., Roth, B.L., Pin, J.-P., Anisman, H., and Ferguson, S.S.G. (2010), 'CRF receptor 1 regulates anxiety behavior via sensitization of 5-HT2 receptor signaling', *Nature Neuroscience*, 13, pp. 622–9.

Magistretti, P.J., Pellerin, L., and Martin, J.-L. (2000), 'Brain energy metabolism: an integrated cellular perspective'. In *Psychopharmacology: The Fourth Generation of Progress*, eds. F.E. Bloom and D.J. Kupfer. Brentwood, TN: American College of Neuropsychopharmacology.

Marder, E. and Taylor, A.L. (2011), 'Multiple models to capture the variability in biological neurons and networks', *Nature Neuroscience*, 14, pp. 133–8.

Maren, S. (2011), 'Seeking a spotless mind: extinction, deconsolidation, and erasure of fear memory', *Neuron*, 70, pp. 830–45.

Martinelli, A.M. (1993), 'Organ donation: barriers, religious aspects', *AORN*, 58, pp. 236–52.

Maserejian, N.N., Shifren, J.L., Parish, S.J., Braunstein, G.D., Gerstenberger, E.P., and Rosen, R.C. (2010), 'The presentation of hypoactive sexual desire disorder in premenopausal women', *The Journal of Sexual Medicine*, 7, pp. 3439–48.

Maslow, A.H. (1966), *The Psychology of Science: A Reconnaissance*. New York: HarperCollins.

McCabe, D.P. and Castel, A.D. (2008), 'Seeing is believing: the effect of brain images on judgments of scientific reasoning', *Cognition*, 107, pp. 343–52.

McCrory, E., De Brito, S.A., and Viding, E. (2010), 'Research review: the neurobiology and genetics of maltreatment and adversity', *Journal of Child Psychology and Psychiatry*, 51, pp. 1079–95.

McDonald, C.R., Thesen, T., Carlson, C., Blumberg, M., Girard, H.M., Trongnetrpunya, A., Sherfey, J.S., Devinsky, O., Kuzniecky, R., Dolye, W.K., Cash, S. S., Leonard, M.K., Hagler, D.J., Jr, Dale, A.M., and Halgren, E. (2010), 'Multimodal imaging of repetition priming: using fMRI, MEG, and intracranial EEG to reveal spatiotemporal profiles of word processing', *Neuroimage*, 53, pp. 707–17.

McDonald, R.I., Green, P., Balk, D., Fekete, B.M., Revenga, C., Todd, M., and Montgomery, M. (2011), 'Urban growth, climate change, and freshwater availability', *Proceedings of the National Academy of Sciences of the United States of America*, 108, pp. 6312–17.

McGowan, P.O., Meaney, M.J., and Szyf, M. (2008), 'Diet and the epigenetic (re) programming of phenotypic differences in behavior', *Brain Research*, 1237, pp. 12–24.

McGowan, P.O., Sasaki, A., D'Alessio, A.C., Dymov, S., Labonte, B., Szyf, M., Turecki, G., and Meaney, M.J. (2009), 'Epigenetic regulation of the glucocorticoid receptor in human brain associates with childhood abuse', *Nature Neuroscience*, 12, pp. 342–8.

McGowan, P.O. and Szyf, M. (2010), 'The epigenetics of social adversity in early life: implications for mental health outcomes', *Neurobiology of Disease*, 39, pp. 66–72.

McNaughton, P.A. and Robbins, T.W. (2011), 'Neuroscience cuts will hurt key areas', *Nature*, 471, pp. 36–7.

Medina, F.J. and Tunez, I. (2010), 'Huntington's disease: the value of transcranial meganetic stimulation', *Current Medicinal Chemistry*, 17, pp. 2482–91.

Mélik-Parsadaniantz, S. and Rostène, W. (2008), 'Chemokines and neuromodulation', *Journal of Neuroimmunology*, 198, pp. 62–8.

Mendelsohn, A., Furman, O., and Dudai, Y. (2010), 'Signatures of memory: brain coactivations during retrieval distinguish correct from incorrect recollection', *Frontiers in Behavioral Neuroscience*, 4, doi: 10.3389.fnbeh.2010.00018.

Michel, J.-B., Shen, Y.K., Aiden, A.P., Veres, A., Gray, M.K., The Google Books Team, Pickett, J.P., Hoiberg, D., Clancy, D., Norvig, P., Orwant, J., Pinker, S., Nowak, M.A., and Aiden, E.L. (2011), 'Quantitative analysis of culture using millions of digitized books', *Science*, 331, pp. 176–82.

Michelson, A. (1902). *Light Waves and their Uses*. Chicago: University of Chicago Press.

Mikhail, J. (2007), 'Universal moral grammar: theory, evidence and the future', *Trends in Cognitive Sciences*, 11, pp. 143–52.

Milgram, S. (1963), 'Behavioral study of obedience', *Journal of Abnormal and Social Psychology*, 67, pp. 371–8.

Milgram, S. (1997), *Obedience to Authority*. London: Pinter and Martin.

Millan, M.J., Lejeune, F., and Gobert, A. (2000), 'Reciprocal autoreceptor and heteroreceptor control of serotonergic, dopaminergic and noradrenergic transmission in the frontal cortex: relevance to the actions of antidepressant agents', *Journal of Psychopharmacology*, 14, pp. 114–38.

Miller, G. (2010), 'fMRI lie detection fails a legal test', *Science*, 328, pp. 1336–7.

Miller, G. (2011), 'The rise of animal law', *Science*, 332, pp. 28–31.

Minogue, K. and Marshall, E. (2010), 'Guatemala study from 1940s reflects a "dark chapter" in medicine', *Science*, 330, pp. 160.

Miranda, E.R., Magee, W.L., Wilson, J.J., Eaton, J., and Palaniappan, R. (2011), 'Brain-computer music interfacing (BCMI): from basic research to the real world of special needs', *Music and Medicine*, 3, pp. 134–40.

Miyake, A., Kost-Smith, L.E., Finkelstein, N.D., Pollock, S.J., Cohen, G.L., and Ito, T.A. (2010), 'Reducing the gender achievement gap in college science: a classroom study of values affirmation', *Science*, 330, pp. 1234–7.

Moll, J., De Oliveira-Souza, R., and Zahn, R. (2008), 'The neural basis of moral cognition: sentiments, concepts, and values', *Annals of the New York Academy of Sciences*, 1124, pp. 161–80.

Monti, M.M., Vanhaudenhuyse, A., Coleman, M.R., Boly, M., Pickard, J.D., Tshibanda, L., Owen, A.M., and Laureys, S. (2010), 'Willful modulation of brain activity in disorders of consciousness', *New England Journal of Medicine*, 362, pp. 579–89.

Morecraft, R.J., Geula, C., and Mesulam, M.M. (1992), 'Cytoarchitecture and neural afferents of orbitofrontal cortex in the brain of the monkey', *Journal of Comparative Neurology*, 323, pp. 341–58.

Morgan III, C.A., Rasmusson, A., Pietrzak, R.H., Coric, V., and Southwick, S.M. (2009), 'Relationships among plasma dehydroepiandrosterone and dehydroepiandrosterone sulfate, cortisol, symptoms of dissociation, and objective performance in humans exposed to underwater navigation stress', *Biological Psychiatry*, 66, pp. 334–40.

Movassagh, M., Choy, M.K., Goddard, M., Bennett, M.R., Down, T.A., and Foo, R.S. (2010), 'Differential DNA methylation correlates with differential expression of angiogenic factors in human heart failure', *PLoS ONE*, 5, p. e8564.

Muller-Hill, B. (2001), 'Genetics of susceptibility to tuberculosis: Mengele's experiments in Auschwitz', *Nature Reviews Genetics*, 2, pp. 631–4.

Munro, G.D. (2010), 'The scientific impotence excuse: discounting belief-threatening scientific abstracts', *Journal of Applied Social Psychology*, 40, pp. 579–600.

Murakami, S. and Okada, Y. (2006), 'Contributions of principal neocortical neurons to magnetoencephalography and electroencephalography signals', *Journal of Physiology*, 575, pp. 925–36.

Murgatroyd, C., Patchev, A.V., Wu, Y., Micale, V., Bockmuhl, Y., Fischer, D., Holsboer, F., Wotjak, C.T., Almeida, O.F.X., and Spengler, D. (2009), 'Dynamic DNA methylation programs persistent adverse effects of early-life stress', *Nature Neuroscience*, 12, pp. 1559–66.

Nader, K. and Einarsson, E.Ö. (2010), 'Memory reconsolidation: an update', *Annals of the New York Academy of Sciences*, 1191, pp. 27–41.

Nagel, G., Szellas, T., Huhn, W., Kateriya, S., Adeishvili, N., Berthold, P., Ollig, D., Hegemann, P., and Bamberg, E. (2003), 'Channelrhodopsin-2, a directly light-gated cation-selective membrane channel', *Proceedings of the National Academy of Sciences of the United States of America*, 100, pp. 13940–5.

Nagel, T. (1974). 'What is it like to be a bat?', *The Philosophical Review*, 83, pp. 435–50.

Nahrendorf, M., Keliher, E., Marinelli, B., Waterman, P., Feruglio, P.F., Fexon, L., Pivovarov, M., Swirski, F.K., Pittet, M.J., Vinegoni, C., and Weissleder, R. (2010), 'Hybrid PET-optical imaging using targeted probes', *Proceedings of the National Academy of Sciences of the United States of America*, 107, pp. 7910–15.

Nandam, L.S., Hester, R., Wagner, J., Cummins, T.D., Garner, K., Dean, A.J., Kim, B.N., Nathan, P.J., Mattingley, J.B., and Bellgrove, M.A. (2010), 'Methylphenidate but not atomoxetine or citalopram modulates inhibitory control and response time variability', *Biological Psychiatry*, 69, pp. 902–4.

Naselaris, T., Prenger, R.J., Kay, K.N., Oliver, M., and Gallant, J.L. (2009), 'Bayesian reconstruction of natural images from human brain activity', *Neuron*, 63, pp. 902–15.

Nature Editorial (2010a), 'Putting gender on the agenda', *Nature*, 465, p. 665.

Nature Editorial (2010b), 'Unknown quantities', *Nature*, 465, pp. 665–6.

Nature Editorial (2011), 'Best is yet to come', *Nature*, 470, p. 140.

Neher, A. (2009), 'Christopher Wren, Thomas Willis and the depiction of the brain and nerves', *Journal of Medical Humanities*, 30, pp. 191–200.

Nekhendzy, V., Lemmens, H.J., Tingle, M., Nekhendzy, M., and Angst, M.S. (2010), 'The analgesic and antihyperalgesic effects of transcranial electrostimulation with combined direct and alternating current in healthy volunteers', *Anesthesia and Analgesia*, 111, pp. 1301–7.

Nemani, A.K., Atkinson, I.C., and Thulborn, K.R. (2009), 'Investigating the consistency of brain activation using individual trial analysis of high-resolution fMRI in the human primary visual cortex', *Neuroimage*, 47, pp. 1417–24.

Newman-Norlund, R.D., Ganesh, S., van Schie, H.T., De Bruijn, E.R.A., and Bekkering, H. (2009), 'Self-identification and empathy modulate error-related brain activity during the observation of penalty shots between friend and foe', *Social Cognitive and Affective Neuroscience*, 4, pp. 10–22.

Niedermeyer, E. and Lopes Da Silva, F.H., eds. (2004), *Electroencephalography: Basic Principles, Clinical Applications and Related Fields*, 5th edition. Philadelphia: Lippincott Williams and Wilkins.

Nili, U., Goldberg, H., Weizman, A., and Dudai, Y. (2010), 'Fear thou not: activity of frontal and temporal circuits in moments of real-life courage', *Neuron*, 66, pp. 949–62.

Nitsche, M.A., Boggio, P.S., Fregni, F., and Pascual-Leone, A. (2009), 'Treatment of depression with transcranial direct current stimulation (tDCS): a review', *Experimental Neurology*, 219, pp. 14–19.

Northoff, G., Qin, P., and Nakao, T. (2010), 'Rest–stimulus interaction in the brain: a review', *Trends in Neurosciences*, 33, pp. 277–84.

Nowak, N.T., Woodard, T.L., Moffat, S.D., Tancer, M., Balon, R., and Diamond, M.P. (2010), 'Brain activation during viewing of sexually explicit videos in women with normal sexual desire and women with hypoactive sexual desire disorder', abstract presentation *Neuroscience 2010*.

O'Connell, N.E., Wand, B.M., Marston, L., Spencer, S., and DeSouza, L.H. (2010), 'Non-invasive brain stimulation techniques for chronic pain', *Cochrane Database of Systematic Reviews*, CD008208.

O'Connor, J.P.B. (2003), 'Thomas Willis and the background to Cerebri Anatome', *Journal of the Royal Society of Medicine*, 96, pp. 139–43.

O'Reardon, J.P., Solvason, H.B., Janicak, P.G., Sampson, S., Isenberg, K.E., Nahas, Z., McDonald, W.M., Avery, D., Fitzgerald, P.B., Loo, C., Demitrack, M.A., George, M.S., and Sackeim, H.A. (2007), 'Efficacy and safety of transcranial magnetic stimulation in the acute treatment of major depression: a multisite randomized controlled trial', *Biological Psychiatry*, 62, pp. 1208–16.

Ou, W., Nissilä, I., Radhakrishnan, H., Boas, D.A., Hämäläinen, M.S., and Franceschini, M.A. (2009), 'Study of neurovascular coupling in humans via simultaneous magnetoencephalography and diffuse optical imaging acquisition', *Neuroimage*, 46, pp. 624–32.

Ou, W., Nummenmaa, A., Ahveninen, J., Belliveau, J.W., Hamalainen, M.S., and Golland, P. (2010), 'Multimodal functional imaging using fMRI-informed regional EEG/MEG source estimation', *Neuroimage*, 52, pp. 97–108.

Outram, S.M. (2010), 'The use of methylphenidate among students: the future of enhancement?', *Journal of Medical Ethics*, 36, pp. 198–202.

Owen, S.L., Green, A.L., Stein, J.F., and Aziz, T.Z. (2006), 'Deep brain stimulation for the alleviation of post-stroke neuropathic pain', *Pain*, 120, pp. 202–6.

Owen, S.L., Heath, J., Kringelbach, M.L., Stein, J.F., and Aziz, T.Z. (2007), 'Preoperative DTI and probabilistic tractography in an amputee with deep brain stimulation for lower limb stump pain', *British Journal of Neurosurgery*, 21, pp. 485–90.

Ozen, S., Sirota, A., Belluscio, M.A., Anastassiou, C.A., Stark, E., Koch, C., and Buzsaki, G. (2010), 'Transcranial electric stimulation entrains cortical neuronal populations in rats', *Journal of Neuroscience*, 30, pp. 11476–85.

Palacios, S. (2010), 'Hypoactive Sexual Desire Disorder and current pharmacotherapeutic options in women', *Women's Health*, 7, pp. 95–107.

Palade, G.E. and Palay, S.L. (1954), 'Electron microscope observations of interneuronal and neuromuscular synapses', *Anatomical Record*, 118, p. 335.

Parks, C.L., Robinson, P.S., Sibille, E., Shenk, T., and Toth, M. (1998), 'Increased anxiety of mice lacking the serotonin1A receptor', *Proceedings of the National Academy of Sciences of the United States of America*, 95, pp. 10734–9.

Pastrana, E. (2011), 'Brain function marries anatomy', *Nature Methods*, 8, pp. 369–69.

Paur, I., Balstad, T.R., and Blomhoff, R. (2010), 'Degree of roasting is the main determinant of the effects of coffee on NF-kappaB and EpRE', *Free Radical Biology and Medicine*, 48, pp. 1218–27.

Penfield, W. and Erickson, T.C. (1941), *Epilepsy and Cerebral Localization: a Study of the Mechanism, Treatment and Prevention of Epileptic Seizures*. London: Baillière, Tindall and Cox.

Pereira, E.A., Wang, S., Paterson, D.J., Stein, J.F., Aziz, T.Z., and Green, A.L. (2010), 'Sustained reduction of hypertension by deep brain stimulation', *Journal of Clinical Neuroscience*, 17, pp. 124–7.

Persson, I. and Savulescu, J. (2008), 'The perils of cognitive enhancement and the urgent imperative to enhance the moral character of humanity', *Journal of Applied Philosophy*, 25, pp. 162–77.

Peters, J. and Büchel, C. (2010), 'Episodic future thinking reduces reward delay discounting through an enhancement of prefrontal-mediotemporal interactions', *Neuron*, 66, pp. 138–48.

Pettit, D.L., Wang, S.S.H., Gee, K.R., and Augustine, G.J. (1997), 'Chemical two-photon uncaging: a novel approach to mapping glutamate receptors', *Neuron*, 19, pp. 465–71.

Pinker, S. (2011), *The Better Angels of our Nature: the Decline of Violence in History and its Causes*. London: Allen Lane.

Pinteaux, E., Trotter, P., and Simi, A. (2009), 'Cell-specific and concentration-dependent actions of interleukin-1 in acute brain inflammation', *Cytokine*, 45, pp. 1–7.

Plis, S.M., Calhoun, V.D., Eichele, T., Weisend, M.P., and Lane, T. (2010), 'MEG and fMRI fusion for nonlinear estimation of neural and BOLD signal changes', *Frontiers in Neuroinformatics*, 4, doi: 10.3389/fninf.2010.00114.

Poliseno, L., Salmena, L., Zhang, J., Carver, B., Haveman, W.J., and Pandolfi, P.P. (2010), 'A coding-independent function of gene and pseudogene mRNAs regulates tumour biology', *Nature*, 465, pp. 1033–8.

Ponseti, J., Granert, O., Jansen, O., Wolff, S., Beier, K., Neutze, J., Deuschl, G., Mehdorn, H., Siebner, H., and Bosinski, H. (2012), 'Assessment of pedophilia using hemodynamic brain response to sexual stimuli', *Archives of General Psychiatry*, 69, pp. 187–94.

Porter, R. (2001), *Enlightenment: Britain and the Creation of the Modern World*. London: Penguin.

Pravdich-Neminsky, V.V. (1913), 'Ein versuch der registrierung der elektrischen gehirnerscheinungen (approximate translation: an attempt at the registration of the electrical features of the brain)', *Zentralblatt für Physiologie*, 27, pp. 951–60.

Pressman, J.D. (1998), *Last Resort: Psychosurgery and the Limits of Medicine*. New York: Cambridge University Press.

Priori, A., Hallett, M., and Rothwell, J.C. (2009), 'Repetitive transcranial magnetic stimulation or transcranial direct current stimulation?', *Brain Stimulation*, 2, pp. 241–5.

Pyysiäinen, I. and Hauser, M. (2010), 'The origins of religion: evolved adaptation or by-product?', *Trends in Cognitive Sciences*, 14, pp. 104–9.

Quinkert, A.W., Schiff, N.D., and Pfaff, D.W. (2010), 'Temporal patterning of pulses during deep brain stimulation affects central nervous system arousal', *Behavioural Brain Research*, 214, pp. 377–85.

Quirk, G.J. and Milad, M.R. (2010), 'Editing out fear', *Nature*, 463, pp. 36–7.

Rai, T.S. and Fiske, A. (2010), 'ODD (observation- and description-deprived) psychological research', *Behavioral and Brain Sciences*, 33, pp. 106–7.

Raichle, M.E. (2009), 'A brief history of human brain mapping', *Trends in Neurosciences*, 32, pp. 118–26.

Raichle, M.E. and Gusnard, D.A. (2002), 'Appraising the brain's energy budget', *Proceedings of the National Academy of Sciences of the United States of America*, 99, pp. 10237–9.

Raine, A. (2008), 'From genes to brain to antisocial behavior', *Current Directions in Psychological Science*, 17, pp. 323–8.

Raine, A. and Yang, Y. (2006), 'Neural foundations to moral reasoning and antisocial behavior', *Social Cognitive and Affective Neuroscience*, 1, pp. 203–13.

Rajkowska, G. and Goldman-Rakic, P.S. (1995), 'Cytoarchitectonic definition of prefrontal areas in the normal human cortex: II. Variability in locations of areas 9 and 46 and relationship to the Talairach coordinate system', *Cerebral Cortex*, 5, pp. 323–37.

Ramachandran, V.S. (2011), *The Tell-tale Brain: Unlocking the Mystery of Human Nature*. London: William Heinemann.

Ramboz, S., Oosting, R., Amara, D.A., Kung, H.F., Blier, P., Mendelsohn, M., Mann, J.J., Brunner, D., and Hen, R. (1998), 'Serotonin receptor 1A knockout: an animal model of anxiety-related disorder', *Proceedings of the National Academy of Sciences of the United States of America*, 95, pp. 14476–81.

Rancz, E.A., Franks, K.M., Schwarz, M.K., Pichler, B., Schaefer, A.T., and Margrie, T.W. (2011), 'Transfection via whole-cell recording *in vivo*: bridging single-cell physiology, genetics and connectomics', *Nature Neuroscience*, 14, pp. 527–32.

Rauch, S.L., Dougherty, D.D., Malone, D., Rezai, A., Friehs, G., Fischman, A.J., Alpert, N.M., Haber, S.N., Stypulkowski, P.H., Rise, M.T., Rasmussen, S.A., and Greenberg, B.D. (2006), 'A functional neuroimaging investigation of deep brain stimulation in patients with obsessive-compulsive disorder', *Journal of Neurosurgery*, 104, pp. 558–65.

Ray, N.J., Jenkinson, N., Kringelbach, M.L., Hansen, P.C., Pereira, E.A., Brittain, J.S., Holland, P., Holliday, I.E., Owen, S., Stein, J., and Aziz, T. (2009), 'Abnormal thalamocortical dynamics may be altered by deep brain stimulation: using magnetoencephalography to study phantom limb pain', *Journal of Clinical Neuroscience*, 16, pp. 32–6.

Ray, N.J., Jenkinson, N., Wang, S., Holland, P., Brittain, J.S., Joint, C., Stein, J.F., and Aziz, T. (2008), 'Local field potential beta activity in the subthalamic nucleus of patients with Parkinson's disease is associated with improvements in bradykinesia after dopamine and deep brain stimulation', *Experimental Neurology*, 213, pp. 108–13.

Richardson-Jones, J.W., Craige, C.P., Guiard, B.P., Stephen, A., Metzger, K.L., Kung, H.F., Gardier, A.M., Dranovsky, A., David, D.J., Beck, S.G., Hen, R., and Leonardo, E.D. (2010), '5-HT1A autoreceptor levels determine vulnerability to stress and response to antidepressants', *Neuron*, 65, pp. 40–52.

Richardson-Jones, J.W., Craige, C.P., Nguyen, T.H., Kung, H.F., Gardier, A.M., Dranovsky, A., David, D.J., Guiard, B.P., Beck, S.G., Hen, R., and Leonardo, E.D. (2011), 'Serotonin-1A autoreceptors are necessary and sufficient for the normal formation of circuits underlying innate anxiety', *Journal of Neuroscience*, 31, pp. 6008–18.

Ringler, R., Greiner, M., Kohlloeffel, L., Handwerker, H.O., and Forster, C. (2003), 'BOLD effects in different areas of the cerebral cortex during painful mechanical stimulation', *Pain*, 105, pp. 445–53.

Rissman, J., Greely, H.T., and Wagner, A.D. (2010), 'Detecting individual memories through the neural decoding of memory states and past experience', *Proceedings of the National Academy of Sciences of the United States of America*, 107, pp. 9849–54.

Robertson, J.D. (1953), 'Ultrastructure of two invertebrate synapses', *Proceedings of the Society for Experimental Biology and Medicine*, 82, pp. 219–23.

Robinson, T.R. (2010), *Genetics For Dummies*, 2nd edition. New York: Wiley.

Rockstrom, J., Steffen, W., Noone, K., Persson, A., Chapin, F.S., Lambin, E.F., Lenton, T.M., Scheffer, M., Folke, C., Schellnhuber, H.J., Nykvist, B., de Wit, C. A., Hughes, T., van der Leeuw, S., Rodhe, H., Sorlin, S., Snyder, P.K., Costanza, R., Svedin, U., Falkenmark, M., Karlberg, L., Corell, R.W., Fabry, V.J., Hansen, J., Walker, B., Liverman, D., Richardson, K., Crutzen, P., and Foley, J.A. (2009), 'A safe operating space for humanity', *Nature*, 461, pp. 472–5.

Rodrigues, S.M., Saslow, L.R., Garcia, N., John, O.P., and Keltner, D. (2009), 'Oxytocin receptor genetic variation relates to empathy and stress reactivity in humans', *Proceedings of the National Academy of Sciences of the United States of America*, 106, pp. 21437–41.

Romei, V., Driver, J., Schyns, P.G., and Thut, G. (2011), 'Rhythmic TMS over parietal cortex links distinct brain frequencies to global versus local visual processing', *Current Biology*, 21, pp. 334–7.

Rossato, J.I., Bevilaqua, L.R., Izquierdo, I., Medina, J.H., and Cammarota, M. (2010), 'Retrieval induces reconsolidation of fear extinction memory', *Proceedings of the National Academy of Sciences of the United States of America*, 107, pp. 21801–5.

Rothwell, J.C. (1997), 'Techniques and mechanisms of action of transcranial stimulation of the human motor cortex', *Journal of Neuroscience Methods*, 74, pp. 113–22.

Rouaud, T., Lardeux, S., Panayotis, N., Paleressompoulle, D., Cador, M., and Baunez, C. (2010), 'Reducing the desire for cocaine with subthalamic nucleus deep brain stimulation', *Proceedings of the National Academy of Sciences of the United States of America*, 107, pp. 1196–200.

Royal Society (2011), 'Brain waves module 1: neuroscience, society and policy', *Brain Waves*, London: Royal Society.

Rummel, R.J. (1997), *Death by Government: Genocide and Mass Murder Since 1900* Piscataway, NJ: Transaction.

Rydell, R.J., McConnell, A.R., and Beilock, S.L. (2009). 'Multiple social identities and stereotype threat: imbalance, accessibility, and working memory.' *Journal of Personality and Social Psychology*, 96, pp. 949–66.

Rydell, R.J., Shiffrin, R.M., Boucher, K.L., Van Loo, K., and Rydell, M.T. (2010), 'Stereotype threat prevents perceptual learning', *Proceedings of the National Academy of Sciences of the United States of America*, 107, pp. 14042–7.

Sabia, S., Gueguen, A., Marmot, M.G., Shipley, M.J., Ankri, J., and Singh-Manoux, A. (2010), 'Does cognition predict mortality in midlife? Results from the Whitehall II cohort study', *Neurobiology of Aging*, 31, pp. 688–95.

Sacktor, T.C. (2011), 'How does PKMζ maintain long-term memory?', *Nature Reviews Neuroscience*, 12, pp. 9–15.

Sahakian, B.J. and Morein-Zamir, S. (2011), 'Neuroethical issues in cognitive enhancement', *Journal of Psychopharmacology*, 25, pp. 197–204.

Salimpoor, V.N., Benovoy, M., Larcher, K., Dagher, A., and Zatorre, R.J. (2011), 'Anatomically distinct dopamine release during anticipation and experience of peak emotion to music', *Nature Neuroscience*, 14, pp. 257–62.

Sandovici, I., Smith, N.H., Nitert, M.D., Ackers-Johnson, M., Uribe-Lewis, S., Ito, Y., Jones, R.H., Marquez, V.E., Cairns, W., Tadayyon, M., O'Neill, L.P., Murrell, A., Ling, C., Constância, M., and Ozanne, S.E. (2011), 'Maternal diet and aging alter the epigenetic control of a promoter–enhancer interaction at the Hnf4a gene in rat pancreatic islets', *Proceedings of the National Academy of Sciences of the United States of America*, 108, pp. 5449–54.

Sandrini, M., Umiltà, C., and Rusconi, E. (2010), 'The use of transcranial magnetic stimulation in cognitive neuroscience: a new synthesis of methodological issues', *Neuroscience and Biobehavioral Reviews*, 35, pp. 516–36.

Saper, C.B. (2011), 'Animal behaviour: the nexus of sex and violence', *Nature*, 470, pp. 179–81.

Sasaki, T., Matsuki, N., and Ikegaya, Y. (2011), 'Action-potential modulation during axonal conduction', *Science*, 331, pp. 599–601.

Sato, M. and Stryker, M.P. (2010), 'Genomic imprinting of experience-dependent cortical plasticity by the ubiquitin ligase gene *Ube3a*', *Proceedings of the National Academy of Sciences of the United States of America*, 107, pp. 5611–16.

Savulescu, J. (2006), 'Genetic interventions and the ethics of enhancement of human beings'. In *The Oxford Handbook on Bioethics*, ed. B. Steinbock. Oxford: Oxford University Press, pp. 516–35.

Schalkwyk, L.C., Meaburn, E.L., Smith, R., Dempster, E.L., Jeffries, A.R., Davies, M.N., Plomin, R., and Mill, J. (2010), 'Allelic skewing of DNA methylation is widespread across the genome', *American Journal of Human Genetics*, 86, pp. 196–212.

Schauer, F. (2010), 'Neuroscience, lie-detection, and the law: contrary to the prevailing view, the suitability of brain-based lie-detection for courtroom or forensic use should be determined according to legal and not scientific standards', *Trends in Cognitive Sciences*, 14, pp. 101–3.

Schiller, D., Monfils, M.-H., Raio, C.M., Johnson, D.C., LeDoux, J.E., and Phelps, E.A. (2010), 'Preventing the return of fear in humans using reconsolidation update mechanisms', *Nature*, 463, pp. 49–53.

Schmeck Jr, H.M. (1987), 'Potent tool fashioned to probe inherited ills: scientists near completion of crucial map of human genes', *The New York Times*, August 11.

Schnall, S., Haidt, J., Clore, G.L., and Jordan, A.H. (2008), 'Disgust as embodied moral judgment', *Personality and Social Psychology Bulletin*, 34, pp. 1096–109.

Schölvinck, M.L., Maier, A., Ye, F.Q., Duyn, J.H., and Leopold, D.A. (2010), 'Neural basis of global resting-state fMRI activity', *Proceedings of the National Academy of Sciences of the United States of America*, 107, pp. 10238–43.

Schoonover, C.E. (2010), *Portraits of the Mind: Visualizing the Brain from Antiquity to the 21st Century*. New York: Harry N. Abrams.

Schrödinger, E. (1926), 'An undulatory theory of the mechanics of atoms and molecules', *Physical Review*, 28, p. 1049.

Schrödinger, E. (1935), 'Die gegenwärtige situation in der quantenmechanik', *Naturwissenschaften*, 23, pp. 807–12.

Schulz, D., Southekal, S., Junnarkar, S.S., Pratte, J.-F., Purschke, M.L., Stoll, S.P., Ravindranath, B., Maramraju, S.H., Krishnamoorthy, S., Henn, F.A., O'Connor, P., Woody, C.L., Schlyer, D.J., and Vaska, P. (2011), 'Simultaneous assessment of rodent behavior and neurochemistry using a miniature positron emission tomograph', *Nature Methods*, 8, pp. 347–52.

Schumacher, V. and Martin, M. (2009), 'Comparing age effects in normally and extremely highly educated and intellectually engaged 65–80 year-olds:

potential protection from deficit through educational and intellectual activities across the lifespan', *Current Aging Science*, 2, pp. 200–4.

Schurger, A., Pereira, F., Treisman, A., and Cohen, J.D. (2010), 'Reproducibility distinguishes conscious from nonconscious neural representations', *Science*, 327, pp. 97–9.

Schwarzkopf, D.S. and Rees, G. (2010), 'Brain activity to rely on?', *Science*, 327, pp. 43–4.

Shalom, D.B. (2009), 'The medial prefrontal cortex and integration in autism', *Neuroscientist*, 15, pp. 589–98.

Shapiro, J. (2002), *Radiation Protection: a Guide for Scientists, Regulators, and Physicians*, 4th revised edition. Cambridge, MA: Harvard University Press.

Sheffield, M.E.J., Best, T.K., Mensh, B.D., Kath, W.L., and Spruston, N. (2011), 'Slow integration leads to persistent action potential firing in distal axons of coupled interneurons', *Nature Neuroscience*, 14, pp. 200–7.

Shema, R., Sacktor, T.C., and Dudai, Y. (2007), 'Rapid erasure of long-term memory associations in the cortex by an inhibitor of PKMζ', *Science*, 317, pp. 951–3.

Shetty, B.S.K., Kanchan, T., Shetty, M., Naik, R., Menezes, R.G., Sameer, K.S.M., and Hasan, F. (2010), 'Fatal electrocution by a support metal wire', *Journal of Forensic Sciences*, 55, pp. 830–1.

Shin, J.W., Wang, J.H., Kang, J.K., and Son, C.G. (2010), 'Experimental evidence for the protective effects of coffee against liver fibrosis in SD rats', *Journal of the Science of Food and Agriculture*, 90, pp. 450–5.

Shirtcliff, E.A., Vitacco, M.J., Graf, A.R., Gostisha, A.J., Merz, J.L., and Zahn-Waxler, C. (2009), 'Neurobiology of empathy and callousness: implications for the development of antisocial behavior', *Behavioral Sciences and the Law*, 27, pp. 137–71.

Silvanto, J. and Cattaneo, Z. (2010), 'Transcranial magnetic stimulation reveals the content of visual short-term memory in the visual cortex', *Neuroimage*, 50, pp. 1683–9.

Silvia, P.J. (2008), 'Another look at creativity and intelligence: exploring higher-order models and probable confounds', *Personality and Individual Differences*, 44, pp. 1012–21.

Singer, C. (1956), 'Brain dissection before Vesalius', *Journal of the History of Medicine and Allied Sciences*, 11, pp. 261–74.

Singer, T. (2006), 'The neuronal basis and ontogeny of empathy and mind reading: review of literature and implications for future research', *Neuroscience and Biobehavioral Reviews*, 30, pp. 855–63.

Singer, T. and Lamm, C. (2009), 'The social neuroscience of empathy', *Annals of the New York Academy of Sciences*, 1156, pp. 81–96.

Singer, T., Seymour, B., O'Doherty, J.P., Stephan, K.E., Dolan, R.J., and Frith, C.D. (2006), 'Empathic neural responses are modulated by the perceived fairness of others', *Nature*, 439, pp. 466–9.

Skuban, T., Hardenacke, K., Woopen, C., and Kuhn, J. (2011), 'Informed consent in deep brain stimulation—ethical considerations in a stress field of pride and prejudice', *Frontiers in Integrative Neuroscience*, 5, doi: 10.3389/fnint.2011.00007.

Snapp, S.S., Blackie, M.J., Gilbert, R.A., Bezner-Kerr, R., and Kanyama-Phiri, G.Y. (2010), 'Biodiversity can support a greener revolution in Africa', *Proceedings of the National Academy of Sciences of the United States of America*, 107, pp. 20840–5.

Spence, S.A. (2008), 'Playing devil's advocate: the case against fMRI lie detection', *Legal and Criminological Psychology*, 13, pp. 11–25.

Spulber, S. and Schultzberg, M. (2010), 'Connection between inflammatory processes and transmittor function—modulatory effects of interleukin-1', *Progress in Neurobiology*, 90, pp. 256–62.

Stefanko, D.P., Barrett, R.M., Ly, A.R., Reolon, G.K., and Wood, M.A. (2009), 'Modulation of long-term memory for object recognition via HDAC inhibition', *Proceedings of the National Academy of Sciences of the United States of America*, 106, pp. 9447–52.

Steinbock, B. (2006), *The Oxford Handbook on Bioethics*. Oxford: Oxford University Press.

Steiner, G. (2010), 'The cultural significance of Rembrandt's "Anatomy Lesson of Dr Nicolaas Tulp"', *History of European Ideas*, 36, pp. 273–9.

Stephens, M. (2011), 'Animal research: replacing the lab rat', *Nature*, 471, pp. 449–49.

Stevens, M.C. (2009), 'The developmental cognitive neuroscience of functional connectivity', *Brain and Cognition*, 70, pp. 1–12.

Stevenson, I.H. and Kording, K.P. (2011), 'How advances in neural recording affect data analysis', *Nature Neuroscience*, 14, pp. 139–42.

Stirman, J.N., Crane, M.M., Husson, S.J., Wabnig, S., Schultheis, C., Gottschalk, A., and Lu, H. (2011), 'Real-time multimodal optical control of neurons and muscles in freely behaving *Caenorhabditis elegans*', *Nature Methods*, 8, pp. 153–8.

Stoeckel, L.E., Weller, R.E., Cook, 3rd, E.W., Twieg, D.B., Knowlton, R.C., and Cox, J.E. (2008), 'Widespread reward-system activation in obese women in response to pictures of high-calorie foods', *Neuroimage*, 41, pp. 636–47.

Straube, T., Schmidt, S., Weiss, T., Mentzel, H.J., and Miltner, W.H.R. (2009), 'Sex differences in brain activation to anticipated and experienced pain in the medial prefrontal cortex', *Human Brain Mapping*, 30, pp. 689–98.

Sugama, S. and Conti, B. (2008), 'Interleukin-18 and stress', *Brain Research Reviews*, 58, pp. 85–95.

Sutherland, S. (2007), *Irrationality*. London: Pinter and Martin.

Suzuki, A., Stern, S.A., Bozdagi, O., Huntley, G.W., Walker, R.H., Magistretti, P. J., and Alberini, C.M. (2011), 'Astrocyte-neuron lactate transport is required for long-term memory formation', *Cell*, 144, pp. 810–23.

Swanson, L.W. (1995), 'Mapping the human brain: past, present, and future', *Trends in Neurosciences*, 18, pp. 471–4.

Synofzik, M. and Schlaepfer, T.E. (2011), 'Electrodes in the brain—ethical criteria for research and treatment with deep brain stimulation for neuropsychiatric disorders', *Brain Stimulation*, 4, pp. 7–16.

Takahashi, H., Kato, M., Matsuura, M., Koeda, M., Yahata, N., Suhara, T., and Okubo, Y. (2008), 'Neural correlates of human virtue judgment', *Cerebral Cortex*, 18, pp. 1886–91.

Talairach, J. and Tournoux, P. (1988), *Co-planar Stereotaxic Atlas of the Human Brain*. New York: Thieme.

Tanriverdi, F., Karaca, Z., Unluhizarci, K., and Kelestimur, F. (2007), 'The hypothalamo-pituitary-adrenal axis in chronic fatigue syndrome and fibromyalgia syndrome', *Stress*, 10, pp. 13–25.

Tanriverdi, T., Ajlan, A., Poulin, N., and Olivier, A. (2009), 'Morbidity in epilepsy surgery: an experience based on 2,449 epilepsy surgery procedures from a single institution', *Journal of Neurosurgery*, 110, pp. 1111–23.

Tao, K.S., Wang, W., Wang, L., Cao, D.Y., Li, Y.Q., Wu, S.X., and Dou, K. F. (2008), 'The multifaceted mechanisms for coffee's anti-tumorigenic effect on liver', *Medical Hypotheses*, 71, pp. 730–6.

Taylor, K. (2006), *Brainwashing: the Science of Thought Control*, paperback edition. Oxford: Oxford University Press.

Taylor, K. (2009), *Cruelty: Human Evil and the Human Brain*. Oxford: Oxford University Press.

Taylor, K.E. (2000), 'A data-donor scheme for brain researchers', *Lancet*, 355, pp. 849–50.

Taylor, K.E. (2001), 'Applying continuous modelling to consciousness', *Journal of Consciousness Studies*, 8, pp. 45–60.

Tecuapetla, F., Patel, J.C., Xenias, H., English, D., Tadros, I., Shah, F., Berlin, J., Deisseroth, K., Rice, M.E., Tepper, J.M., and Koos, T. (2010), 'Glutamatergic signaling by mesolimbic dopamine neurons in the nucleus accumbens', *Journal of Neuroscience*, 30, pp. 7105–10.

Teter, C.J., McCabe, S.E., Boyd, C.J., and Guthrie, S.K. (2003), 'Illicit methylphenidate use in an undergraduate student sample: prevalence and risk factors', *Pharmacotherapy*, 23, pp. 609–17.

Theis, T., Ganssle, P., Kervern, G., Knappe, S., Kitching, J., Ledbetter, M.P., Budker, D., and Pines, A. (2011), 'Parahydrogen-enhanced zero-field nuclear magnetic resonance', *Nature Physics*, 7, pp. 571–5.

Thirion, B. (2007), 'Analysis of a large fMRI cohort: statistical and methodological issues for group analyses', *Neuroimage*, 35, pp. 105–20.

Thomson Reuters (2004–2009), Journal Citation Reports® (Thomson Reuters, 2010).

Thyssen, A., Hirnet, D., Wolburg, H., Schmalzing, G.n., Deitmer, J.W., and Lohr, C. (2010), 'Ectopic vesicular neurotransmitter release along sensory axons mediates neurovascular coupling via glial calcium signaling', *Proceedings of the National Academy of Sciences of the United States of America*, 107, pp. 15258–63.

Tian, P., Teng, I.C., May, L.D., Kurz, R., Lu, K., Scadeng, M., Hillman, E.M.C., De Crespigny, A.J., D'Arceuil, H.E., Mandeville, J.B., Marota, J.J.A., Rosen, B.R., Liu, T.T., Boas, D.A., Buxton, R.B., Dale, A.M., and Devor, A. (2010), 'Cortical depth-specific microvascular dilation underlies laminar differences in blood oxygenation level-dependent functional MRI signal', *Proceedings of the National Academy of Sciences of the United States of America*, 107, pp. 15246–51.

Tomasi, D. and Volkow, N.D. (2010), 'Functional connectivity density mapping', *Proceedings of the National Academy of Sciences of the United States of America*, 107, pp. 9885–90.

Tracey, K.J. (2011), 'Ancient neurons regulate immunity', *Science*, 332, pp. 673–4.

Tufail, Y., Matyushov, A., Baldwin, N., Tauchmann, M.L., Georges, J., Yoshihiro, A., Tillery, S.I., and Tyler, W.J. (2010), 'Transcranial pulsed ultrasound stimulates intact brain circuits', *Neuron*, 66, pp. 681–94.

Turkle, S. (2011), *Alone Together: Why We Expect More from Technology and Less from Each Other*. New York: Basic Books.

Turner, D.C., Clark, L., Dowson, J., Robbins, T.W., and Sahakian, B.J. (2004), 'Modafinil improves cognition and response inhibition in adult attention-deficit/hyperactivity disorder', *Biological Psychiatry*, 55, pp. 1031–40.

Urban, N.B.L., Kegeles, L.S., Slifstein, M., Xu, X., Martinez, D., Sakr, E., Castillo, F., Moadel, T., O'Malley, S.S., Krystal, J.H., and Abi-Dargham, A. (2010), 'Sex differences in striatal dopamine release in young adults after oral alcohol challenge: a positron emission tomography imaging study with [11C]raclopride', *Biological Psychiatry*, 68, pp. 689–96.

Urgesi, C., Aglioti, S.M., Skrap, M., and Fabbro, F. (2010), 'The spiritual brain: selective cortical lesions modulate human self-transcendence', *Neuron*, 65, pp. 309–19.

Urry, H.L., van Reekum, C.M., Johnstone, T., and Davidson, R.J. (2009), 'Individual differences in some (but not all) medial prefrontal regions reflect cognitive demand while regulating unpleasant emotion', *Neuroimage*, 47, pp. 852–63.

Uto-Kondo, H., Ayaori, M., Ogura, M., Nakaya, K., Ito, M., Suzuki, A., Takiguchi, S., Yakushiji, E., Terao, Y., Ozasa, H., Hisada, T., Sasaki, M., Ohsuzu, F., and Ikewaki, K. (2010), 'Coffee consumption enhances high-density lipoprotein-mediated cholesterol efflux in macrophages', *Circulation Research*, 106, pp. 779–87.

van den Heuvel, M.P. and Hulshoff Pol, H.E. (2010), 'Exploring the brain network: a review on resting-state fMRI functional connectivity', *European Neuropsychopharmacology*, 20, pp. 519–34.

van Veen, V., Krug, M.K., Schooler, J.W., and Carter, C.S. (2009), 'Neural activity predicts attitude change in cognitive dissonance', *Nature Neuroscience*, 12, pp. 1469–74.

Veenema, A.H. (2009), 'Early life stress, the development of aggression and neuroendocrine and neurobiological correlates: what can we learn from animal models?', *Frontiers in Neuroendocrinology*, 30, pp. 497–518.

Vesper, J., Steinhoff, B., Rona, S., Wille, C., Bilic, S., Nikkhah, G., and Ostertag, C. (2007), 'Chronic high-frequency deep brain stimulation of the STN/SNr for progressive myoclonic epilepsy', *Epilepsia*, 48, pp. 1984–9.

Vinge, V. (1993), 'The coming technological singularity: how to survive in the post-human era', *VISION-21 Symposium*.

Vitaglione, P., Morisco, F., Mazzone, G., Amoruso, D.C., Ribecco, M.T., Romano, A., Fogliano, V., Caporaso, N., and D'Argenio, G. (2010), 'Coffee reduces liver damage in a rat model of steatohepatitis: the underlying mechanisms and the role of polyphenols and melanoidins', *Hepatology*, 52, pp. 1652–61.

Volz, K.G., Kessler, T., and von Cramon, D.Y. (2009), 'In-group as part of the self: in-group favoritism is mediated by medial prefrontal cortex activation', *Social Neuroscience*, 4, pp. 244–60.

Vucetic, Z., Kimmel, J., Totoki, K., Hollenbeck, E., and Reyes, T.M. (2010), 'Maternal high-fat diet alters methylation and gene expression of dopamine and opioid-related genes', *Endocrinology*, 151, pp. 4756–64.

Wald, C. and Wu, C. (2010), 'Biomedical research. Of mice and women: the bias in animal models', *Science*, 327, pp. 1571–2.

Wallace, M., ed. (2008), *The Way We Will Be 50 Years from Today: 60 of the World's Greatest Minds Share Their Visions of the Next Half Century*. Nashville, TN: Thomas Nelson.

Walsh, J.K., Randazzo, A.C., Stone, K.L., and Schweitzer, P.K. (2004), 'Modafinil improves alertness, vigilance, and executive function during simulated night shifts', *Sleep*, 27, pp. 434–9.

Weaver, I.C. (2007), 'Epigenetic programming by maternal behavior and pharmacological intervention. Nature versus nurture: let's call the whole thing off', *Epigenetics*, 2, pp. 22–8.

Weisberg, D.S., Keil, F.C., Goodstein, J., Rawson, E., and Gray, J.R. (2008), 'The seductive allure of neuroscience explanations', *Journal of Cognitive Neuroscience*, 20, pp. 470–7.

Weiss, A., Gale, C.R., Batty, G.D., and Deary, I.J. (2009), 'Emotionally stable, intelligent men live longer: the Vietnam Experience Study cohort', *Psychosomatic Medicine*, 71, pp. 385–94.

West, C.E., Videky, D.J., and Prescott, S.L. (2010), 'Role of diet in the development of immune tolerance in the context of allergic disease', *Current Opinion in Pediatrics*, 22, pp. 635–41.

Wheat, K.L., Cornelissen, P.L., Frost, S.J., and Hansen, P.C. (2010), 'During visual word recognition, phonology is accessed within 100 ms and may be mediated by a speech production code: evidence from magnetoencephalography', *Journal of Neuroscience*, 30, pp. 5229–33.

Wheatley, T. and Haidt, J. (2005), 'Hypnotic disgust makes moral judgments more severe', *Psychological Science*, 16, pp. 780–4.

Wheless, J.W., Castillo, E., Maggio, V., Kim, H.L., Breier, J.I., Simos, P.G., and Papanicolaou, A.C. (2004), 'Magnetoencephalography (MEG) and magnetic source imaging (MSI)', *Neurologist*, 10, pp. 138–53.

Whittingstall, K. and Logothetis, N.K. (2009), 'Frequency-band coupling in surface EEG reflects spiking activity in monkey visual cortex', *Neuron*, 64, pp. 281–9.

Williams, J.A., Imamura, M., and Fregni, F. (2009), 'Updates on the use of non-invasive brain stimulation in physical and rehabilitation medicine', *Journal of Rehabilitation Medicine*, 41, pp. 305–11.

Wilson, T. (2002), *Strangers to Ourselves: Discovering the Adaptive Unconscious*. Cambridge, MA: Harvard University Press.

Wittgenstein, L. (1974), *Philosophical Investigations*, trans. G.E.M. Anscombe, 3rd edition. Oxford: Blackwell.

Wittmann, M., van Wassenhove, V., Craig, A.D., and Paulus, M.P. (2010), 'The neural substrates of subjective time dilation', *Frontiers in Human Neuroscience*, 4, doi: 10.3389/neuro.09.002.2010.

Wolf, S.M. (2008), 'Neurolaw: the big question', *American Journal of Bioethics*, 8, pp. 21–2.

Wooffitt, R. (2007), 'Communication and laboratory performance in parapsychology experiments: demand characteristics and the social organization of interaction', *British Journal of Social Psychology*, 46, pp. 477–98.

Wu, C.W.H., Vasalatiy, O., Liu, N., Wu, H., Cheal, S., Chen, D.-Y., Koretsky, A.P., Griffiths, G.L., Tootell, R.B.H., and Ungerleider, L.G. (2011), 'Development of a MR-visible compound for tracing neuroanatomical connections *in vivo*', *Neuron*, 70, pp. 229–43.

Wu, H.-M., Wang, X.-L., Chang, C.-W., Li, N., Gao, L., Geng, N., Ma, J.-H., Zhao, W., and Gao, G.-D. (2010), 'Preliminary findings in ablating the nucleus accumbens using stereotactic surgery for alleviating psychological dependence on alcohol', *Neuroscience Letters*, 473, pp. 77–81.

Wyndham, J. (1960), *The Midwich Cuckoos*. Harmondsworth: Penguin.

Wyndham, J. (1973), *The Chrysalids*. Harmondsworth: Penguin.

Xu, T.-X. and Yao, W.-D. (2010), 'D1 and D2 dopamine receptors in separate circuits cooperate to drive associative long-term potentiation in the prefrontal cortex', *Proceedings of the National Academy of Sciences of the United States of America*, 107, pp. 16366–71.

Xue, G., Lu, Z., Levin, I.P., Weller, J.A., Li, X., and Bechara, A. (2009), 'Functional dissociations of risk and reward processing in the medial prefrontal cortex', *Cerebral Cortex*, 19, pp. 1019–27.

Yang, Y., Glenn, A.L., and Raine, A. (2008), 'Brain abnormalities in antisocial individuals: implications for the law', *Behavioral Sciences and the Law*, 26, pp. 65–83.

Yarkoni, T., Poldrack, R.A., Van Essen, D.C., and Wager, T.D. (2010), 'Cognitive neuroscience 2.0: building a cumulative science of human brain function', *Trends in Cognitive Sciences*, 14, pp. 489–96.

Ye, S., Zaitseva, E., Caltabiano, G., Schertler, G.F.X., Sakmar, T.P., Deupi, X., and Vogel, R. (2010), 'Tracking G-protein-coupled receptor activation using genetically encoded infrared probes', *Nature*, 464, pp. 1386–9.

Yoshida, M. and Hirano, R. (2010), 'Effects of local anesthesia of the cerebellum on classical fear conditioning in goldfish', *Behavioral and Brain Functions*, 6, doi:10.1186/1744-9081-6-20.

Young, E. and Korszun, A. (2010), 'Sex, trauma, stress hormones and depression', *Molecular Psychiatry*, 15, pp. 23–8.

Youngentob, S.L. and Glendinning, J.I. (2009), 'Fetal ethanol exposure increases ethanol intake by making it smell and taste better', *Proceedings of the National Academy of Sciences of the United States of America*, 106, pp. 5359–64.

Zanto, T.P., Rubens, M.T., Thangavel, A., and Gazzaley, A. (2011), 'Causal role of the prefrontal cortex in top-down modulation of visual processing and working memory', *Nature Neuroscience*, 14, pp. 656–61.

Zaranek, A.W., Levanon, E.Y., Zecharia, T., Clegg, T., and Church, G.M. (2010), 'A survey of genomic traces reveals a common sequencing error, RNA editing, and DNA editing', *PLoS Genetics*, 6, p. e1000954.

Zhang, F., Gradinaru, V., Adamantidis, A.R., Durand, R., Airan, R.D., de Lecea, L., and Deisseroth, K. (2010), 'Optogenetic interrogation of neural circuits: technology for probing mammalian brain structures', *Nature Protocols*, 5, pp. 439–56.

Zhang, F., Wang, L.P., Brauner, M., Liewald, J.F., Kay, K., Watzke, N., Wood, P. G., Bamberg, E., Nagel, G., Gottschalk, A., and Deisseroth, K. (2007), 'Multimodal fast optical interrogation of neural circuitry', *Nature*, 446, pp. 633–9.

Zhou, H., Xu, J., and Jiang, J. (2011), 'Deep brain stimulation of nucleus accumbens on heroin-seeking behaviors: a case report', *Biological Psychiatry*, 69, pp. e41–e42.

Zhu, P., Narita, Y., Bundschuh, S.T., Fajardo, O., Schärer, Y.-P.Z., Chattopadhyaya, B., Bouldoires, E.A., Stepien, A.E., Deisseroth, K., Arber, S., Sprengel, R., Rijli, F.M., and Friedrich, R.W. (2009), 'Optogenetic dissection of neuronal circuits in zebrafish using viral gene transfer and the tet system', *Frontiers in Neural Circuits*, 3, doi: 10.3389/neuro.04.021.2009.

Zilles, K. and Amunts, K. (2010), 'Centenary of Brodmann's map—conception and fate', *Nature Reviews Neuroscience*, 11, pp. 139–45.

Zotev, V.S., Matlashov, A.N., Volegov, P.L., Savukov, I.M., Espy, M.A., Mosher, J.C., Gomez, J.J., and Kraus Jr, R.H. (2008a), 'Microtesla MRI of the human brain combined with MEG', *Journal of Magnetic Resonance*, 194, pp. 115–20.

Zotev, V.S., Volegov, P.L., Matlashov, A.N., Espy, M.A., Mosher, J.C., and Kraus Jr, R.H. (2008b), 'Parallel MRI at microtesla fields', *Journal of Magnetic Resonance*, 192, pp. 197–208.

INDEX